Clinical Toxicology
of Drugs:
Principles and Practice

Clinical Toxicology of Drugs:

Principles and Practice

VASILIOS A. SKOUTAKIS, PHARM.D.

Associate Professor and Vice Chairman
Department of Drug and Material Toxicology
Director, Division of Clinical Toxicology
College of Pharmacy
University of Tennessee Center for the Health Sciences
Memphis, Tennessee
Editor and Publisher, *Clinical Toxicology Consultant*

LEA & FEBIGER
Philadelphia 1982

WARNER MEMORIAL LIBRARY
EASTERN COLLEGE
ST. DAVIDS, PA. 19087

4-15-86

LEA & FEBIGER
600 Washington Square
Phila PA 19106
U.S.A.

RA 1238 .C54 1982

Clinical toxicology of drug

Library of Congress Cataloging in Publication Data
Main entry under title:

Clinical toxicology of drugs.

  Bibliography: p.
  Includes index.
  1. Drugs—Toxicology. I. Skoutakis, Vasilios A.
[DNLM: 1. Poisoning.   QV 600 C6415]
RA1238.C54   1981   615.9   81–20930
ISBN 0-8121-0807-8   AACR2

Copyright © 1982 by Lea & Febiger. Copyright under the International
Copyright Union. All rights reserved. This book is protected by copyright.
*No part of it may be reproduced in any manner or by any means without
written permission from the publisher.*

PRINTED IN THE UNITED STATES OF AMERICA

Print No. 3   2   1

For her patience, love and support,
this textbook is dedicated to my wife,

Eleni Z. Skoutakis

Foreword

During the past two decades, the practice of pharmacy has emerged into patient services, and clinical aspects of drug therapy and management have become a part of the student's background. A knowledge of the toxicologic problems that drugs and other agents can pose must go hand in hand with the study of the proper and appropriate therapeutic approaches to the treatment of the ill, diseased, or injured patient. At times, only a delicate line separates a clinically desired event from a harmful or toxic manifestation of the drug. Students of pharmacy and the pharmacy practitioner are offered a unique opportunity to become actively involved in the provision of patient-oriented services in clinical toxicology.

The discipline of toxicology, which dates back to ancient times, has currently advanced to an extremely important position in contemporary society. Acute intoxications of children and deliberate suicidal and homicidal overdoses by adults constitute a continuing source of morbidity in the United States and around the world. Similarly, drug abuse, drug addiction, adverse drug effects, chronic drug intoxications, and hazards related to environmental and industrial chemicals all contribute, not only to a number of serious health problems, but to the total cost of national health care. Prevention of toxic events and proper treatment of poisonings can help reduce the tragic consequences of death and suffering while reducing the economic cost to the families of the patients involved.

At the present time, many disciplines are involved in instruction, research, training, and services in toxicology. Physicians, nurses, pharmacologists, dentists, veterinarians, chemists and biochemists, public health scientists, and pharmacists are all contributing to the rapid development of different specialty areas of toxicology. However, there are relatively few trained scientists, educators, and practitioners available to provide patient-oriented services and public health education in the area of clinical toxicology.

The pharmacist, with his or her background in the basic sciences of pharmacology, physiology, biochemistry, and chemistry, as well as clinically oriented courses in drug therapy and adverse drug reactions, is in a unique position to act in the field of clinical toxicology. In fact, in many communities in this nation, the pharmacy may be the only public health center, and thus the pharmacist may become the first person contacted in the event of an intoxication. Through these pharmacies, both in the community and in certain hospital settings, the practicing pharmacist is often called to provide poison information, drug abuse programs, and programs that deal with public health problems.

Presently, most of the colleges of pharmacy in this country can offer one or more courses in toxicology, including clinical toxicology, with rotations of students in poison centers, and even in hospital emergency wards. Through these educational programs and experiences, the emerging pharmacist can become a key figure in all aspects of clinical toxicology.

A number of valuable texts on toxicology have been written to train pharmacists and other health care professionals in the mastery of the cognitive concepts in toxicology. For the most part, these texts have dealt with basic aspects of toxicology. A few texts in the past have dealt with clinical aspects of toxicology; a more modern approach to the subject, however, emphasizing not only principles of toxicology, but dealing also with intoxicated patients and the toxicology laboratory, has not been available.

The textbook, *Clinical Toxicology of Drugs: Principles and Practice*, provides the student, educator, and practitioner with the information needed to pursue and practice patient-oriented toxicology. Dr. Skoutakis has masterfully produced a book of clarity and thoughtful organization, dealing with commonly seen drug-related intoxications. This book will become a valuable addition to the reference library of the pharmacist, whether he or she practices in a community setting or in an institution. The text should also take a prominent position in various other resource centers, such as poison control centers, hospital emergency rooms, public health offices, and centers and institutions dealing with health care. Finally, the text will be an excellent supplement to courses dealing in clinical toxicology.

John Autian, Ph.D.
Dean, College of Pharmacy
University of Tennessee Center for the Health Sciences
Memphis, Tennessee

The physician in almost any branch of medicine today faces the eventuality of being confronted with the drug-intoxicated patient. Such situations frequently are medical emergencies with life-threatening potential, requiring prompt therapeutic measures. In an age when hundreds of new drugs are marketed annually, it has become virtually impossible for the physician to be familiar with the pharmacodynamics of more than a few of these agents.

In addition, clinical toxicology has become a complex subject, involving not only a myriad of drugs with a variety of actions, but also taking into consideration the effects of drug interactions, routes of excretion, and alterations in drug metabolism by such variables as kidney or liver disease. The best approach to the problem for the physician would appear to be the development of fundamental

knowledge of the principles of management of the intoxicated patient, coupled with a readily available reference of the more commonly seen overdosages.

To this extent, *Clinical Toxicology of Drugs: Principles and Practice* succeeds admirably. Dr. Skoutakis is to be commended for not attempting to provide an exhaustive review of all possible agents, better left to the reference library or poison center. Instead, the approach taken here provides the student and physician alike with a clinically oriented and practical text that should prove invaluable to some and useful to all.

Fred E. Hatch, Jr., M.D.
Professor, College of Medicine
University of Tennessee Center for the Health Sciences
Memphis, Tennessee

Preface

Accidental drug ingestions by children and deliberate suicidal and homicidal drug intoxications and overdosages by adults are numerous in this era of drug-oriented society, and such incidents constitute a continuing source of morbidity and mortality. In 1977 in the United States alone, 12,866 people died from accidental, suicidal, and homicidal intoxications.

The management of these patients places a considerable burden on the physician, both inside and outside the hospital, because (1) little time in the medical school curriculum is devoted to clinical toxicology, (2) the number and variety of new chemicals and drugs to which patients can be exposed is unlimited, and frequently the names, characteristics, and toxic effects of these new agents are unfamiliar to physicians, and (3) specific information concerning formulations, toxicity, symptoms, and treatment of intoxicated patients may not be available from the chemical and pharmaceutical industries. Therefore, one of the challenges facing medicine and other health care professions today is to keep up to date with new information regarding current trends and promising developments in the prevention, detection, diagnosis, and treatment of intoxicated patients.

The primary concern of the clinical toxicologist is the rational management of the intoxicated patient. It is from this viewpoint that *Clinical Toxicology of Drugs: Principles and Practice* was written. Portions of the material and/or topics appearing in this textbook were initially published in the *Clinical Toxicology Consultant*, a journal of which I am editor and publisher. The textbook, as its title implies, is clinically oriented and deals with both the general considerations and principles of management of the intoxicated patient (Section I), as well as with the management of specific drug overdosages (Section II). It is designed for students and practitioners of all areas of health care.

For the students, its goal is to assist them (1) to acquire a thorough knowledge and understanding of clinical toxicology through an integrated study of physiology, pathology, pharmacology, and pharmacokinetics, (2) to establish a knowledge base with regard to problem solving; that is, the ability to use data obtained from the patient or laboratory to formulate a reasonable interpretation of the patient's clinical condition, and (3) to develop a rational therapeutic plan for the management and monitoring of intoxicated patients.

As for the practitioners, its goals are (1) to assist them in dealing quickly and effectively with the rational management of intoxicated patients, and (2) to serve them as a reference source in their daily practice.

This book is personal in many ways and carries with it a permanent sense of deep gratitude to many people: To my wife, to whom this book is dedicated, for her patience, love, support, and understanding throughout the years; to my parents, brothers, and sisters for their love, encouragement, and constant support; to those teachers who along the way had the desire, motivation, and skill to urge me to set high academic standards in the pursuit of excellence; to Drs. Sergio R. Acchiardo, Sidney A. Rosenbluth, Domingo R. Martinez, and Gary W. Cripps for their friendship, counsel, wisdom, knowledge, and skill, as well for the educational opportunities they provided for me while I was a student; to the late Dr. James A. Leventis, a true friend, whose memory and influence will always remain with me; to the late Dean of The College of Pharmacy, Dr. Sheldon D. Feurt, for the counsel, educational opportunities, and support he provided for me, both as a student and a faculty member; and last, but not least, to all of my students, residents, and fellows who allowed me the great privilege of teaching them and learning together with them.

In preparation for this book, I imposed on the friendship of many of my colleagues, both for their contributions to specific chapters in their areas of expertise and for their review and criticism of each chapter: Drs. S.R. Acchiardo, G.E. Bass, Jr., J. Bell, G.J. Burckart, P.A. Czajka, B.R. Ekins, J.I. Escobar, R.L. Kingston, W. Klein-Schwartz, A.S. Manoguerra, D.R. Martinez, J.B. Mowry, G.M. Oderda, K. Saxena, L.J. Sioris, I.S. Sketris, S. Ternullo, M.I.B. Thompson, J.C. Veltri, B.D. White, and N. Wojciechowski; their assistance, skill, and willingness to participate are greatly appreciated. My special appreciation also goes to Dr. John Autian, Dean of the College of Pharmacy; Dr. George C. Wood, Chairman, Department of Drug and Material Toxicology; and Dr. Fred E. Hatch, Jr., Professor of Medicine and Nephrology, and Chief, Division of Nephrology, for their support and encouragement in the preparation of this textbook.

My immeasurable gratitude also goes to Ms. Mary R. Harris, Ms. Phyllis King, and Ms. Betty Hudson for their secretarial support and sense of commitment in the preparation of this textbook. The help and editorial assistance of Mr. Martin C. Dallago and Ms. Martha Colgan of Lea & Febiger are also gratefully acknowledged.

Memphis, Tennessee Vasilios A. Skoutakis

Contributors

Sergio R. Acchiardo, M.D.
Professor of Medicine and Nephrology
College of Medicine
University of Tennessee Center for the Health
  Sciences
Director, Memphis Artificial Kidney Center
Memphis, Tennessee

George E. Bass, Jr., Ph.D.
Associate Professor, Departments of Drug and
  Material Toxicology and Psychiatry
Colleges of Pharmacy and Medicine
University of Tennessee Center for the Health
  Sciences
Memphis, Tennessee

Judy Bell, B.Sc., Ph.D. Candidate
Department of Drug and Material Toxicology
College of Pharmacy
University of Tennessee Center for the Health
  Sciences
Memphis, Tennessee

Gilbert J. Burckart, Pharm.D.
Associate Professor, Department of Pharmacy
  Practice
College of Pharmacy
University of Tennessee Center for the Health
  Sciences
Memphis, Tennessee

Peter A. Czajka, Pharm.D.
Assistant Professor, Department of Drug and
  Material Toxicology
University of Tennessee Center for the Health
  Sciences
Director, Southern Poison Center
Memphis, Tennessee

Brent R. Ekins, Pharm.D.
Assistant Professor, Department of Pharmacy
  Practice
College of Pharmacy, University of Utah
Poison Information Pharmacist
Intermountain Regional Poison Control Center
Salt Lake City, Utah

Javier I. Escobar, M.D., M.Sc.
Associate Professor of Psychiatry, College of
  Medicine
University of California at Los Angeles
Los Angeles, California

Richard L. Kingston, Pharm.D.
Assistant Professor, College of Pharmacy
University of Minnesota
Coordinator, Poison Treatment Team
St. Paul, Minnesota

Wendy Klein-Schwartz, Pharm.D.
Assistant Professor, Department of Clinical
  Pharmacy
School of Pharmacy, University of Maryland
Assistant Director, Maryland Poison Center
Baltimore, Maryland

Anthony S. Manoguerra, Pharm.D.
Associate Professor, Departments of Clinical
  Pharmacy and Medicine
University of California–San Diego
Director, Professional Services
San Diego Poison Information Center
San Diego, California

James B. Mowry, Pharm.D.
Director, Indiana Poison Center
Indianapolis, Indiana

Gary M. Oderda, Pharm.D.
Associate Professor, Department of Clinical
   Pharmacy
School of Pharmacy, University of Maryland
Director, Maryland Poison Center
Baltimore, Maryland

Kusum Saxena, M.D.
Medical Director, Poison Treatment Team
Department of Emergency Medicine
St. Paul–Ramsey Medical Center
St. Paul, Minnesota

Leo J. Sioris, Pharm.D.
Clinical Pharmacist, Divine Redeemer
   Memorial Hospital
St. Paul, Minnesota

Ingrid S. Sketris, Pharm.D.
Assistant Professor, College of Pharmacy
Dalhousie University
Halifax, Nova Scotia

Vasilios A. Skoutakis, Pharm.D.
Associate Professor and Vice Chairman
Department of Drug and Material Toxicology
Director, Division of Clinical Toxicology
   College of Pharmacy
University of Tennessee Center for the Health
   Sciences
Memphis, Tennessee

Sharon R. Ternullo, Pharm.D.
Coordinator of Pediatric Pharmacy Services
Medical College of Virginia Hospital
Richmond, Virginia

Marietta I. B. Thompson, Pharm.D.
Fellow, Department of Pharmacy Practice
College of Pharmacy, University of Utah
Salt Lake City, Utah

Joseph C. Veltri, Pharm.D.
Associate Professor, Department of Pharmacy
   Practice
College of Pharmacy, University of Utah
Director, Intermountain Poison Control Center
Salt Lake City, Utah

Contents

FOREWORD: *John Autian* vii
Fred Hatch, Jr. viii

PREFACE: *Vasilios A. Skoutakis* ix

SECTION I

THE INTOXICATED PATIENT

CHAPTER

1   **Toxic Emergencies: Principles of Treatment** 3
     Vasilios A. Skoutakis

2   **The Role of the Toxicology Laboratory** 19
     James B. Mowry and Vasilios A. Skoutakis

3   **Dialysis and Hemoperfusion of Drugs and Toxins** 37
     Ingrid S. Sketris and Vasilios A. Skoutakis

SECTION II

MANAGEMENT OF COMMON DRUG OVERDOSAGES

4   **Barbiturates** 61
     Vasilios A. Skoutakis and Sergio R. Acchiardo

5   **Nonbarbiturates** 77
     Vasilios A. Skoutakis and Sergio R. Acchiardo

6   **Narcotic Analgesics** 101
     Vasilios A. Skoutakis

7   **Tricyclic Antidepressants** 127
    Vasilios A. Skoutakis

8   **Neuroleptics** 137
    Judy Bell, George E. Bass, Jr.,
    Javier I. Escobar, and Vasilios A. Skoutakis

9   **Lithium** 153
    Javier I. Escobar and Vasilios A. Skoutakis

10 **Anticonvulsants** 171
    Gilbert J. Burckart and Sharon R. Ternullo

11 **Central Nervous System Stimulants** 183
    Gary M. Oderda and Wendy Klein-Schwartz

12 **Cocaine** 201
    Gary M. Oderda and Wendy Klein-Schwartz

13 **Phencyclidine (PCP)** 217
    Leo J. Sioris and Vasilios A. Skoutakis

14 **Salicylates** 227
    Joseph C. Veltri and Marietta I. B. Thompson

15 **Digoxin** 245
    Brent R. Ekins

16 **Acetaminophen** 259
    Peter A. Czajka

17 **Iron** 271
    Anthony S. Manoguerra

18 **Isoniazid (INH)** 279
    Richard L. Kingston and Kusum Saxena

    Index 287

Section I

The Intoxicated Patient

Chapter 1

Toxic Emergencies: Principles of Treatment

Vasilios A. Skoutakis

Accidental intoxications by children and deliberate suicidal and homicidal overdosages by adults constitute continuing sources of morbidity and mortality in the United Sates. Recent national statistics attest to this problem. Data from the National Center for Health Statistics, Mortality Statistic Branch, reveal that 12,866 people died in 1977 due to accidental, suicidal, and homicidal intoxications. The deaths of all ages from accidental, suicidal, and homicidal intoxications and from undetermined intent in 1977 are summarized in Table 1–1.[1]

From the reported findings, it is clear that increased efforts must be made to prevent the incidents of accidental overdosages and reduce the morbidity and mortality due to suicidal and homicidal overdosages. However, despite all precautions, accidental, suicidal, and homicidal intoxications/overdosages will continue to remain an important problem in our society, one which every clinician must be prepared to treat promptly and effectively. Furthermore, there are few areas in pediatric and adult medicine in which a patient's survival is more directly correlated with proper management than in cases of intoxication.

When the intoxicated pediatric or adult patient is presented to a clinic or a hospital facility for treatment, he may be asymptomatic, symptomatic but awake, semicomatose, or comatose. The first priority for the clinician in the management of the patient is to assess and treat the patient according to his clinical status and not the intoxicant ingested. Furthermore, the management of pediatric and adult intoxicated patients is similar, except that volumes of fluid or medications administered to

3

Table 1–1. Deaths Due to Ingestions in 1977.

TYPES OF INGESTION	SUBSTANCES INVOLVED	NUMBER OF DEATHS
Accidental in children under 5 years of age	Solid and liquid substances (including drugs)	94
	Gases and vapors	35
Accidental for all ages	Solid and liquid substances (including drugs)	3,374
	Gases and vapors	1,596
Suicidal	Barbiturates	847
	Salicylates and congeners	73
	Antidepressants, tranquilizers, other psychotherapeutic agents	520
	Other drugs	1,685
	Non-drug solid and liquid substances	754
	Gases and vapors	2,608
Undetermined intent for all ages	Barbiturates	118
	Salicylates	31
	Antidepressants, tranquilizers, other psychotherapeutic agents	85
	Other drugs	577
	Total non-drug solid and liquid substances	277
	Total gases and vapors	295
Homicidal	Drugs, other solids, liquids, and gases	46
Total number of deaths in 1977		12,866

pediatric patients must be adjusted to be appropriate to body size and/or weight.

THE ASYMPTOMATIC OR SYMPTOMATIC BUT AWAKE PATIENT

In some cases, when brought to a clinic or an emergency room (ER), the intoxicated patient may be asymptomatic because a sufficient dose or quantity of the intoxicant has not been ingested, or because not enough of the intoxicant has been absorbed to produce significant signs and symptoms. In other cases, the intoxicated patient may have a variety of signs and symptoms but will be awake. The variability of signs and symptoms in such a patient can be attributed to the intoxicant ingested, the time elapsed since ingestion, the amount ingested, the method by which the intoxicant was taken (e.g., orally, intravenously, or through inhalation), and the patient's prior medical history (e.g., diabetes, hepatitis, asthma, heart disease, renal disease, or traumatic experience, particularly to the head).

Therefore, when such an intoxicated pa-

tient is presented to a clinic or an ER, and prior to the initiation of any therapeutic measures, the vital signs (e.g., respiration, blood pressure, pulse rate, and temperature) must be checked and recorded, and a quick physical examination of the head, lungs, heart, abdomen, and central nervous system (CNS) should be performed and evaluated. In addition, pertinent information should be obtained from the patient, if possible, or from the person(s) who brought the patient in for treatment, regarding the patient's past medical history, therapeutic drug history, and intoxicant(s) ingested. Unfortunately, sometimes even when a friend or family member accompanies the intoxicated patient, the history obtained may be unreliable or unknown, or the patient may be uncooperative. In such cases, prior hospital admissions or the use of toxicology laboratory can be of valuable assistance.

EMESIS OR GASTRIC LAVAGE

Once the clinical condition of the intoxicated but alert and awake patient has been assessed and stabilized, the next step should be to remove the toxic ingestant from the patient's stomach before significant absorption can occur. Evacuation of the stomach can be accomplished by the induction of emesis or by gastric lavage. It is now clear that gastric lavage, although more predictable and immediately active, is less effective than emesis in removing the toxic ingestant from a patient's stomach, because the stomach normally traps large quantities of the toxic ingestant in several pouches inaccessible to the lavage tube.[2,3]

Syrup of ipecac. The most effective way to induce emesis is by the administration of syrup of ipecac (not the fluid extract, 14 times more concentrated).[4] The recommended dose of syrup of ipecac is 10 ml orally for children 1 year of age, 15 ml orally for children 1 to 5 years old, and 15 to 30 ml for children over 5 years old. The recommended dose for adults is 30 ml orally. It should be followed by one or two glasses of water, because ipecac only works effectively on a full stomach (administering ipecac on an empty stomach is like squeezing an empty balloon). The emetic action of syrup of ipecac has an average latent period of 20 to 30 minutes and depends in part on gastrointestinal (GI) absorption.[4,5] Therefore, ipecac cannot be used in conjunction with other therapeutic measures intended to minimize absorption of the ingestant. A second dose of ipecac should be administered if no vomiting occurs after 20 to 30 minutes. The initial emesis should be placed in a disposable container and sent to the toxicology laboratory for confirmation of the intoxicant ingested when warranted. Vomiting should be induced even if several hours (4 to 6) have elapsed after ingestion, since many substances when ingested in large quantities not only can remain for a long period in the stomach in

Table 1–2. Commonly Ingested Corrosives and Petroleum Distillates.

CLASSIFICATION		COMMON PRODUCTS	TREATMENT
Corrosives/caustics	Acids	Automobile battery acid Hydrochloric acid Phenol Toilet bowl cleaners	Immediately irrigate all exposed areas or contaminated tissues. Do not induce emesis. Administer orally milk or water or both.

	Bases	Ammonia
		Ammonium hydroxide
		Chemical drain openers
		Chemical oven cleaners
		Copper sulfate, sodium hydroxide
		  (Clinitest tablets)
		Electric dishwasher detergent
		  granules
		Lye
		Potassium hydroxide
		Sodium hypochlorite (active
		  ingredient in household bleach)
			Immediately irrigate all contaminated
			  tissue, or administer orally water or milk
			  or both.
			Do not give acids (e.g., vinegar) to
			  neutralize alkali products or bicarbonate
			  (baking soda) to neutralize acidic
			  products. This method produces heat
			  and more tissue damage.
			Do not induce emesis.
			Do not administer activated charcoal.
			Do not perform gastric lavage.
			Discourage oral administration of large
			  amounts of fluids, since this may induce
			  emesis.

Petroleum distillates
(Hydrocarbons)
		Furniture polish
		Gasoline
		Kerosene
		Mineral seal oil
		Lighter fluid
			Do not induce emesis if ingested dose
			  is not greater than 1 ml/kg of body
			  weight.
			Avoid oral administration of large volumes
			  of fluid. This may cause emesis.
			Avoid administration of oils.
			Obtain chest roentgenogram.
			Implement supportive and symptomatic
			  care as indicated.

the form of mass concentrations but can also decrease GI transit time, resulting in a prolongation of the toxicologic manifestations and increasing the risk of possible complications.

Administration of syrup of ipecac is contraindicated if loss of the gag reflex has occurred and in severely depressed or convulsing patients, because of the danger of tracheal aspiration of vomitus. Syrup of ipecac is also contraindicated in patients who have ingested corrosives, because of tissue damage,[6] or liquid hydrocarbons if the amount ingested is *not* greater that 1 ml/kg of body weight, because they are potent lung irritants.[7] The commonly available and frequently ingested corrosives and petroleum distillate products and their treatment are summarized in Table 1–2. If significant CNS depression intervenes between the administration of syrup of ipecac and the occurrence of vomiting, the airway must be protected by insertion of a cuffed endotracheal tube to avoid aspiration pneumonia. In such cases, the patient should be admitted and treated as in the comatose situation discussed later in the chapter.

Other emetics. Other methods and/or agents that have been used for the induction of emesis are mechanical gagging and administration of apomorphine, copper sulfate, sodium chloride, mustard powder, raw eggs, and soapy water.[8-10] Mechanical induction of vomiting by gagging is not the method of first choice because it is so often ineffective.[8] The administration of apomorphine, 0.06 mg/kg intramuscularly (IM), tends to produce vomiting within 5 minutes, and administration of 0.01 mg/kg intravenously (IV) results in immediate action.[5,9] However, it is not recommended as the agent of choice because of its CNS and respiratory-depressant effects and because it is not readily available. Emetics such as copper sulfate, sodium chloride, mustard powder, raw eggs, and soapy water, are ineffective, potentially dangerous, and should not be used.[10] Again, syrup of ipecac is the drug of choice; it is safe enough for home use and can be purchased without a prescription.

PREVENTION OF ABSORPTION

Since neither emesis nor gastric lavage empties the stomach completely, prevention of absorption by trapping of the ingested intoxicant should be initiated in all intoxicated patients after the induction of emesis.

Activated charcoal. Because it absorbs most intoxicants in the GI tract and prevents their absorption into the blood stream, activated charcoal is the drug of choice.[11-13] The theoretical dose is 5 to 10 times the estimated toxic weight of the ingested intoxicant. However, since in the clinical setting the ingested dose of the intoxicant is usually not known, the activated charcoal dose is 30 to 50 g for adults and 30 g for children, and is administered orally in a slurry with water. The administration of activated charcoal should be carried out slowly over a period of 15 minutes, in order to minimize possible gastric distention and resultant emesis, which can cause the patient to aspirate some of the charcoal contents. Activated charcoal also can serve as a marker of intestinal transit time, and when it appears in the stool, it indicates that further absorption of the intoxicant from the intestinal tract will not occur. There are no known contraindications to the use of activated charcoal. However, substances such as corrosives, petroleum distillates, alcohols, lead, and iron do not adsorb to activated charcoal. Its administration therefore is not recommended in patients who have been intoxicated by any of these substances either alone or in combination with other intoxicants.

Catharsis. Another useful way to prevent further absorption of the ingested intoxicant is to administer a saline cathartic. Saline cathartics promote intestinal evacuation of the ingestant-activated charcoal complex, and thus decrease potential toxic effects. Three agents commonly used as saline cathartics are sodium sulfate, in an oral dose of 250 mg/kg, or 1 ml/kg of 25% solution; magnesium sulfate (Epsom salts), in an oral dose of 250 mg/kg, or 1 ml/kg of 25% solution; and magnesium citrate NF, in an oral dose of 4 ml/kg of body weight. Administration of a saline cathartic is usually recommended for intoxicated patients unless there are specific contraindications.[14-16] The intestinal evacuation action of saline cathartics has an average latent period of 2 to 3 hours. Therefore, prior to the administration of a second dose, confirmation of the presence or absence of bowel sounds is required. Cathartics containing magnesium should be avoided in patients with compromised renal function, because of the danger of CNS-toxic effects due to high serum magnesium levels.

DECONTAMINATION

In cases where the patient has been exposed to substances that are absorbed from or burn the skin (e.g., corrosives, hydrocarbons, pesticides), decontamination of the body surface is essential. Tincture of green soap is recommended because, in addition to alkaline substances that hydrolyze the organophosphates, it contains alcohol, which dissolves hydrocarbons more readily than does plain soap. However, if green soap is not available, plain soap can be used. It is important to clean all exposed body surface areas thoroughly, but caution should be exercised not to abrade the skin, since abrasion increases the absorption of the majority of these chemicals. The personnel decontaminating these patients, particularly patients intoxicated with pesticides, should take extreme precautions not to be contaminated themselves, and should wear disposable gloves, aprons and shoe covers. The use of substances that will neutralize chemical agents is not recommended (e.g., vinegar and lemon juice for alkali, or bicarbonate for corrosive acids, Table 1–2), because they will create an exothermic reaction and burn the exposed body surface or tissue areas.[16] Emollients such as greases or oils also are not recommended, because they are ineffective and make decontamination more difficult.

In case of an eye exposure, irrigation of the eye is the most important aspect of the treatment and must be initiated immediately. Permanent irreversible destruction of the cornea can occur within the first 20 to 30 minutes of exposure. The patient's head should be held back over a sink and a saline solution or plain water poured from a container or liter bottle into the affected eye. The purpose of irrigation is to dilute and remove the agent completely, and therefore, the use of an eyedropper or an irrigating syringe is not recommended. Irrigation should continue for at least 10 to 15 minutes, particularly when the eye has been exposed to an alkaline substance. Once irrigation has been carried out, consultation with an ophthalmologist is imperative.[16,17]

DISCHARGE

After vomiting has been induced, charcoal and a cathartic have been administered or decontamination has been performed, the patient's vital signs and mental status should be checked every 15 minutes to determine whether or not he will continue to have symptoms or become stuporous or comatose. If, after a few hours, it is apparent that the patient's condition is stabilized, he should be directed to the appropriate personnel for consultation (e.g., ophthalmologist, psychiatrist, clinical pharmacist, or social worker) and then should be discharged from the clinic or hospital. If the patient continues to have symptoms, he should be admitted for overnight observation, and supportive and symptomatic care should be carried out as discussed in the following section.

THE SEMICOMATOSE OR COMATOSE PATIENT

When the intoxicated patient is brought to the emergency room in a semicomatose or comatose state, all treatment procedures directed toward the ingested toxic substance are secondary. The first priority should be to assess and treat as necessary any impairment of respiratory and cardiovascular function that may be present. This may appear to state the obvious, but in the heat of the moment many clinicians forget this priority and give their attention to gastric lavage, blood samples for toxicologic analysis, or methods to increase the elimination of the toxic substance ingested. Therefore, life support measures must be instituted at once, in all semicomatose or comatose patients.

RESPIRATORY FUNCTION

The mouth should be examined and all foreign materials (e.g., food, vomit, secretions, dentures) removed. The patient then should be positioned head down on his left side to minimize the risk of aspiration of stomach contents into the lungs. If respiration is absent or inadequate, mechanical ventilation should be provided by mouth-to-mouth resuscitation, manual resuscitation bag, or positive-pressure respirator until the patient is adequately oxygenated. If the patient is comatose or if the gag reflex is absent, a cuffed endotracheal tube should be inserted and bronchial suction performed to clear mucous and foreign materials from the major bronchi. After the procedure has been completed, the placement of the endotracheal tube should be evaluated through a determination of whether or not the chest is being inflated symmetrically and whether breathing sounds are audible bilaterally. In addition, arterial blood should be drawn, to evaluate the degree and adequacy of ventilation, and an x-ray examination performed to further assess the patient's clinical situation, and to serve as a baseline from which future progress can be judged.[16-18]

CARDIOVASCULAR FUNCTION

While one member of the ER staff is assuring adequate ventilation, a second member should be assessing the patient's cardiovascular function by measuring pulse, blood pressure, and temperature (both core and peripheral) and assuring access to the circulation by the insertion of an 18-gauge catheter for the initiation of IV fluid administration. Other therapeutic agents should be used as indicated to support life. If the patient is in shock, the use of vasopressor agents should be initially avoided (Table 1–3), and fluids, plasma protein fraction (Plasmanate), or blood should be administered. In addition, a baseline electrocardiogram (EKG) should be obtained, and blood should be drawn and sent to the clinical chemistry (20 ml) and toxicology laboratories (10 ml) for biochemical, hematologic, and toxicologic determinations.

URINARY CATHETERIZATION

Once procedures to support the vital functions have been implemented, an indwelling urinary catheter should be inserted in all patients who are comatose because of toxic ingestions. Upon insertion of the catheter, the volume of residual urine should be measured, and 100 ml should be sent to both the clinical chemistry and toxicology laboratories for urinalysis, including drug screening and determination of specific gravity and osmolality. Thereafter, strict balance of fluid intake and urinary output should be maintained throughout the patient's hospital course.

Table 1–3.   Commonly Used Vasopressor Agents.*

NAME	PREPARATION	DOSAGE
Isoproterenol (Isuprel)	2 mg added to 1,000 ml of D_5W makes a solution of 2 μg/ml.	Start infusion with 0.1 μg/kg/minute, and slowly increase the dose until the desired effect is obtained. Stop increasing the dose if the heart rate exceeds 180 to 200 beats/minute.
Levarterenol (Levophed)	4 ml vial added to 100 ml of D_5W makes a solution of 4 μg/ml.	Start infusion with 0.1 to 0.2 μg/kg/minute, and increase dose as needed to obtain desired effect.
Metaraminol (Aramine)	Available in 10 mg/ml, in a 10 ml vial. 100 mg added to 1,000 ml of D_5W makes a solution of 100 μg/ml.	Start infusion with 5 μg/kg/minute, and increase dose slowly to obtain desired effect.
Dopamine (Intropin)	1 ampule (5 ml = 200 mg) added to 500 ml normal saline solution or D_5W makes a solution of 400 μg/ml.	Start infusion with 2 to 5 μg/kg/minute, and increase dosage as needed to as high as 50 μg/kg/minute. A dose higher than 50 μg/kg/minute may produce renal shutdown. Ventricular arrhythmias may also occur—decrease infusion rate with increased ectopic beats.

* It is best to avoid vasopressors and to use fluids for correction of hypotension, if possible.
  If the patient dose not respond to the administration of fluids, any of the above vasopressors can be used, depending on the condition of the patient.

HISTORY OF THE COMATOSE PATIENT

To help establish the cause of coma, attempts should be made to obtain a prompt and adequate history of the patient if possible. The person(s) who brought the patient to the emergency room should not be permitted to leave until the maximum amount of historical information can be obtained from them once the patient has received emergency supportive treatment. Inquiry should be made regarding the type and quantity of intoxicant ingested, when and how it was ingested, and the presence of any medical complications (drug- or nondrug-related) that may aggravate or potentiate the toxicologic effects in the patient. Examination of any pill bottles brought in may also be helpful, not only for determination of the drug or drugs involved so an appropriate antidote can be administered, but also to alert the clinician to other medical problems for which the patient is currently being treated. Therefore, information obtained from the history and more detailed

subsequent physical examination generally helps the clinician to establish whether the comatose patient could be treated with specific measures (e.g., antidote, dialysis), or whether the patient should receive supportive management only.

ANTIDOTES

The concept of using an antidote to reverse the toxic effects of an ingestant is popular with both layman and professionals. Unfortunately, specific antidotal therapy is available for only a few ingestants. Names of the toxic ingestants and antidotes available, including dosages, mechanisms of antidotal action, and cautions and contraindications, are summarized in Table 1–4. It must be remembered, however, that antidotes should be used only to improve adequacy of vital functions and should not be relied upon to the exclusion of supportive and symptomatic care. It is also important to remember that the so-called "universal antidote,"

Table 1–4. Available Antidotal Agents.

| TOXIC INGESTANT | ANTIDOTE | DOSE | | CAUTIONS/CONTRAINDICATIONS | MECHANISM OF ANTIDOTAL ACTION |
		PEDIATRIC	ADULT		
Anticholinergics	Physostigmine (Antilirium)	Test dose, 0.5 mg every 5 minutes; maximum dose, 2 mg; administer IV over 2 to 3 minutes; repeat dose at 0.5 mg IV as needed.	Test dose, 2 mg; administer IV over 2 to 3 minutes; repeat dose if needed at 1 to 2 mg.	Physostigmine may cause seizures when administered rapidly by the IV route. Its use is contraindicated in patients with bradycardia, and is possibly contraindicated in patients with asthma or urinary bladder obstruction.	Antidote competes with different intoxicants for essential receptors.
Carbon monoxide	Oxygen	Administer 100% oxygen.	Same as for pediatric patients.	No contraindications are known.	Antidote competes with intoxicant for essential receptors.
Coumarin anticoagulants	Vitamin K	The initial dose should be 2 to 10 mg, depending on amount of ingestion. Thereafter, the dose, frequency of administration, and duration of treatment would depend on the severity of the prothrombin deficiency and should be regulated by repeated determinations of prothrombin time.	The initial dose should be 5 to 25 mg IV, depending on amount of ingestion. Thereafter, the same principles apply as in pediatric patients.	Hypotension may occur if the IV dose exceeds 3 mg/m²/minute.	Antidote competes with intoxicant for essential receptors.
Cyanide	Amyl nitrite pearls	Administer amyl nitrite pearls; break one at a time and hold it under the patient's nose for 20 to 30 seconds every minute.	Same dosage (ml/kg) and route of administration as for pediatric patients.	Observe for hypotension. Excessive doses of amyl nitrite and sodium nitrite can produce methemoglobinemia and death.	Antidote forms complex with intoxicant, making it inactive.
	Sodium nitrite	After stopping amyl nitrite, administer 3% sodium nitrite IV over 3 to 5 minutes in a dose of 6 to 8 ml/m² or 0.2 ml/kg; do not exceed the administration of 10 ml.			
	Sodium thiosulfate	Inject 30 to 40 ml/m² or 1 ml/kg of 25% sodium thiosulfate.	Inject 50 ml of 25% sodium thiosulfate.		Antidote accelerates metabolic conversion of intoxicant to a nontoxic product.
Iron	Deferoxamine (Desferal)	Primary method: 10 to 15 mg/ kg/hr by controlled IV infusion. Alternate method: 90 mg/kg, to a maximum of 1 g; administer IM every 8 hours, for 3 doses.	Dosage regimen and route of administration are similar to the recommendations listed under the pediatric dose.	Hypotension may occur if the recommended IV dose and rate of administration are exceeded. Contraindicated in patients with renal insufficiency.	Antidote forms complex with intoxicant, making it inert.

Intoxicant	Antidote	Pediatric dose	Adult dose	Precautions	Mechanism
Metals (lead, mercury, arsenic)	Dimercaprol (BAL)	3 to 5 mg/kg/dose, deep IM every 4 hours for 2 days; then every 4 to 12 hours for up to an additional 7 days.	Similar to pediatric listing.	Observe patient for hypotension, hyperpyrexia, and urticaria. Agents are contraindicated in patients with renal insufficiency. Meticulous monitoring of serum and urinary electrolytes is needed.	Antidotes form complexes with intoxicants, making them inert.
	Calcium disodium edetate (EDTA)	75 mg/kg/24 hours, deep IM or slow IV infusion, given in 3 to 6 divided doses for up to 5 days.	Similar to pediatric listing.		
	D-Penicillamine	100 mg/kg/day for 5 to 10 days orally in 4 equally divided doses.	250 mg orally, 4 times daily for 5 to 10 days.		
Alcohols Methyl alcohol Ethylene glycol	Ethyl alcohol in conjunction with dialysis	1 ml/kg of 100% ethanol initially in glucose solution. Thereafter, maintain blood ethanol level at 100 mg/dl.	Similar to pediatric listing.	Glucose should be administered to prevent hypoglycemia. Dialysis should be initiated in patients with compromised renal function.	Antidote blocks metabolic formation of intoxicants, forming less toxic precursors.
Nitrites	Methylene blue	0.2 ml/kg of 1% solution IV over 3 to 5 minutes.	Same as pediatric dose.	This therapy is contraindicated if methemoglobin is greater than 30%. Care must be exercised when repeated doses are required, as excess methylene blue may cause an increase in methemoglobin.	Antidote restores normal body function by repairing or bypassing effect of intoxicant.
Narcotics (including propoxyphene)	Naloxone (Narcan)	0.01 mg/kg push; 2 to 3 consecutive doses may be needed within 5 to 10 minutes to produce a desirable response.	0.48 to 0.8 mg IV push; sometimes 3 to 5 consecutive doses may be required during the first 5 to 10 minutes to produce a desirable response.	No contraindications are known.	Antidote competes with intoxicants for essential receptors.
Organophosphates and carbamate insecticides	Atropine	Test dose, 0.05 mg/kg; administer IV over 1 to 2 minutes. Maintenance dose, 0.05 mg/kg as needed to keep patient atropinized.	Test dose, 2 mg; administer IV over 1 to 2 minutes. Maintenance dose at 2 mg as needed to keep patient atropinized.	Excessive atropine administration can cause hallucinations and tachycardia. Furthermore, its use is contraindicated in patients with tachycardia.	Antidote blocks receptors that are responsible for toxic effects.
	Pralidoxime (2 PAM, Protopam)	20 to 50 mg/kg; administer over 15 to 30 minutes as IV infusion in 100 ml of normal saline solution. May repeat dose every 4 to 12 hours as needed for muscle twitching and weakness.	1 to 2 g; administer over 15 to 20 minutes as IV infusion in 100 ml of normal saline solution. May repeat dose every 4 to 12 hours as needed for muscle twitching and weakness.	Concurrent use of atropine with pralidoxime may require reduction of the atropine dose. The use of atropine is possibly contraindicated in patients with myasthenia gravis.	Antidote forms complex with intoxicant, making it inert.

which consists of a mixture of charcoal, magnesium oxide, and tannic acid and has been used in the treatment of intoxications, is not only ineffective but could itself give rise to intoxications.[13,19]

PREVENTION OF ABSORPTION

Once the vital functions have been determined to be adequate, or procedures to support life have been implemented, gastric lavage should be performed. Gastric lavage is indicated for the patient in whom emesis cannot be performed or is contraindicated (e.g., a patient who is comatose, semicomatose, convulsing, or has a depressed or absent gag reflex). The purpose of gastric lavage is to dilute and remove any unabsorbed amount of the ingested intoxicant from the patient's stomach, and it should be carried out if it can be determined that the intoxicant was ingested 4 to 6 hours before treatment. Furthermore, in patients in whom there are no audible bowel sounds, gastric lavage should be carried out regardless of the time that has elapsed between ingestion of strong corrosives such as mineral acids and alkali, because of the danger of perforating injured tissues.[6]

Prior to the initiation of gastric lavage, a cuffed endotracheal tube should be inserted in all intoxicated patients when tolerated, for the prevention of possible pulmonary aspiration of stomach contents. Where insertion of a cuffed endotracheal tube is not possible or practical (e.g., the semicomatose patient or a young child), gastric lavage is also indicated and, when properly performed, carries little risk of aspiration of gastric contents into the lungs. Furthermore, the advantage of removing the unabsorbed intoxicant from the stomach usually outweighs the danger of possible pulmonary aspiration that may occur during the lavage procedure.

The patient should be positioned head down on his left side, and the largest tolerable nasogastric or orogastric tube (e.g., 18 French for children, and at least 32 French for adults), should be used. Small tubes do not permit a fluid flow rapid enough to remove particulate matter and should **not** be used. Once the nasogastric or orogastric tube has been inserted, 100 to 200 ml of gastric contents

Table 1–5.   Lavage Solutions for Specific Intoxications.

LAVAGE SOLUTION	CONCENTRATION	TYPE OF INTOXICATION	COMMENTS/CAUTIONS
Ammonium acetate	5 mg/500 ml of water	Formaldehyde	Forms nontoxic methenamine
Calcium gluconate	15 to 30 g in 1 L of water	Oxalic acid, fluorides	Calcium acts as precipitate
Cornstarch	75 to 80 g in 1 L of water	Iodine	Administer lavage until return is no longer blue
Normal saline	0.9% solution	Silver nitrate; solution of choice for flushing eyes	Do not use as an emetic
Potassium permanganate	1:5,000 or 1:10,000 solution	Alkaloids, mushroom	Severe irritant; should not be used in stronger concentration, or with undissolved particles in solution
Sodium bicarbonate	Dilute sodium bicarbonate with tap water to make 1.5% solution	Ferrous sulfate	Forms an insoluble complex with iron in the gastrointestinal tract and decreases absorption of iron into the bloodstream
Sodium biphosphate and sodium phosphate (Fleet Phospho-soda)	Dilute 1 part Fleet Phospho-soda enema with 3 parts tap water, or 1 part oral Fleet Phospho-soda solution with 11 parts tap water		Administration of large amounts of sodium bicarbonate or Fleet Phospho-soda may promote the development of hypocalcemia

should be aspirated prior to lavage, and saved in case the toxicology laboratory has to be used for identification and analysis of the ingested intoxicant.

Thereafter, gastric lavage should be performed in cycles by administration of normal saline solution or lukewarm water in doses of 200 to 300 ml in adults and 100 to 150 ml in young children. Normal saline solution or tap water will suffice as a lavage fluid in the majority of intoxications. Table 1–5, however, lists the names, concentrations, and comments or cautions for a limited number of other lavage solutions, whose use may be more desirable than normal saline or tap water in some specific types of intoxications.

Regardless of the type of intoxication, the lavage fluid should be administered slowly over a period of 2 to 3 minutes, left in place for approximately 1 minute, and drained by gravity over a period of 3 to 4 minutes. It is also important to administer only the previously recommended amounts of fluid at each washing time interval, in order to prevent the promotion of the ingested intoxicant into the intestines. Gastric lavage should be continued until the aspirate becomes clear. Generally, the total amount of lavage fluid required is 3 to 4 L for a child and 6 to 8 L for an adult.

INTERFERENCE WITH GASTROINTESTINAL ABSORPTION

Administration of activated charcoal and a saline cathartic via the nasogastric or orogastric tube should follow the gastric lavage procedure. Dosages and rationale for use of these agents have been discussed in the preceding section.

REMOVAL OF ABSORBED INTOXICANT

Toxic ingestants or their active metabolites are usually excreted from the body in expired air by the lungs, in bile by the liver, and in urine by the kidneys.[20,21] Any

therapeutic approach that can accelerate the effectiveness of these mechanisms will shorten the biologic half-life of the intoxicant, thereby reducing the duration and severity of the toxicologic effects. Selection of the therapeutic approach and mechanism to be used by the clinician depends on the patient's condition and urgency of the situation, the amount of the intoxicant present in the body, the pharmacokinetic properties of the intoxicant, and availability of trained personnel and equipment.

Lung excretion. Many toxic substances used as inhalants are excreted in expired air. This route of excretion, however, cannot be significantly modified or accelerated by therapeutic interventions beyond those necessary to assure that the patient has an adequate ventilation. Carbon monoxide intoxication is an exception, however, because increases in the percentage of oxygen in inspired air significantly decrease the half-life of carboxyhemoglobin and hence decrease the severity of the intoxication.[20]

Biliary excretion. Although certain intoxicants (or their active metabolites) with organic acid properties are secreted into the bile against large concentration gradients (e.g., cardiac glycosides, tricyclic antidepressants, phenothiazines, glutethimide),[22,23] modification or acceleration of this process is not possible at the present time. However, intestinal reabsorption of ingested intoxicants (or their active metabolites already secreted into the bile or undergoing enterohepatic or hepatoenteric circulation) can be decreased by the continuous administration of activated charcoal every 4 to 6 hours and the toxicity of the ingested intoxicant consequently minimized.

Urinary excretion. The renal excretion of many toxic ingestants depends on glomerular filtration, active tubular secretion, and passive tubular reabsorption.[24–26] Therefore, modification or alteration of these excretory processes could lead to an increase in the renal excretion of the toxic ingestants and a resulting decrease in the duration and severity of the toxicologic effects. Unfortunately, when different therapeutic interventions are applied to accelerate or promote the renal excretion of the toxic ingestants, only modification of the passive tubular reabsorption process has been found significantly effective.[25-28] The passive reabsorption process is the one primarily involved in urinary excretion because it plays an important role in the prolongation of the toxicologic actions of toxic ingestants.

Passive reabsorption of most filtered intoxicants takes place largely in the proximal tubules, because the concentration of the intoxicants in the filtrate increases as salt and water are reabsorbed. The administration of an osmotic diuretic such as mannitol or the intravenous infusion of furosemide would inhibit water and sodium reabsorption, and consequently would accelerate the renal excretion of the toxic ingestants. Therefore, forced diuresis (3 to 6 ml of urine per kg of body weight every hour), using intravenous fluids and diuretics, is potentially applicable to all toxic ingestants that undergo glomerular filtration and are passively reabsorbed. The adult dose and rate of administration of mannitol is 25 g, infused continuously as long as clinically indicated, or until a maximum dose of 150 g/day has been given. The pediatric dose and rate of administration of mannitol is 1 g/kg of body weight, infused continuously as clinically indicated, or until a maximum of 25 g/day has been administered. The adult and pediatric dose and rate of administration of furosemide is 1 mg/kg of body weight IV, initially. Thereafter, the dosage and rate of administration vary with the patient's fluid and electrolyte balance, urinary volume, and clinical signs and symptoms.

Alteration of the urinary pH can also inhibit back-diffusion of some intoxicants and, as a result, can accelerate their renal excretion.[24,25,27,28] This can be accomplished because weak organic acids and bases diffuse readily out of the tubular fluid in their nonionized form, but are trapped in this fluid when ionized. Therefore, alkalinization of the urine greatly increases the ionization in the tubular fluid of such organic acids as phenobarbital, salicylates, arsenic, isoniazid, lithium, meprobamate, and naphthalene, and decreases their back-diffusion through the renal tubular epithelium cells.[24,25,28-31] This therapeutic intervention therefore increases the excretion of these weak acids. Alkalinization of the urine can be achieved with the administration of sodium bicarbonate at an initial dose of 3 to 5 mEq/kg of body weight, infused over a period of 2 to 3 hours. Thereafter, the dose and rate of the continuous administration of sodium bicarbonate should be determined by measurements of urinary and blood pH. The endpoint of urinary alkalinization is a pH of 8.0.

Acidification of the urine also greatly increases the ionization in the tubular fluid of such organic bases as amphetamines, phencyclidine, strychnine, phosphorus, quinine, and quinidine, and thus accelerates their excretion.[24,25,28,31,32] Acidification of the urine can be accomplished with the intravenous infusion or oral administration of ascorbic acid or ammonium chloride. The initial dose and rate of administration of ascorbic acid is 500 mg to 2 g orally or intravenously as needed to obtain an acidic urine. The initial dose and rate of administration of ammonium chloride is 2 to 6 g/day, or 75 mg/kg/dose in four divided doses. Ascorbic acid and ammonium chloride are available as IV solutions, and also in tablets and syrup preparations. The endpoint of urinary acidification with both of these agents is a pH of 4.5 to 5.5.

In summary, urinary excretory mechanisms are commonly the focus of therapeutic intervention or modification in an effort to treat the intoxicated patient more efficiently and effectively. A combination of osmotic diuresis and alteration of urinary pH is even more effective than any single type of manipulation alone. It must be remembered, however, that any form of forced diuresis demands careful hourly monitoring of fluid intake, urine output, and blood and urine electrolytes and pH. Pulmonary edema, water intoxication, cerebral edema, and acid-base and fluid and electrolyte disturbances are well-recognized complications. Therefore, forced alkalinized or acidified diuresis should be undertaken only in the presence of high-quality intensive care facilities and should be used only for those ingestants whose excretion is significantly altered by these procedures and when there is no possibility that the patient's cardiovascular and renal functions will be compromised.

DIALYSIS AND HEMOPERFUSION

In cases where the intoxicated patient with life-threatening symptoms is not responsive to conventional treatment, or develops renal failure or severe acid-base and fluid and electrolyte disturbances, dialysis or hemoperfusion can be used. The three dialytic procedures available to the clinician are peritoneal dialysis, hemodialysis, and charcoal or resin hemoperfusion. Although these procedures are described in more detail in Chapter 3, they will be discussed briefly here.

Peritoneal dialysis. The paramount advantage of peritoneal dialysis is its simplicity. Its disadvantages are its inefficiency and complications (e.g., peritoneal infection, intra-abdominal trauma, pulmonary complications). This procedure is valuable for the removal of intoxicants only in preschool children, or if renal function is impaired, forced diuresis cannot be implemented, hemodialysis or hemoperfusion procedures cannot be carried out, or the patient cannot be transferred to a tertiary care facility where hemodialysis and hemoperfusion procedures and trained personnel are available.[33-34]

Hemodialysis. This procedure is 5 to 10 times more effective than peritoneal dialysis for the removal of water-soluble toxic ingestants that are not highly protein bound. Furthermore, addition of albumin or lipids to the dialysate solution promotes the removal of greater quantities not only of water-soluble, non-highly protein-bound intoxicants, but protein-bound, highly lipophilic intoxicants as well. Its major disadvantages are medical complications (e.g., extracorporeal clotting, infection, blood loss, hematomas, shock), and complex apparatus and skilled personnel, which are not readily available in all institutions.[35-37]

Charcoal or resin hemoperfusion. In recent years, the limitations of hemodialysis in the removal of high-molecular-weight toxins, as well as highly protein-bound, lipophilic intoxicants has led to the development of alternative approaches for the treatment of the intoxicated patient. Perfusion of blood through activated charcoal or an exchange resin achieves removal of higher quantities of intoxicants, even those with high molecular weights, or those that are highly lipophilic and distributed throughout body tissues. However, both of these techniques are inadequate if the intoxicant is highly protein bound, and their application in the clinical setting has been hampered because of damage to blood components and risks of sorbent embolization.[37-40]

Toxic ingestants that may be actively removed by dialysis or hemoperfusion are listed under various chemical and pharmacologic titles in Chapter 3, Table 3-3.

SUPPORTIVE AND SYMPTOMATIC CARE

The majority of toxic ingestions result in reversible, self-limited disease states. The use of skillful supportive and symptomatic care remains the cornerstone of treatment, particularly when the ingested intoxicant has no specific antidote available. It must be remembered, however, that in all cases, even when an antidote is available, the patient must be treated first, and not the intoxicant. In addition, with anticipation of the possible needs of the patient, recognition of potential toxic effects that can be produced by the intoxicant, and an understanding of how these toxic effects can be managed, the outcome cannot be

Table 1–6.   Physiologic Disturbances Commonly Seen in Intoxicated Patients.

PHYSIOLOGIC DISTURBANCES	CAUSES	THERAPEUTIC INTERVENTIONS
CNS depression	Direct depressant effect of the reticular activating system Depression of the medullary centers	Support of vital functions by mechanical means Most intoxicated patients will emerge from coma as from prolonged anesthesia Avoidance of CNS stimulants or analeptics
Convulsion	Specific excitatory effects Hypoxia Hypoglycemia Metabolic disturbances Cerebral edema	Short-acting barbiturates Diazepam
Cerebral edema	Increased capillary permeability Hypoxia	Symptomatic treatment with adrenocortical steroids, hypertonic solutions (mannitol or urea)
Pulmonary edema	Depressed myocardial contractibility Alveolar injury from irritant gases or direct toxic effect Alveolar injury from aspirate fluids	Continued suctioning. Administration of high concentration of oxygen under positive pressure Bronchodilators Adrenocortical steroids
Hypotension	Depression of medullary vasomotor Blockage of autonomic ganglia or adrenergic receptors Decreased myocardial contractility Depression of the tone of arterial or venous smooth muscle Cardiac arrhythmias	Correction of abnormalities, if possible When central venous pressure is low, fluid replacement should be the first therapeutic approach Use of vasoactive drugs only if patient is not responsive to fluid administration
Cardiac arrhythmias	Specific effects on the electrical properties of cardiac fibers Myocardial hypoxia Metabolic disturbances	Administration of antiarrhythmic agents as indicated by the nature of the arrhythmia present
Hypoxia	Central respiratory depression Muscular paralysis Obstruction of airway Pulmonary edema Shock Anemia, methemoglobinemia, Carboxyhemoglobinemia Depression of cellular oxidation	(Depending on the degree of hypoxia): Maintenance of an adequate airway Frequent suctioning Insertion of an oropharyngeal airway or endotracheal tube, or a tracheostomy Administration of high concentrations of oxygen Combined administration of oxygen with artificial ventilation Hyperbaric oxygenation
Fluid and electrolyte abnormalities	Ingestion of intoxicant and treatment through vomiting, diarrhea, diuresis, catharsis, impaired or inadequate fluid and electrolyte administration, or retention of fluid and electrolytes due to renal insufficiency	Meticulous attention to fluid and electrolyte balance Evaluation of each patient in terms of pre-existing deficits or excesses, as well as continuous losses Determination of the integrity of cardiac and renal function

anything but successful. Table 1–6 briefly summarizes the physiologic disturbances commonly seen in intoxicated patients, as well as their etiologic factors and initial therapeutic interventions.[14,16,18,41] Detailed information regarding physiologic disturbances and approaches to therapeutic management for specific intoxicants or pharmacologic classes of intoxicants are described elsewhere in this text.

Once all the initial technical tasks have been performed and the patient has been kept for observation or admitted for hospitalization, good nursing care is the single most important factor in the reduction of mortality and morbidity rates from toxic ingestions. This includes turning of the comatose patient, suctioning of the upper respiratory tract, dressing of bullous lesions, maintenance of adequate eye care, catheter care, and continued monitoring of vital signs, state of consciousness, arterial blood gases, and serum and urinary electrolytes. These tasks are of the greatest importance and can determine the difference between the patient who will have multiple complications and the one who will walk out of the hospital 3 to 4 days postadmission.

Accidental ingestions and/or deliberate drug intoxications constitute a common and serious medical problem. Although accidental intoxications have increased during the last decade, the most significant rise has occurred in intentionally self-administered overdosages. Because of the increased numbers of patients admitted to emergency rooms because of overdosages, the clinician must be ever cognizant of the general considerations and principles of management of these patients.

REFERENCES

1. Anon: Poisoning deaths in the United States. *National Clgh Poison Control Center Bull*, 24(2):2–7, 1980.

2. Arnold FJ, Hodges JB, and Barta RA: Evaluation of the efficacy of lavage and induced emesis in treatment of salicylate poisoning. *Pediatrics*, 23:286, 1959.

3. Boxer L, Anderson FP, and Rowe DS: Comparison of ipecac-induced emesis with gastric lavage in the treatment of acute salicylate ingestion. *J Pediatr*, 74:800–803, 1969.

4. Manoguerra AS, and Krenzelok EP: Rapid emesis from high-dose ipecac syrup in adult and children intoxicated with antiemetics or other drugs. *Am J Hosp Pharm*, 34:1360-1363, 1978.

5. MacLean WC: A comparison of ipecac syrup and apomorphine in the immediate treatment of ingestion of poisons. *J Pediatr*, 82:121–124, 1973.

6. Scher LA, and Maull KI: Emergency management and sequelae of acid ingestion. *JACEP*, 7:206–208, 1978.

7. Ng RC, Darwish H, and Stewart DA: Emergency treatment of petroleum distillate and turpentine ingestion. *Can Med Assoc J*, 111:537–539, 1974.

8. Dabbous IA, German AB, and Paterson WO: The ineffectiveness of mechanically induced vomiting. *J Pediatr*, 66:952–954, 1965

9. Schofferman JA: A clinical comparison of syrup of ipecac and apomorphine use in adults. *JACEP*, 5:22–25, 1976.

10. Barer J, Hill LL, and Martinez RM: Fatal poisoning from salt used as an emetic. *Am J Dis Child*, 125:889–890, 1973.

11. Corby DG, Decker WH: Management of acute poisoning with activated charcoal. *Pediatrics*, 54:324–328, 1974.

12. Picchioni AL, Chin L, and Laird HE: Activated charcoal preparation—relative antidotal activity. *Clin Toxicol*, 7:97–108, 1974.

13. Decker WJ, Combs HF, and Corby DG: Absorption of drugs and poisons by activated charcoal. *Toxicol Appl Pharmacol*, 13:454–460, 1968.

14. Friedman PA: Chemical intoxication: General considerations and principles of management. In *Harrison's Principles of Internal Medicine*. 9th Ed. Edited by KJ Isselbacher, et al. New York, McGraw-Hill, 1980, pp. 949–990.

15. Czajka PA, and Duffy JP (eds): Drugs for the management of acute poisonings. In *Poisoning Emergencies*. St. Louis, C.V. Mosby, 1980, pp. 14–21.

16. Rumack BH: Management of acute poisoning and overdose. In *Management of the Poisoned Patient*. Edited by BH Rumack and AR Temple. Princeton, N.J., Science Press, 1977, pp. 250–280.

17. Gosselin RE, Hodge HC, Smith RP, and Gleason MN (eds): Section 1. First aid and emergency treatment. In *Clinical Toxicology of Commercial Products*. 4th ed. Baltimore, Williams and Wilkins, 1976, pp. 1–6.

18. Comstock EG: Guide to management of drug overdose. In *Physicians' Desk Reference*. 34th Ed. Oradell, NJ, Medical Economics Co., 1980.

19. Picchioni AL, et al: Activated charcoal vs. "universal antidote" as an antidote for poisons. *Toxicol Appl Pharmacol*, 8:447–454, 1966.

20. Klaasan CD: Absorption, distribution, and excretion of toxicants. In *Toxicology: The Basic*

Sciences of Poisons. Edited by LJ Casarett and D Doull. New York, Macmillan, 1975, pp. 26–44.

21. Whorton MD: Carbon monoxide intoxication: A review of 14 patients. *JACEP*, 5:505–509, 1976.

22. Smith RL: The biliary excretion and enterohepatic circulation of drugs and other organic compounds. *Fortschr Arzneimiltelforsch*, 9:229–360, 1966.

23. Gard HD, et al: Studies on the disposition of amitriptylline and other tricyclic antidepressant drugs in man as it relates to the management of the overdosed patient. *Adv Biochem Psychopharmacol*, 7:95–105, 1973.

24. Sir D Black (ed): Renal excretion and nephrotoxicity of drugs. In *Renal Disease.* 3rd Ed. London, Blackwell Scientific Publications, 1972, pp. 591–613.

25. Weiner IM: Mechanisms of drug absorption and excretion: The renal excretion of drugs and related compounds. *Annu Rev Pharmacol*, 7:39–56, 1967.

26. Pitts RF (eds): *Physiology of The Kidney and Body Fluids.* 2nd Ed. Chicago, The Year Book Medical Publishers, Inc., 1970.

27. Cafruny EJ: Renal pharmacology. *Annu Rev Pharmacol*, 8:131:150, 1968.

28. Levine RR (ed): *Pharmacology: Drug Actions and Reactions.* 1st ed. Boston, Little, Brown, 1973, pp. 113–134.

29. Sjoquist F, et al: The pH-dependent excretion of monomethylated tricyclic antidepressants. *Clin Pharmacol Ther*, 10:826–833, 1969.

30. Sperber I: Secretion of organic acids in the formation of urine and bile. *Pharmacol Rev*, 11:109–134, 1959.

31. Weiner IM, and Mudge GH: Renal tubular mechanisms for excretion of organic acids and bases. *Am J Med*, 36:743–762, 1964.

32. Peters L: Renal tubular excretion of organic bases. *Pharmacol Rev*, 12:1–35, 1960.

33. Nolph KD: Peritoneal dialysis. In *Replacement of Renal Function by Dialysis.* 2nd Ed. Edited by W Drukker, FM Parsons and JF Maher. The Hague, Netherlands, Martinus Nijhoff Publishers, 1979, pp. 277–321.

34. Maxwell MH, Rokney RE, and Kleeman CR: Peritoneal dialysis. 1. Technique and application. *JAMA*, 170:917–929, 1959.

35. Schreiner GE: The role of hemodialysis (artificial kidney) in acute poisoning. *Arch Intern Med*, 102:896–913, 1958.

36. Blagg CR: Acute complications associated with hemodialysis. In *Replacement of Renal Function by Dialysis.* 2nd Ed. Edited by W Drukker, FM Parsons, and JF Maher. The Hague, Netherlands, Martinus Nijhoff, Publishers, 1979, pp. 486–503.

37. Winchester JF, et al: Dialysis and hemoperfusion of poisons and drugs-update. *Trans Am Soc Artif Intern Organs*, 23:762–842, 1977.

38. Rosenbaum JL, et al: Hemoperfusion for acute drug intoxication. *Arch Intern Med*, 136:263–266, 1976.

39. DeMyttenaere MH, Maher JR, and Schreiner GE: Hemoperfusion through a charcoal column for glutethimide poisoning. *Trans Am Soc Artif Intern Organs*, 13:190, 1967.

40. Hagstam K, Larsson L, and Thysell H: Experimental studies on charcoal hemoperfusion in phenobarbital intoxication and uremia. *Acta Med Scand*, 180:593–603, 1966.

41. Gosselin RE, Hodge HC, Smith RP, and Gleason MN (eds): Section IV. Supportive treatment in acute chemical poisoning. In *Clinical Toxicology of Commercial Products.* 4th Ed. Baltimore, Williams and Wilkins, 1976, pp. 1–86.

Chapter 2

The Role of the Toxicology Laboratory

James B. Mowry
Vasilios A. Skoutakis

An increasing problem in any hospital emergency room throughout the United States is the frequency with which patients are admitted because of accidental drug ingestions, deliberate drug overdosages, and chronic drug abuse problems. Consequently, the toxicology laboratory is frequently asked by many clinicians to provide rapid, accurate analyses of biologic fluids to assist in the management of these patients. Our experiences and those reported by others, however, suggest that although many clinicians tend to utilize the toxicology laboratory for assistance, particularly when dealing with a patient who has ingested an unknown intoxicant, the majority of clinicians do not have a functional knowledge of the appropriate use of the laboratory for the management of these patients.[1-3]

The purpose of this chapter is to familiarize the clinician and/or student with some basic principles regarding the use of the toxicology laboratory and how the results obtained from the laboratory can assist in effective management of these patients.

ROLE AND APPROPRIATE USE OF THE TOXICOLOGY LABORATORY

Presently there is a controversy as to whether or not the toxicology laboratory emergency measurements are needed in the management of intoxicated patients,[2] since the key to therapy in the vast majority of these patients is supportive and symptomatic care. Opponents of the use of emergency toxicologic measurements believe that (1) in acute intoxications, the intoxicant involved is usually known, and the laboratory merely confirms its presence, (2) treatment in many cases has started long before the laboratory results are available, thereby nullifying the need for specific identification of the intoxicant, (3) the therapeutic approaches in treatment of these patients will be essentially the same regardless of the intoxicant, and (4) emergency toxicologic measurements can be costly to the patient.

Proponents of the use of the toxicology laboratory for the treatment of intoxicated patients believe, however, that the value of the emergency toxicology measurements is not in the provision of the diagnosis for the clinician, but in (1) confirmation of the suspected diagnosis so other diagnostic tests will not be done, (2) identification of the specific intoxicant responsible, to enable specific therapeutic approaches to be implemented based on the properties of the intoxicant, (3) assessment of the severity of the intoxication so that the therapeutic approaches can be altered if necessary, (4) prediction of the patient's outcome and the chances for survival, (5) recognition of symptoms caused by the intoxicant as distinguished from those of other disease states, and (6) follow-up of the patient's progress to prevent recurrent toxicologic complications.

It is most important that the clinician and the laboratory personnel each appreciate the others' capabilities and limitations if meaningful emergency toxicologic determinations are to be made. Therefore, prior to initiation of an order for a general toxicologic screen or for a specific toxicologic analysis, the clinician should be knowledgeable about the assessment of the intoxicated patient, the time needed to analyze results, and the use of biologic fluids.

ASSESSMENT OF THE INTOXICATED PATIENT

The laboratory geared to emergency operations can provide quick and accurate verification or identification of the drugs or chemicals ingested only if the clinician can provide some clues from the patient's history and/or clinical findings. In many cases, unless the patient is in a comatose state, some knowledge of the ingested intoxicant can be obtained. In such cases, if the patient's history is judged reliable, a full toxicologic screen would not be necessary. In the case of a comatose patient, information can be obtained from relatives, friends, prescription medications and, most importantly, from the clinical condition of the patient.

If the symptoms of the patient are incompatible with the known toxic effects of the suspected intoxicant, a broader search for the identification of the intoxicant is warranted. Conversely, if the patient's clinical condition is consistent with the history, the laboratory can provide quick confirmation of the diagnosis and can help assess the potential severity of the situation. If a history is unobtainable, the patient's clinical findings may suggest a certain intoxicant, and again the laboratory can provide confirmation. It must be remembered that, without a good clinical evaluation and appreciation of the clinical findings, the laboratory personnel will be simply looking blindfolded for the proverbial needle in the haystack.

TIME NEEDED TO ANALYZE RESULTS

For optimal utilization of an emergency toxicologic determination, the turn around time (TAT), or the interval between the time when the sample is received in the laboratory and when the results are reported, is important. A particular assay may be simple or quickly performed, but if it is not given emergency service status, the results will not be received in time to influence the therapy. Conversely, an assay itself may be lengthy and may require several hours for the results to be reported. For example, serum assays for most narcotics will have a TAT of more than 24 hours. However, a provocative challenge of the patient with a specific narcotic antagonist such as naloxone can yield an immediate answer.

USE OF BIOLOGIC FLUIDS

Many clinicians commonly ask what type of biologic fluids should be sent for analysis to the toxicology laboratory. Different information can be obtained depending on the type of biologic fluid used for toxicologic analysis. We will briefly discuss the most commonly used biologic fluids (e.g., gastric contents, urine, and blood or serum) according to their practicality, timing of collection, and usable information.

GASTRIC CONTENTS

The analysis of gastric contents is frequently overlooked by many clinicians, but it can provide valuable information. Gastric contents, whether obtained by emesis or gastric lavage, obviously will be of value neither in an overdose with an intoxicant that has been injected, nor if obtained 24 to 36 hours after an ingestion in most cases. Therefore, gastric samples are best utilized within a reasonable time after ingestion, before absorption or gastric emptying has occurred. The usefulness of analysis of gastric contents is three-fold. First, such an analysis aids in the initial determination of whether the patient has actually ingested the suspected intoxicant. Secondly, gastric samples can be used to roughly quantitate the amount of intoxicant the patient has taken, if the

volume of the gastric sample is known. Thirdly, when the amount ingested is roughly known, gastric analysis is useful in quantitating the amount of intoxicant removed from the GI tract, so that the adequacy of lavage or emesis can be assessed.[3] These last two uses are more theoretical, however, than practical.

URINE

Urine samples are frequently used because they are easy to obtain, simple to prepare as samples for analysis, and suitable for screening procedures. Urine samples, however, have their limitation. They are of no value if obtained immediately after ingestion, because sufficient time must be allowed for absorption, metabolism, and excretion to occur. Therefore, a sample obtained 15 to 30 minutes after an ingestion, for example, usually will not reveal the intoxicant unless its absorption, metabolism, and excretion are rapid. Furthermore, if only the metabolites of the intoxicant and not the intoxicant itself were renally excreted, urine specimens may not be helpful unless the assay also detects the specific metabolites of the intoxicant. Fortunately, the principal substances measured in many of the available assays are the metabolites of the parent intoxicant, since many of the intoxicants commonly involved in overdoses are metabolized before excretion. In any case, the information received by an analysis of the urine sample is only of a confirmatory nature. Some indication of the severity of an intoxication can be obtained by measurement of the relative amount of the intoxicant or its metabolites, but the results can be used only as a rough guide and at best can be regarded as semiquantitative.[4]

BLOOD

Blood and serum samples are the most reliable samples for the detection of an

Table 2–1. Compendium of Common Intoxicants in Human Biofluids.

CHEMICAL CLASS	THERAPEUTIC LEVELS[3,12-15,47-49]	TOXIC/LETHAL LEVELS[3,12-15,47-49]	LETHAL DOSE *toxic dose	ASSAY TECHNIQUES	SPECIMEN	TYPE	TAT (HR)	COMMENTS
ANALGESICS								
Acetaminophen	10–20 µg/ml	400 µg/ml	>10–15 g[56,58-61]	GLC,[19] S_{UV}[38]	SERUM	QUANT	4	toxic levels @ 4 hrs serial levels rec for t½[6]
Codeine	25 ng/ml	1500 µg/ml	>140 mg/kg*[59]	C,[1] HPLC[59] TLC,[38] GLC[38] EMIT[39]	URINE	S-QUANT	>24	
Narcotics	—	20–300 ng/ml	>5–15 mg/kg*[84]	TLC[38,42] GLC[19,28,42] EMIT[1,39]	URINE	S-QUANT	>24	measures codeine, morphine, meperidine, chlorpromazine, DM
Pentazocine	0.14–0.6 µg/ml	2–5 µg/ml 10–20 µg/ml	—	TLC,[38] GLC[38]	URINE	S-QUANT	>24	
Propoxyphene	50–200 ng/ml	5–20 µg/ml 57 µg/ml	10.7 mg/kg*[74] > 35 mg/kg[74]	GLC[19,38] TLC,[38] EMIT[39]	URINE	S-QUANT	>24	EMIT includes metabolite, McBay lethal-2 µg/ml
Salicylates	10–30 mg/dl	30–50 mg/dl 50–80 mg/dl	>240 mg/kg*	C[38]	SERUM	QUANT	4	
ALCOHOLS								
Ethanol	100 mg/dl	100–200 mg/dl >350 mg/dl	>3 g/kg (child)[62] >5–8 g/kg (adult)	GLC[19,38]	SERUM	QUANT	4	(a)
Ethylene glycol	—	150 mg/dl	>2 ml/kg[67]	GLC[19,38]	SERUM	QUANT	4	
Isopropanol	—	200–400 mg/dl 340 mg/dl	>100 ml (adult)[67] >700 ml* of 100%	GLC[19,38]	SERUM	QUANT	4	
Methanol	—	20–80 mg/dl 75–125 mg/dl	10–60 ml of 100%	GLC[19,38]	SERUM	QUANT	4	
TRICYCLIC ANTIDEPRESSANTS	50–300 ng/ml	300–1000 ng/ml >1000–2000 ng/ml	10–20 mg/kg[50]	GLC[38] GC-MS[40]	SERUM URINE URINE	QUANT S-QUANT QUAL	>24	(b)
AMPHETAMINES	20–30 ng/ml	2.0 µg/ml	20–25 mg/kg[50]	GLC[19,28,42] TLC[38,42] EMIT[4]	URINE	QUANT	4	(a), (c) McBay lethal-500–600 ng/ml. Fatality at 5 mg/kg.
ANTICONVULSANTS								
Phenytoin	5–22 µg/ml	20–50 µg/ml 100 µg/ml	100, 160 mg/kg[55] 36–300 mg/kg*[55]	S_{UV},[38] GLC[40] EMIT[19,39]	SERUM	QUANT	4	36–300 mg/kg with survival. McBay lethal-70 µg/ml
Primidone	5–12 µg/ml	50–80 µg/ml 100 µg/ml	20–30 g[81]	GLC[38] EMIT[19,39]	SERUM	QUANT	4	
ANTIHISTAMINES								
Diphenhydramine	5 µg/ml	10 µg/ml	100–500 mg (< 3 yrs. old)[64]	TLC[38] GLC[38]	URINE	S-QUANT	>24	
Methapyrilene	2 ng/ml	30–50 µg/ml >50 µg/ml	20–40 mg/kg[83] 0.95–1.8 g[83]	TLC[38] GLC[38]	URINE	S-QUANT	>24	survival with 2.5 g[83]

	Therapeutic	Toxic	Lethal/Dose	Method	Specimen	Quant	TAT (hr)	Comments
CARDIOVASCULAR								
Digoxin	0.6–1.3 ng/ml	2.9 ng/ml	>5–23 mg*	EMIT[39] RIA[40]	SERUM	QUANT	>24	EMIT-4 hr TAT
Disopyramide	2–8 µg/ml	—	>6 g[85]	GLC, HPLC, S[88]	SERUM	QUANT		
Procainamide	3–8 µg/ml	8.5–114 µg/ml >8–12 µg/ml	>7–19 g*[57]	GLC,[19] S[38] EMIT[39]	SERUM	QUANT	4	
Propranolol	50–100 ng/ml	—	>3.6 g[75] (1 case)	GLC[87]	SERUM	QUANT	>24	survival with 5.1 g[76]
Quinidine	2–6 µg/ml	>6–10 µg/ml 30–50 µg/ml	>4 g	GLC[40] EMIT[39]	SERUM	QUANT	4	survival with 8 g[63]
METALS								
Arsenic	0–20 ng/ml	1.0 µg/ml 15 µg/ml	1 mg–10 g*	AA[19]	URINE	S-QUANT	4	
Iron	50–150 µg/dl	500–600 µg/dl	400–5000 mg[69] >60 mg/kg*	Bathophenan-troline[38]	SERUM	QUANT	4	
Lead	0.05–1.3 µg/ml	0.7 µg/ml >2 µg/ml	>1.5 mg/dl*	AA[19]	SERUM URINE	QUANT S-QUANT	4 >24	24-hr urine collection needed
Lithium	0.5–1.5 mEq/L	2 mEq/L 2–5 mEq/L	>140–1620 mEq*[70]	AA[19]	SERUM	QUANT	4	
Mercury	60–120 ng/ml	—	1–4 g[71]	AA[40]	SERUM URINE	QUANT S-QUANT	>24	
SEDATIVES HYPNOTICS								
Barbiturates (Long-acting)	10–25 µg/ml	40–60 µg/ml 80–150 µg/ml	>8 mg/kg* >5 g[50]	EMIT[19,39] GLC[19,41] S_{UV}[38,41]	SERUM URINE	QUANT S-QUANT	4	(a). $EMIT_U$–no differentiation. $EMIT_S$-phenobarb. only.
Barbiturates (Short-acting)	0.1–1 µg/ml	7–20 µg/ml >10–30 µg/ml	>5–8 mg/kg* >3 g[50]	EMIT[19,39] GLC[19,41] S_{UV}[38,41]	SERUM URINE	QUANT S-QUANT	4 4	$EMIT_U$–no differentiation, false pos. with high-glutethimide conc.
Chloral hydrate	10 µg/ml	100 µg/ml 250 µg/ml	4 g (1 case) 10 g*	GLC[38,45] Pyridine Rx[38]	SERUM URINE	QUANT S-QUANT	>24 4	(a)
Ethchlorvynol	5 µg/ml	20 µg/ml 150 µg/ml	>10 g[50]	GLC[19,43,45] S[38,44,45]	SERUM	QUANT	>24	(a). death with 2.5 g
Glutethimide	0.2 µg/ml	10–80 µg/ml 30–100 µg/ml	>5–28 g[51]	GLC[19,45] S_{UV}[38,45]	SERUM	QUANT	4	(a). 1 death–5 g. 1 survival–28 g
Methyprylon	10 µg/ml	30–60 µg/ml 100 µg/ml	>6 g[50,54]	GLC[38,45]	SERUM	QUANT	>24	(a). 1 death 6 g survival with 30 g
Methaqualone	5 µg/ml	10–30 µg/ml >30 µg/ml	>5–7.5 g[52,53]	GLC[19,38,45] S_{UV}[38,45]	SERUM	QUANT	4	McBay lethal-5 µg/ml
STREET DRUGS								
Cocaine	—	—	20–1200 mg	EMIT[39] TLC[38]	URINE	S-QUANT	4	EMIT measures metabolite, (a)
Phencyclidine	—	<0.5 µg/ml 1.0 µg/ml	mild: 5–10 mg*[72] moderate: 10–20 mg* severe: >20 mg*	GLC[19,38,44] EMIT[39]	SERUM URINE	QUANT S-QUANT	>24 4	(d), deaths with 150–200 mg[86]

Table 2–1.   Compendium of Common Intoxicants in Human Biofluids (Continued).

CHEMICAL CLASS	THERAPEUTIC LEVELS[3,12-15,47-49]	TOXIC/LETHAL LEVELS[3,12-15,47-49]	LETHAL DOSE *toxic dose	ASSAY TECHNIQUES	SPECIMEN	TYPE	TAT (HR)	COMMENTS
TRANQUILIZERS								
Benzodiazepines	0.5–6 µg/ml	5–30 µg/ml / 50 µg/ml	not known[50]	GLC[19,45] / S_{UV}[38,45] / EMIT[39]	SERUM / URINE	QUANT / S-QUANT	>24 / 4	(a), (e) EMIT for both serum and urine
Meprobamate	5–30 µg/ml	50–100 µg/ml / 200 µg/ml	>50 mg/kg,* 8–12 g[79], 12–20 g[81]	GLC[19,45] / S[38]	SERUM	QUANT	4	(a), death-12 g[77] survival-40 g[78] McBay lethal-50 µg/ml
Chlorpromazine	0.1–0.5 µg/ml	1–2 µg/ml / 3–12 µg/ml	20–74 mg/kg[73] (children)	C[38,46]	URINE	S-QUANT	4	
Thioridazine	1–1.5 µg/ml	10 µg/ml / 20–80 µg/ml	1.5–8 g[73] (adults)	C[38,46]	URINE	S-QUANT	4	
MISCELLANEOUS								
Caffeine	—	— / 100 µg/ml	>5–10 g[66] / 1 g*	GLC[38]	URINE	S-QUANT	>24	
Isoniazid	—	—	80–150 mg/kg[68]	S_{UV}[38]	SERUM	QUANT	>24	
Theophylline	10–20 µg/ml	>50 µg/ml / —	—	GLC[19] / EMIT[39]	SERUM	QUANT	4	
Warfarin	1.0–10 µg/ml	—	—	S_{UV}[38]	SERUM	QUANT	>24	Not routinely performed

THERAPEUTIC TOXIC and LETHAL DOSES: approximate values, for guideline use only.[3,12-15,47-49]

TOXIC/LETHAL LEVELS: top number = toxic level(s); bottom number = lethal level(s).

ASSAYS: GLC = gas-liquid chromatography
TLC = thin layer chromatography
EMIT = enzyme-multiplied immunoassay technique
S = spectrophotometric
S_{UV} = ultraviolet spectrophotometry
C = colorimetric
AA = atomic absorption
RIA = radioimmunoassay
GC-MS = gas chromatography/mass spectrometry
HPLC = high performance liquid chromatography

TYPE: QUANT = quantitative
S-QUANT = semiquantitative
QUAL = qualitative

SPECIMEN and TYPE: examples of those commonly used at USC Section of Pathology and Laboratories

TAT: Turn around time for USC Section of Pathology and Laboratories

COMMENTS: (a) = tolerance can occur

(b) = Amitriptyline	Child	Adult
DEATH	375–500 mg	1750 mg[80]
SURVIVAL	500 mg	3925 mg

(c) = EMIT measures methamphetamine, cyclopentamine, mephentermine, nylidin, phenmetrazine, high concentrations of ephedrine and phenylpropanolamine

(d) = EMIT measures metabolites and analogs of PCP and high concentrations of morphine, meperidine, chlorpromazine, promethazine and dextromethorphan (DM)

(e) = EMIT urine measures oxazepam
EMIT serum measures clonazepam, clorazepate, flurazepam, medazepam, prazepam, chlordiazepoxide, diazepam, lorazepam, oxazepam plus metabolites

intoxicant, since the intoxicant must be absorbed into the blood stream before it can reach its target tissue and produce an effect. Several factors, however, play a role in the interpretation of blood or serum concentrations in the overdose situation.

Blood or serum, in contrast to gastric or urine specimens, can be taken at multiple times to test for continued absorption and elimination of the intoxicant. As an example, digoxin has been shown in overdose situations to reach its peak as late as 34 hours after ingestion.[5] In addition, for acetaminophen, the half-life determination after completion of absorption has been used as a prognosticator of the seriousness of the intoxication.[6]

When an intoxicant is taken in a single massive dose, as in the overdose situation, there is for many intoxicants little correlation between the serum concentration and the effect of the intoxicant.[7] If the sample is drawn too soon after the ingestion, there may be insufficient time for absorption and distribution of the intoxicant and the result will be a false low or high serum concentration. For example, in acute digoxin intoxications, if the blood is drawn earlier than 6 to 12 hours after ingestion, an erroneously high value is obtained because of incomplete distribution.[8] In the case of an anticholinergic intoxication, if the blood is drawn too soon after the ingestion, a low serum concentration may be obtained, owing to decreased GI motility, which results in delayed absorption. The effect of an intoxicant may also be delayed by physiologic mechanisms, as with warfarin intoxication, in which the clinical effects of severe anticoagulation take at least 36 to 48 hours to appear, because of the time necessary for the degradation of existing clotting factors.[9]

Another pitfall, which is typically associated with sedative-hypnotics, is the occurrence of tolerance. In these cases, the blood concentration can be far in excess of the normally established toxic range, with little or no serious toxicity to the patient.[10] Other factors that can hinder the interpretation of blood or plasma concentrations are differences in protein binding and target organ sensitivity among patients. It is also possible that a metabolite that cannot be measured, rather than the parent compound, could be responsible for the damage incurred from the overdose. This can be seen in acetaminophen intoxication, in which the major toxic result, hepatic necrosis, is mediated by a toxic metabolite.[11] Various authors have tabulated therapeutic, toxic and lethal blood levels for certain compounds,[3,12-15] which will be discussed later (see Table 2–1).

METHODS FOR QUALITATIVE OR QUANTITATIVE ANALYSIS OF INTOXICANTS

Although many clinicians use the toxicology laboratory for assistance in the management of intoxicated patients, in the majority of cases, only the results of a determination are reported from the laboratory. As a consequence, many clinicians have an inadequate knowledge and understanding of the scope and limitations of the assay techniques used for the determination of these results, particularly when the results obtained do not correlate with the patients' symptoms. For this reason, we will review and evaluate here the major techniques for assaying biologic fluids.

COLOR TESTS

Color or spot tests in many cases are preliminary, rough screening aids used in many toxicology laboratories. They are simple to perform, require little or no special equipment, and can be carried out by personnel with minimal laboratory experience. Two classic examples of color tests are the Reinsch test for heavy metals and the Forrest test for phenothiazines. In the Reinsch test, 5 to 10 ml of urine or stomach contents are mixed with an equal amount of 10% HCI; a coil of copper wire or a thoroughly cleaned penny is added, and the mixture is heated on a water bath for 10 minutes. The copper wire or penny is then examined for a dark stain. If no stain appears in 1 hour, the test is negative.

In the Forrest test, 1 ml of urine is mixed with 1 ml of FPN reagent (5% ferric chloride, 20% perchloric acid, 50% nitric acid in a 1:9:10 ratio) and observed for a pink or violet color within 10 seconds, depending on the phenothiazine present (see Table 8–3). This technique utilizes samples of urine or stomach contents, which can be either assayed intact or extracted and then assayed. The proper reagents are added, with or without heating, and the resulting color is observed. If a characteristic change in the color occurs initially, additional tests can be used to confirm the result. Controls or blanks are used throughout the procedure to decrease the number of false positives, although Fitzgerald and Walaszek have circumvented this process by the use of multiple reagents to classify some intoxicants.[16]

The limitations to this technique include a lack of specificity, which results in false positive results owing to cross reactivity and subjective interpretation. False negative findings occur frequently and can be the result of rapid color changes, low sensitivity, metabolites that do not react as the parent compound does, and color interferences by other substances.[17] For these reasons, color tests should be used only as a preliminary indication of the ingested substance and should be followed by a more specific form of analysis.

IMMUNOASSAY TECHNIQUES

The immunoassay techniques include enzyme multiplied immunoassay technique (EMIT), hemagglutination inhibi-tion (HI), free radical assay technique (FRAT), and radioimmunoassay (RIA). The general theory behind each of these four methods is that a labeled drug is competitively displaced from an antibody complex by an unlabeled drug in the sample. The amount of labeled drug displaced from the antibody is proportional to the amount of unlabeled drug in the sample.[18]

In general, the immunoassays show high sensitivity with relative specificity, allow for direct analysis of the sample without prior extraction, and can be rapidly performed. The main disadvantages of these techniques are that the specificity is not absolute, there is a great deal of cross reactivity with substances of similar chemical structure, and they are not well suited to simultaneous screening of a sample for the presence of several drugs. Therefore, because of the cross reactivity and lack of specificity, all positive results should be confirmed by a nonimmunological method, such as chromatography or spectrophotometry.[18–21]

The four available methods differ in the manner in which the drug is labeled, and in the method of detection of the displaced labeled drug. The first three assays mentioned above are "homogeneous" assays, in that they do not require that the drug bound to the antibody be physically separated from the unbound drug.[22] Radioimmunoassay involves physical separation before analysis and is therefore called "nonhomogeneous."

Enzyme multiplied immunoassay technique. In the EMIT system, the drug is labeled with the enzyme lysozyme, which is capable of lysing bacterial cell walls by catalyzing the hydrolysis of the mucopolysaccharide component of cell walls.[18–20] Drug molecules bound to the enzyme do not disturb its enzymatic activity, whereas antibodies bound to the drug-enzyme complex sterically hinder the enzyme from reaching the bacterial cell wall. The unlabeled drug can displace some of the antibody-labeled drug from the enzyme, thereby releasing a portion of the enzyme, which results in increased enzyme activity. The increase in enzyme activity is measured by spectrophotometry as a decrease in the cloudiness (optical density) of a solution of bacteria as a function of time.

Automated systems measure the optical density at 0 and 40 seconds after the addition of the sample, giving a sensitivity of about 0.4 μg/ml in standard use, with results in less than 1 minute.[18,23] This sensitivity can be increased by a lengthening of the time over which the change in the optical density is measured. False positive results have occurred in approximately 2% of the samples in one series,[21] and may be due to natural lysozyme in some urine samples. Therefore, with low positive findings, background lysosomal activity should be measured by omission of the labeled drug from an otherwise identical assay.[18,20]

Advantages of the EMIT system include rapid TAT, objective results, minimal technical skill required, and no sample preparation.[20,23] Disadvantages include the number of false positives, pH dependence in some aged samples, cost of the instrumentation, and a relative lack of sensitivity and specificity compared to other methods.[20]

Free radical assay technique. The label in the free radical assay technique (FRAT) is a stable free radical, nitroxide. The nitroxide is termed a spin-labeled hapten, because of its unpaired electrons, which can provide electron-spin resonance (ESR) spectra when exposed to a magnetic field.[18-20] When the labeled hapten forms a complex with an antibody, there is a decrease in the tumbling or spin of the complex, producing a low, broad ESR spectra. Free drug in the sample will compete with and displace some of the spin-labeled hapten, resulting in a higher, more sharply defined ESR spectra. The magnitude of the peak of the spectra is proportional to the quantity of the free

drug in the sample.[18,19] These ESR spectra are measured in a special spectrophotometer,[23] and unknown concentrations are determined by comparison with preconstructed calibration charts. The sensitivity of this method, approximately 250 ng/ml, is greater than that of the EMIT system, whereas the time for each analysis, between 30 and 60 seconds, is comparable.[18,20,23] The advantages and disadvantages of this system are similar to those of the EMIT system, with the exception that the instrumentation is more costly.[20]

Hemagglutination inhibition. In the hemagglutination inhibition method (HI), several molecules of the drug are bound to the label, which is a red blood cell (RBC) stabilized by pretreatment with formaldehyde.[18] When antibodies specific to the drug are added to the specimen, crosslinking can occur between two of the RBCs coated with the drug, as a result of the two binding sites for the drug on each antibody.[18-20] This agglutination appears as a diffuse, reddish-brown settling pattern in the well of a microtitre tray.[20] When free drug is added to the antibody-RBC-drug complex in the form of a specimen, competitive binding properties allow some of the RBC-drug complexes to be displaced from the antibody by the free drug, thereby inhibiting crosslinking and stopping agglutination. As this occurs, a sharp pellet of RBCs forms in the bottom of the well. In practice, the sample and the antibody are added to the microtitre tray, the drug-labeled RBCs are added, and the reaction is read with the naked eye at between 1 and 3 hours.[19,20] Sensitivity in the 10- to 50-ng/ml range can be achieved by a variation of the amount of antibody used in the procedure, but there is a high risk of false positives owing to loss of antibody binding capacity at these levels.[18,19] A decrease in the sensitivity to 100 to 200 ng/ml obviates this problem.

The main advantages of this system are

that no instrumentation is required, the technique is simple, the sensitivity can be easily adjusted if desired, and it is relatively inexpensive. Disadvantages include longer assay time, subjective reading of the results, urinary sediment obscuring readings in some urine samples, variability in the quality of available reagents, and lack of specificity.

Radioimmunoassay. The radioimmunoassay (RIA) uses a radioactive isotope such as ^{3}H, ^{14}C, or ^{125}I as the label for the drug in question.[18-20] For polypeptide hormones, ^{125}I is the label used, whereas ^{3}H is used for the smaller drug molecules.[24] The unlabeled drug is added to the isotope-labeled drug, and the mixture is allowed to equilibrate for 10 to 15 minutes. In order for the radioactivity of the displaced labeled drug to be analyzed, it must be physically separated from the antibody-bound labeled drug. This is usually done by precipitation of the entire antibody pool with ammonium sulfate. The unbound portion of the labeled drug remains in the supernatant liquid, where an aliquot can be measured for radioactivity of the label by liquid scintillation spectrometry or gamma scintillation counting, depending on the label used.[18,20] By comparison of the radioactivity of the unknown solution to a standard calibration curve, the concentration of the unknown solution can be found. The specificity of this method is high with morphine (as low as 5 ng/ml with confidence),[18] although the time for this analysis is relatively slow (1 to 2 hours).[18,20,21,24] If the isotope-labeled drug has a high specific radioactivity, its concentration can be determined with high precision even in dilute solutions.

Advantages of RIA include objective results, high sensitivity, and the versatility of the equipment, which can be used for other assays as they are developed.[20,21,24] The disadvantages are the time required for analysis, sophisticated technical skills necessary for handling radioactive material, high cost and variability in the quality of reagents, and moderately high cost of instrumentation.[20,21,24]

In summary, all of the immunoassay techniques use the principle of displacing a bound, labeled drug by the nonlabeled specimen drug. They differ in the type of label used and the method of detection. In general, the immunoassays show high sensitivity, with a relatively lower order of specificity, and they may be performed rapidly.

CHROMATOGRAPHY

Chromatography is a general term denoting the separation of closely related compounds by adsorption from a solution to an adsorbent medium.[25,26] The two types commonly used in the analysis of drugs and poisons are thin layer chromatography (TLC) and gas-liquid chromatography (GLC).

Thin layer chromatography. TLC is the simplest and most widely used qualitative and semiquantitative method for the analysis of intoxicants. TLC is an inexpensive, adaptable method, able to provide useful information about drug mixtures in biologic samples. The relatively simple equipment consists of glass or plastic plates, usually coated with aluminum oxide or silica gel as an adsorbent, a liquid solvent system, and a development chamber.[26]

All TLC is performed with the same basic technique. Biologic samples are extracted by acidic, neutral, or basic buffer systems and then concentrated. The concentrated specimen is then deposited onto the TLC plate, along with appropriate standard solutions, and allowed to dry after the site of deposition is marked on the plate. The plate is then placed on end in the developing tank, which contains a mixture of different organic solvents selected by the properties of the compounds being identified. The solvent mixture is then allowed to travel up the plate, carrying the compounds with it. Elution or deposition of the compound at a certain point on the plate is determined by the adsorption affinity of the compound, which depends on the structural properties of the compound.[25] At the point where it has a greater affinity for the plate adsorbant than for the solvent, the compound will elute from the organic solvent mixture and adsorb to the chromatographic plate. Once the solvent front has progressed to the other end, the plate is removed from the tank, the solvent front marked, and the plate dried. The separated drugs and standards are then visualized through the use of ultraviolet light and sequential chromatographic spraying.[19] The distance from the point of origin of the solvent front to the drug spots is determined, and an R_f value is calculated with the following formula:[26]

$$R_f = \frac{\text{distance traveled by spot}}{\text{distance traveled by solvent front}}$$

The R_f values for the unknown compounds are compared to the R_f values for the standards, and the compounds can be accurately identified by a combination of the R_f value and color reactions.

Another value that can be calculated is the R_r value, given by the following equation:[26]

analyzed by GLC or spectrophotometry.[19,27]

The main advantages of TLC are low cost, ability to detect multiple drugs present in a sample, and ease of use. The disadvantages are the time required (2 to 4 hrs), multiple extractions needed, subjective interpretation of the data (R_f, R_r, and color) and a lack of sensitivity for low concentrations of substances.[19] The R_f and R_r values can be influenced by the composition of the solvent mixture, distance traveled by the solvent front, concentration of the solution, presence of other substances, and temperature at the time of development.[25] Two different compounds could possibly have the same R_f values and be represented by the same spot on the plate.

Gas-liquid chromatography. The principle behind gas-liquid chromatography is analogous to that of thin layer chromatography. The carrier vehicle or mobile phase is an inert gas such as helium or nitrogen, instead of a liquid solvent mixture, and the stationary phase is a suitable liquid instead of a solid. The selection of the carrier gas depends on the mode of detection used. A thermal conductivity detector requires helium as the carrier gas, and an argon-methane mixture is necessary for an electron capture detector.[26,28] A flame ionizing detector uses

$$R_r = \frac{\text{distance traveled by unknown compound}}{\text{distance traveled by known compound}}$$

The closer this value is to unity, the higher the probability that the unknown is the reference compound. Since the R_r is an index of the positions of compounds relative to each other on the TLC plate, it should not be used as the only criterion for identification, but should always be combined with the sequential color reactions.[25] If further analysis is desired, the spots can be scraped off the plate and

helium as the carrier and a hydrogen-oxygen mixture as fuel.[28]

The liquid phase used in GLC must have a low vapor pressure, high boiling point, and definite selectivity, with high resolving power.[26,28] The liquid should not be eluted from the column under the operating temperature used, and the compounds sought after should come off the column with sufficient space between them for identification and quantification. The carrier gas is forced (pressurized) over the adsorbant liquid, which is supported in either a standard or capillary chromatography column.

The standard column is packed with an inert solid support material, which is coated with the liquid phase. The typical column is about 1.25 m in length, with a 5-mm internal diameter.[26] The capillary column uses no packing, since the walls of the column provide the support for the stationary liquid phase. The typical capillary column is 50 to 250 m in length, with an internal diameter of 0.2 mm.[26] Both columns can be in the shape of a "U," "W," or a coil; the coil is the most practical, since it fits easily into a small, thermostatically controlled compartment, with one end of the column at the injector part and the other at the detector. The oven can be set at a constant temperature or programmed to increase linearly, with time allowed for the compounds to be eluted in order of their molecular structure.[29]

The sample is extracted in a manner similar to that in thin layer chromatography to allow for analysis and is then injected into the column, where it is immediately volatilized and carried through the column by the carrier gas. Since the compound is analyzed in the gaseous state, any compound to be analyzed must volatilize at high temperatures without decomposition.[19] As the sample enters the column, separation occurs when the sample is partitioned between the gas and liquid phases. As each successive compound is eluted from the column by the carrier gas, it is detected and recorded as a peak on the recorder.[19,25,26,28]

The time between injection and emergence of the peak is called the retention time. Different compounds have different retention times for a specific GLC setup and can thus be differentiated. The concentration of the sample can be determined by measurement of either the peak height or the area under the curve, as compared with a standard curve based on known quantities.[28] It should be noted, however, that even with the increased specificity of this method, occasionally two compounds will have the same retention time, so that for medico-legal purposes, the results of GLC can be confirmed by an alternative method.[19] The accuracy for a typical gas-liquid chromatograph can be expected to be ± 2%, with a lower sensitivity limit of approximately 1 to 5 μg/ml.[26]

The advantages of GLC over TLC include improved separation of closely related compounds with a single extraction, short analysis time, detection of solute quantities of less than 1 μg, and the ability to make analyses over a wide range of temperatures.[25]

SPECTROPHOTOMETRIC METHODS

Spectrophotometry measures the ability of a substance to absorb electromagnetic radiation.[30] A beam of monochromatic light is passed through a solution of an unknown compound and the absorbance or percent transmittance recorded for various wavelengths of light. The wavelengths of maximum absorbance and the shape and pattern of the absorbance spectrum identify the compound. Once the compound is identified, standards can be run with different concentrations of the compound, to determine the sample concentration by comparison of the intensities of the absorbances. Spectrophotometric analysis of drugs in biologic fluids is hampered by the lengthy purification and extraction techniques needed to reduce interference.[20]

Visual spectrophotometry will be discussed only briefly here, since it has been replaced by better techniques in many laboratories. In general, the compound is extracted with inorganic solvents, and the percent absorbance at a particular wavelength of light is measured. Many compounds, such as salicylates and iron, must react with a reagent known as a chromophore to produce a color in the sample. The absorbance of this compound is then measured in the visible light spectrophotometer.

Concentration of the sample is found by comparison to a calibration curve of percent absorbance versus concentration to quantitate the result. The main advantages to this method are ease of use and relatively rapid results, Disadvantages include low sensitivity and specificity due to interference with other substances, although this is the method of choice for salicylates and iron, two of the most common overdoses. Of the other types of spectrophotometric techniques, the most useful are ultraviolet and infrared spectrophotometry, spectrofluorometry, and atomic absorption spectrophotometry.

Ultraviolet (UV) spectrophotometry. The major role of UV spectrophotometry in toxicology is the analysis of weak acids, neutral compounds, and certain weak bases in blood.[31] The advantages of UV spectrophotometry are ease of use, short setup time for instruments, rapid analysis time after sample preparation, qualitative and quantitative data, and with a few exceptions, the nondestructive nature of the procedure. The disadvantages are four-fold:[31] (1) drugs which do not have a sufficiently strong ultraviolet spectrum cannot be analyzed, (2) the procedure lacks sensitivity, in that concentrations of less than 2 μg/ml cannot be measured accurately, (3) mixtures of drugs with overlapping absorption spectra cannot be resolved, and (4) some spectra obtained may be similar enough to prohibit identification.

Infrared (IR) absorption. Infrared absorption spectrophotometry involves the same basic principles as UV or visible spectrophotometry, but with some differences.[32] The total analysis can take as few as 10 minutes. The sample is not destroyed by the infrared radiation, since the energy absorbed in infrared spectrophotometry affects only the vibrational energy of the molecule.[33] The frequency of an absorption peak is directly related to the energy of the motion observed for different chemical functional groups.

The spectrum of absorption peaks for a compound is unique for that compound owing to the many motions possible in polyatomic molecules,[32] and it acts as a fingerprint for the compound. Quantitative analysis can also be performed, since the intensity of the absorption peaks is proportional to the amount of drug present.[32,33] Owing to the extremely complex nature of IR spectra in mixtures of compounds, TLC and GLC can be used before IR analysis for purification, and also afterwards, to further aid in identification of the compound.[33]

Fluorometry. In fluorometry, the relative fluorescent intensity of a compound is measured after the compound is exposed to an exciting light source. Drugs with natural fluorescence such as quinine and imipramine, and those with fluorescent derivatives such as phenothiazines and benzodiazepines, can be identified by this method.[19,33] The main advantages of fluorometry are that it is at least 10 to 1000 times more sensitive than visible spectrophotometry and that it increases specificity because it measures both the maximum absorption and fluorescent wavelength, instead of the maximum absorption alone.[32,33]

Atomic absorption. Atomic absorption spectrophotometry, used for the analytic determination of approximately 67 elements including lead, arsenic, and mercury, is essentially free of spectral interference, with only a few chemical interferences.[32] The element is dissociated from its chemical bonds to the unexcited, nonionized ground state. In a low energy state, the atom can absorb monochromatic light at characteristic wavelengths for the element being searched for, in amounts proportional to the number of atoms present in the sample. This method is capable of high precision, with a sensitivity of approximately 100 times that of flame emission spectrophotometry, a method previously used.[32,33]

The spectrophotometric methods of drug analysis are diverse in nature, although they all follow the general principle of absorbing some type of electromagnetic radiation (from infrared to ultraviolet) by the target compound. The differences in sensitivity and specificity depend directly on the methods used and their relationship to the chemical properties they are designed to identify. In general, these assays are widely used in the toxicology laboratory for a great variety of compounds.

MASS SPECTROMETRY

The most advanced toxicologic instrumentation includes a mass spectrometer coupled with a gas-liquid chromatograph. As the compounds are separated by the GLC, they are introduced directly into the mass spectrometer for further analysis. The advantages of the mass spectrometer are rapidity, accuracy, high sensitivity, and applicability to a wide number of compounds, with retention of almost 100% specificity for individual drugs that are closely related in structure.[34,35] Disadvantages are the extremely high cost of the instrument and the lengthy and meticulous maintenance needed.[36]

The mass spectrometer functions on the principle that an electrical field can be produced that causes ionized particles of a particular mass to oscillate in phase.[34] Only the particles oscillating in phase can reach the detector, which in essence separates them from all other particles. Since there are numerous compounds of the same mass in serum or urine, bombardment of the ionized molecules with electrons will fragment some of the compounds into their respective chemical groups before ionization. Each of these groups can then be ionized and separated by the oscillating electric field.

Every compound has a highly reproducible, specific fragmentation pattern, so that a compound can be positively identified.[34] The peak heights of the individual molecules or groups of molecules are proportional to the concentrations of these molecules or groups in the compound. Once the identities of the large peaks for a specific compound are determined, an identification of the compound can be made, either manually or by a computer, by comparison with a published reference list of the mass spectra of 133 compounds and their metabolites.[37] With this technique, the time from acquisition of samples to reporting of the results may be from 30 minutes to 2 hours.[35,36]

Table 2–1 summarizes 43 of the most commonly ingested or abused drugs under various chemical and/or pharmacologic titles. It also includes the approximate therapeutic, toxic, and lethal serum concentrations, approximate lethal dose in acute situations, assay techniques commonly used for detection of each compound, required biologic fluid or specimen, type of analysis performed, TAT required for results to be obtained, comments, and a key as to how the table should be used. It should be kept in mind, however, that the values or parameters listed are not absolute; they can vary from laboratory to laboratory, and are intended to be used only as a guide in the assessment of the severity of the intoxication. In addition, it must be remembered that a negative result from the laboratory for an intoxicant does not mean that the intoxicant was not ingested, only that it was not detected. For example, it is possible that the concentration of the intoxicant was below the sensitivity range of the assay used, or that the sampling time was not optimal. The patient's clinical condition should be the final determining step at all times with regards to severity of acute or chronic intoxications.

If meaningful and accurate emergency toxicologic determinations are to be made, the clinician and the laboratory personnel must appreciate each others' capabilities and limitations. Our experiences have been that the toxicology laboratory, if properly utilized, can play an important supportive role, and is of great value to the clinician in assessing the intoxicated patient and guiding his therapy.

REFERENCES

1. Walberg CB, Pantlik VA, and Lundberg GD: Toxicology test ordering patterns in a large urban general hospital during five years: An update. *Clin Chem*, 24:507–511, 1978.
2. Wiltbank TB, Sine HE, and Brody BB: Are emergency toxicology measurements really used? *Clin Chem*, 20:116–120, 1974.
3. Winek CL: Laboratory criteria for the adequacy of treatment and significance of blood levels. *Clin Toxicol*, 3:541–549, 1970.
4. Lundberg GD, Walberg CB, and Gupta RC: The patient-focused approach to organization of a clinical toxicology laboratory. *Lab Med*, 3:14–16, 1972.
5. Hobson JD, and Zettner A: Digoxin serum half-life following suicidal digoxin poisoning. *JAMA*, 223:147–149, 1973.
6. Prescott LF, et al: Plasma paracetamol half-life and hepatic necrosis in patients with paracetamol overdosage. *Lancet*, 1:519–522, 1971.
7. Rawlins MD, Davies DM, and Routledge PA: Toxicity in relation to blood levels. In *Clinical Toxicology*. Edited by WA Duncan and BJ Leonard. Amsterdam, Excerpta Medica, 1977, pp. 41–49.
8. Doherty JE: The clinical pharmacology of digitalis glycosides: A review. *Am J Med Sci*, 255:382–414, 1968.
9. Levy G: Relationship between pharmacological effects and plasma or tissue concentrations of drugs in man. In *Biological Effects of Drugs in Relation to Their Plasma Concentrations*. Edited by DS Davis and BNC Pritchard. London, The Macmillan Press LTD, 1973, pp. 83–95.
10. Newton RW: Acute poisoning and the laboratory. In *The Poisoned Patient: The Role of the Laboratory*. Ciba Foundation Symposium, Vol. 26, 1974, p. 9.
11. Czajka PA: Management of acute acetaminophen overdosage. *Clin Toxicol Consult*, 1:33–49, 1979.
12. Winek CL: A role for the hospital pharmacist in toxicology and drug blood level information. *Am J Hosp Pharm*, 28:351–356, 1971.
13. Winek CL: Tabulation of therapeutic, toxic and lethal concentrations of drugs and chemicals in blood. *Clin Chem*, 22:832–836, 1976.
14. Niyogi SK: Drug levels in cases of poisoning. *Forensic Sci*, 2:67–98, 1973.
15. McBay AT: Toxicological findings in fatal poisonings. *Clin Chem*, 19:361-365, 1973.
16. Fitzgerald TJ, and Walaszek ET: Drug detection with color tests. *Clin Toxicol*, 6(4):599–605, 1973.
17. Decker WJ, and Treuting JJ: Spot tests for rapid diagnosis of poisoning. *Clin Toxicol*, 4(1):89–97, 1971.
18. Brattin WJ, and Sunshine I: Immunological assays for drugs in biological samples. *Am J Med Tech*, 39(6):223–230, 1973.
19. Curtis EG, and Patel JA: Pharmacy based analytical toxicology service. *Am J Hosp Pharm*, 32:685–693, 1975.
20. Bidanset JH: Drug analysis by immunoassays. *J Chromatograph Sci*, 12:293–296, 1974.
21. Mule SJ, Bastos ML, and Jukofsky D: Evaluation of immunoassay methods for detection, in urine, of drugs subject to abuse. *Clin Chem*, 20(2):243–248, 1974.
22. Rubenstein KE, Schneider RS, and Ullman EF: Homogeneous enzyme immunoassay: A new immunochemical technique. *Biochem Biophys Res Commun*, 47(4):846–856, 1972.
23. Bastiani RJ, et al: Homogeneous immunochemical drug assays. *Am J Med Tech*, 39(6):211–216, 1973.
24. Kostenbauder HB, Foster TS, and McGovern JP: Radio-immunoassay in pharmacy practice. *Am J Hosp Pharm*, 31:763–770, 1974.
25. Wynter CI (ed): *Chemical Analysis for Medical Technologists*. Springfield, IL., Charles C Thomas, 1975, pp. 69–83.
26. Perlman P (ed): "Chromatography." In *General Laboratory Techniques*. Englewood, NJ, Franklin Publ. Co., 1964, pp. 272–333.
27. Sunshine I: Use of thin layer chromatography in the diagnosis of poisoning. *Am J Clin Pathol*, 40(6):576–588, 1963.
28. Patel JA: Gas chromatography: A handy tool in the hospital pharmacy assay and control laboratory. *Am J Hosp Pharm*, 27:411–414, 1970.
29. Graham JW, and Plutchak LB: Screening for the non-barbiturate sedative hypnotic drugs. *Lab Med*, 3:20–21, 1972.
30. Perlman P (ed): "Colorimetry and Spectrophotometry". In *General Laboratory Techniques*. Englewood, NJ, Franklin Publ. Co., 1964, pp. 181–194.
31. Jatlow P: Ultraviolet spectrophotometric analysis of drugs in biological fluids. *Am J Med Tech*, 39:231–236, 1973.
32. Wynter, CI (ed): *Chemical Analysis for Medical Technologists*. Springfield, IL, Charles C Thomas, 1975, pp. 84–100.
33. Sunshine I (ed): *Handbook of Analytical Toxicology*. Boca Raton, FL, CRC Press, 1969, p. 909.
34. Sannella JJ: Drugs and the clinical laboratory. *J Tenn Med Assoc*, 68 (9):715, 1975.
35. Billets S, et al: Rapid identification of acute drug intoxications. *Johns Hopkins Med J*, 133:148–155, 1973.
36. Law N: A modern approach for drug identification. *Am J Med Tech*, 39(6):237–243, 1973.

37. Finkle BS, and Taylor DM: A GC/MS reference data system for the identification of drugs of abuse. *J Chromatogr Sci*, 10:312–333, 1972.

38. Lundberg GD, Walberg CB, and Pantlik VA: Frequency of clinical toxicology test ordering (primarily overdose cases) and results in a large urban general hospital. *Clin Chem*, 20:121–125, 1974.

39. Product information, 1979, Syva Company, Palo Alto, CA.

40. Personal communication: Stafford DT, Director, Toxicology Laboratory, Department of Pathology, University of Tennessee Center for the Health Sciences.

41. Kananen G, Osrewicz R, and Sunshine I: Barbiturate analysis—A current assessment. *J Chromatogr Sci*, 10:283–287, 1972.

42. Mule SJ: Methods for the analysis of narcotic analgesics and amphetamines. *J Chromatogr Sci*, 10:275–282, 1972.

43. Evenson MA, and Poquette MA: Rapid gas chromatographic method for quantitation of ethchlorvynol ("Placidyl") in serum. *Clin Chem*, 20:212–216, 1974.

44. Wallace JE, et al: Spectrophotometric determination of ethchlorvynol in biologic specimens. *Clin Chem*, 20:159–162, 1974.

45. Cravey RH, and Jain NC: The identification of non-barbiturate hypnotics from biological specimens. *J Chromatogr Sci*, 128:237–245, 1974.

46. Cimbara G: Review of methods of analysis for phenothiazine drugs. *J Chromatogr Sci*, 10:287–293, 1972.

47. Sine HE, et al: Emergency drug analysis. *J Chromatogr Sci*, 10:297–302, 1972.

48. Avery, GS (ed): *Drug treatment: Principles and Practice of Clinical Pharmacology and Therapeutics.* Sydney, Australia, ADIS Press, 1976, pp. 32, 450.

49. Knoben JE, Anderson PO, and Watanabe AS (eds): *Handbook of Clinical Drug Data.* 4th Ed. Hamilton, IL, Drug Intelligence Publications, 1978.

50. Winchester JF, et al: Dialysis and hemoperfusion of poisons and drugs—update. *Trans Am Soc Artif Intern Organs*, 23:762–841, 1977.

51. Kamisaka Y, et al: Inhibition of glutethimide absorption. *Arch Toxicol*, 28:12–23, 1971.

52. Cardis DT, McAndrew GM, and Matheson NA: Hemodialysis in poisoning with methaqualone and diphenhydramine. *Lancet*, 1:51–52, 1967.

53. Wallace AE: Recovery after massive overdose of diphenhydramine and methaqualone. *Lancet*, 2:1247–1248, 1968.

54. Yudis M, et al: Hemodialysis for methyprylon (Noludar) poisoning. *Ann Intern Med*, 68:1301–1304, 1968.

55. Lubsher FA: Fatal hydantoin poisoning. *JAMA*, 198:1120–1121, 1966.

56. Thompson RPH, et al: Hepatic damage from paracetamol. *Gut*, 13:836, 1972.

57. Atkinson AJ, et al: Hemodialysis for severe procainamide toxicity: Clinical and pharmacokinetic observations. *Clin Pharmacol Ther*, 20:585–592, 1976.

58. Prescott LF: Hepatotoxic dose of paracetamol. *Lancet*, 2:142, 1977.

59. Petersen RG, and Rumack BH: Toxicity of acetaminophen overdose. *JACEP*, 7:202–205, 1978.

60. Protocol on the management of acetaminophen overdose with N-acetylcysteine (1979), McNeil Consumer Products Company, Fort Washington, PA.

61. Ambre J, and Alexander M: Liver toxicity after APAP ingestion: Inadequacy of the dose estimation as an index of risk. *JAMA*, 238:500–501, 1977.

62. Sellers EM, and Kalant H: Alcohol intoxication and withdrawal. *N Engl J Med*, 294:757–762, 1976.

63. Shub C, et al: The management of acute quinidine intoxication. *Chest*, 73:173–178, 1978.

64. Hestand HE, and Teske DW: Diphenhydramine hydrochloride intoxication. *J Pediatr*, 90:1017–1018, 1977.

65. Berger R, Green G, and Malnick A: Cardiac arrest caused by oral diazepam intoxication. *Clin Pediatr*, 14:842–844, 1975.

66. Turner JE, and Cravey RH: A fatal ingestion of caffeine. *Clin Toxicol*, 10:341–344, 1977.

67. Moriarity RW, and McDonald RH: The spectrum of ethylene glycol poisoning. *Clin Toxicol*, 7:583–596, 1974.

68. Sievers ML, and Herrier RN: Treatment of acute isoniazid toxicity. *Am J Hosp Pharm*, 32:202–206, 1975.

69. Manoguerra AS: Iron poisoning: Report of a fatal case in an adult. *Am J Hosp Pharm*, 33:1088–1090, 1976.

70. Hansen HE, and Andisen A: Lithium intoxication—Report of 23 cases and review of 100 cases from the literature. *Q J Med*, 47:123–144, 1978.

71. Arena JM: Treatment of mercury poisoning. *Mod Treatment*, 8:619–625, 1971.

72. Burns SR, et al: Phencyclidine—Status of acute intoxication and fatalities. *West J Med*, 123:345–349, 1975.

73. Davis JM, Bartlett E, and Termini BA: Overdoses of psychotropic drugs: A review. Part 1: Major and minor tranquilizers. *Dis Nerv Syst*, 29:157–164, 1968.

74. Lovejoy FH, Mitchell AA, and Goldman P: The management of propoxyphene poisonings. *J Pediatr*, 85:98–100, 1974.

75. Kristinsson J, and Johannesson T: A case of fatal propranolol intoxication. *Acta Pharmacol Toxicol*, 41:190–192, 1977.

76. Lagerfelt J, and Matell G: Attempted suicide with 5.1 gm of propranol. *Acta Med Scand*, 199:517–518, 1976.

77. Blumbetg HG, Roselt HL, and Dobrow A: Severe hypotensive reaction following meprobamate overdosage. *Ann Intern Med*, 51:607–612, 1959.

78. Selling LS: Clinical study of a new tranquilizer drug. *JAMA*, 157:1594–1596, 1955.

79. Allen MD, Greenblatt DJ, and Noel BJ: Meprobamate overdosage: A continuing problem. *Clin Toxicol*, 11:501–515, 1977.

80. Manoguerra AS, and Weaver LC: Poisoning with tricyclic antidepressant drugs. *Clin Toxicol*, 10:149–158, 1977.

81. Baily DN, and Jatlow PI: Chemical analysis of massive crystalluria following primidone overdose. *Am J Clin Pathol*, 58:583–589, 1972.
82. Ferguson MJ, Germanos S, and Grace WT: Meprobamate overdosage. *Arch Intern Med*, 106:237–239, 1960.
83. Winek CL, et al: Methaprylene toxicity. *Clin Toxicol*, 11:287–294, 1977.
84. Von Muhlendahl KE, et al: Codeine intoxication in children. *Lancet*, 2:303–305, 1976.
85. Hayler AM, Holt PW, and Volans GN: Fatal overdosage with disopyramide. *Lancet*, 1:968–969, 1978.
86. Personal communication: Searcy C, Clincal associate professor, College of Pharmacy, University of Illinois.
87. Walle T: GLC determination of propranolol, other B-blocking drugs and metabolites in biological fluids and tissues. *J Pharm Sci*, 63:1885–1891, 1974.
88. Broussand CA, and Frings CS: Quantitative high performance liquid chromatographic method for determining disopyramide (Norpace) in serum. *Clin Toxicol*, 14(5):579–586, 1979.

Chapter 3

Dialysis and Hemoperfusion of Drugs and Toxins

Ingrid S. Sketris
Vasilios A. Skoutakis

Approximately 10% of all medical admissions to hospitals are due to accidental poisonings and deliberate drug overdosages.[1] The overall mortality rate for such patients is low when appropriate therapeutic modalities are carried out and is usually less than 1% of those patients admitted.[2] However, in severe cases of intoxications (e.g., Grade 4 coma), the reported mortality figures vary from 5% to 38%.[3,4] Furthermore, these reports indicate that the length of time a patient remains in coma directly affects the development of complications and mortality.[4] As a result, implementation of methods that will reduce the duration of coma can decrease the development of complications, and at the same time increase the probability of the patient's survival. In view of these reported findings, the active removal by the use of various dialytic procedures of intoxicants present owing to acute or chronic toxic exposures can be a useful therapeutic adjunct to the management of severely intoxicated patients.

DIALYTIC PROCEDURES

The dialytic procedures most commonly used for the treatment of accidental ingestions and deliberate drug overdosages are hemodialysis (HD), peritoneal dialysis (PD), and charcoal hemoperfusion (CHP) or resin hemoperfusion (RHP).

HEMODIALYSIS

The use of the artificial kidney for the management of severely intoxicated patients who have ingested specific intoxicants (e.g., alcohols), or who are not responding to standard therapeutic management, has been a valuable aid to the clinician. The fundamental physiologic principle in hemodialysis involves the transfer of a solute or toxin across a semipermeable membrane in a direction and at a rate consistent with concentration gradients.[5,6]

Procedure. Hemodialyzers in current clinical use may be divided into four main categories: (1) nondisposable flat plate dialyzers, (2) disposable flat plate dialyzers, (3) disposable coil dialyzers, and (4) disposable fiber dialyzers. The procedure for a coil dialyzer will be briefly discussed as a prototype and is shown in Figure 3–1. The assembly of plate dialyzers and hollow fiber dialyzers has been described and illustrated in detail by other practitioners.[6,7]

Initially, the technique involves establishment of access to the patient's circulation. This is usually accomplished by a simple surgical procedure, which includes the aseptic insertion of Shaldon catheters, 2 inches apart, into the patient's femoral vein. After insertion of the Shaldon catheters, the coil dialyzer is placed in its cannister and connected to devices to monitor pressure within the system.[7] Dialysate concentrate is added to a tub filled with water at 37°C to produce a wash solution that resembles extracellular body fluids. The system is primed with heparinized saline solution, the arterial and venous lines are connected to the Shaldon catheters, and dialysis is begun. Generally, total heparin administration requirements are found to be between 1000 to 2000 IU per hour of dialysis. Heparin is given as a prime dose when dialysis is begun (1500 to 2000 IU) and then

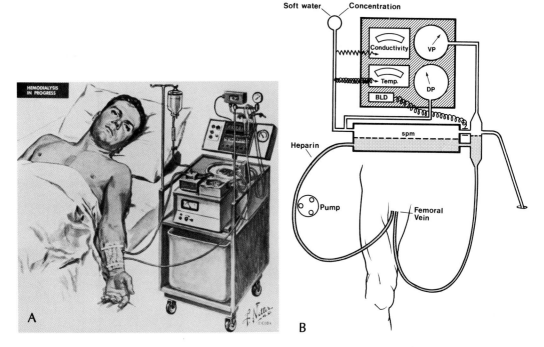

Fig. 3–1. Principles of hemodialysis (A) and of the monitoring equipment. B, The correct composition (i.e., total electrical conductivity), temperature, and pressure of the dialysis fluid (DP) are monitored prior to passage of the fluid through the kidney. After use, the fluid passes through a blood leak detector (BLD). Blood pressure in the extracorporeal blood circuit (VP) is monitored at the bubble trap. (Adapted from Wing AJ, and Magowan M [eds.]: *The Renal Unit.* 1st Ed. Philadelphia, Lippincott, 1975.)

throughout dialysis, either by intermittent injections or by continuous infusion at a rate of 1000 IU per hour. Further adjustments are made according to clotting times.

Blood is pumped at a rate of 200 to 250 ml/min, and the outflow pressure is regulated according to the amount of ultrafiltration (water removal) desired. The dialysate bath is changed every 2 to 3 hours, and dialysis is continued for 6 to 8 hours.

Efficacy. Hemodialyzers vary with respect to their membrane surface area, membrane porosity, residual blood volume, range of ultrafiltration, and diffusion characteristics.[6,8,9,10] These properties influence the blood and dialysate flow rates, as well as the ability of the hemodialyzers to remove intoxicants from the body. Recirculation of the dialysate through activated charcoal may enhance the removal of some toxins.[11]

Complications. The complications commonly encountered during the HD procedure are those of a technical nature (e.g., membrane rupture, clotting in the coil, leakage from connections, poor arterial supply, venous obstruction, dialyzer distention),[13] and those of a medical nature (e.g., hypotension, convulsions, arrhythmias, hematologic defects, anticoagulation rebound, infections, and fluid and electrolyte abnormalities).[13,14] Therefore, close monitoring of both the dialysis system and the patient is essential.

PERITONEAL DIALYSIS

Both peritoneal dialysis and hemodialysis are based on the same physiologic principle. They differ mainly in that PD makes use of an in vivo biologic membrane and is generally less efficient than HD.[14]

Procedure. The technique of PD is essentially a matter of abdominal paracentesis and is usually performed at the bedside. Prior to the initiation of peritoneal dialysis, preparation of the patient includes weighing, emptying of the bladder, aseptic cleansing of the abdomen as in any surgical procedure, placement of the patient in a supine or semisupine position, and administration of local anesthesia around the catheter insertion site and down to the peritoneal cavity.

Thereafter, a nylon catheter with its metal stylet is inserted into the peritoneal cavity through a small incision in the middle of the abdomen, about one third of the distance from the umbilicus to the pubic bone. As soon as the peritoneum is entered, the tip of the stylet is withdrawn and the catheter is aimed down into the pelvis. The catheter is passed as far as it will comfortably go, usually on the right side of the pelvis. Eventually, the tip should lie in the pelvis, and all the side perforations should be inside the peritoneal cavity. In thin individuals and in children, the risk of perforating the bowel may be reduced by the instillation of dialysis fluid (0.4 to 1.0 L in children and 2 L in adults) through a 14-gauge lumbar puncture needle, prior to the insertion of the catheter.[15,16]

While the catheter is inserted, the nurse primes the dialysis tubing set with the first 2 L of dialysis fluid and connects the drainage bag to the drainage side arm. As soon as the catheter is placed into the peritoneal cavity and a gauze dressing with adhesive strapping is applied, the dialysis tubing set is connected to the catheter, and the dialysis cycle is begun at either inflow or outflow by gravity, depending on whether or not the peritoneum was filled with dialysis solution prior to the insertion of the catheter. If dialysis solution was not instilled prior to the catheter insertion, dialysis fluid (2 L in adults and 0.4 to 1.0 L in children) is permitted to flow into the abdominal cavity as rapidly as possible, ordinarily requiring between 5 to 10 minutes for completion.

When the bottles are empty but the

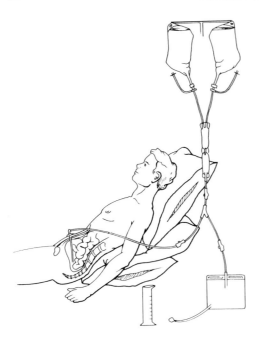

Fig. 3–2. Peritoneal dialysis. (Adapted from Wing AJ, and Magowan M [eds.]: *The Renal Unit.* 1st Ed. Philadelphia, Lippincott, 1975.)

tubing is still filled with fluid, the tubing is clamped and the bottles are placed on the floor beside the patient's bed. The fluid is permitted to remain within the abdominal cavity for 45 to 60 minutes for equilibration to take place, after which the clamp is removed and the abdomen is drained through the closed system back into the two original bottles. Before drainage is begun an additional 2 L of dialysis solution and fresh tubing are prepared, so that as soon as drainage ceases, a new infusion can be started. This process is repeated continuously, depending on the severity of the intoxication and the clinical condition of the patient. Usually, between 20 to 30 L of dialysis solution are changed. The overriding principle in the handling of the tubing set and collecting bottles is to keep the system closed to prevent bacterial invasion.[14,15,16] The complete system is shown in Fig. 3–2.

Dialysis solutions. The PD solutions commercially available vary in composi-

tion but generally contain electrolytes in concentrations approaching those of extracellular body fluids. The solutions also contain either 1.5% or 4.5% dextrose, which are hypertonic relative to plasma glucose. Therefore, excessive fluid loss may occur particularly in patients receiving recurrent PD. Furthermore, the dialysate solutions do not contain potassium and should therefore be chosen after consideration of the patient's serum osmolality and fluid status, sodium, potassium, and bicarbonate concentrations, in order to prevent complications.[14,17]

Efficacy. In acute and chronic intoxications, the rate of removal of a dialyzable intoxicant is usually 5 to 10 times less efficient with PD as compared to HD.[14,18,19] Thus, 6 hours of HD are roughly equivalent to 36 to 72 hours of PD.

The membrane of the capillary wall is usually the major cellular barrier in the delivery of the intoxicant present in the blood to the peritoneal cavity. As a result, the rate of diffusion of an intoxicant becomes a function of splanchnic blood flow, the concentration gradient between the blood and dialysate fluid, and the degree of mixing of solutes with the intoxicant, which occurs during the period of equilibration in the peritoneal cavity. The effectiveness of PD, therefore, can be accelerated by a number of methods, such as increasing the dialysate exchange volume, decreasing the length of time the dialysate stays in the peritoneal cavity, increasing the temperature of the dialysate solution, adding hypertonic saline solution, glucose, or albumin to the dialysate solution, or recirculating the dialysate solution through a charcoal or resin hemoperfusion column.[17,18,19,20]

Complications. Although peritoneal dialysis is generally considered a safe procedure, a wide variety of complications has been reported.[13–17] These include (1) technical hazards, e.g., perforation of the bowel, bladder, aorta, iliac vessels, liver or spleen, (2) fluid and electrolyte abnormalities, e.g., persistent positive fluid balance due to inadequate drainage or to leakage of dialysis fluid into the tissues, and hypotension due to over-zealous administration of hypertonic dialysis solutions, (3) pulmonary complications, e.g., atelectasis, pneumonia, acute purulent bronchitis and pleural effusions due to elevation of the diaphragm, leading to partial collapse of the lower lobe, (4) peritonitis, e.g., peritoneal infection due to contamination of the peritoneal dialysis system, (5) protein loss, e.g., increased protein loss due to duration of dialysis, or increased capillary permeability due to peritoneal inflammation, and (6) pain, e.g., complaints of abdominal pain due to the insertion of the catheter or the administration of hypertonic solutions.

CHARCOAL OR RESIN HEMOPERFUSION

Charcoal hemoperfusion and resin hemoperfusion allow the blood to pass

Table 3–1. Typical sorbents used in hemoperfusion devices for drug intoxication. (Reprinted from Winchester JF, Gelfand MC, and Tilstone WJ: Hemoperfusion in drug intoxication: Clinical and laboratory aspects. *Drug Metab Rev* [FJ DiCarlo, ed.], 8[1]:69, 1978, by courtesy of Marcel Dekker, Inc.)

Activated charcoal	Uncoated granular charcoal (loose bed or fixed bed)
	Coated granular charcoal
	Spherical (petroleum-based) charcoal
	Extruded charcoal
Ion-exchange resins	Amberlite series
	Zerolit 225
Nonionic resins	Polystyrene amberlite series (XAD-2, XAD-4)

directly over an adsorbing surface and are not limited by a dialysis membrane. The various sorbents available for hemoperfusion are summarized in Table 3–1, and manufacturers' instructions should be followed closely. A typical CHP circuit is shown in Figure 3–3, and will be de-

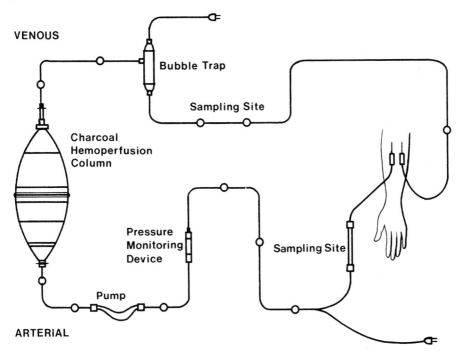

Fig. 3–3. Circuit for clinical hemoperfusion. (From Gelfand MC et al: Treatment of severe drug overdosage with charcoal hemoperfusion. *Trans Am Soc Artif Intern Organs,* 23:599, 1977.)

scribed briefly. The sterilized columns usually contain 300 g of activated charcoal. Before it is connected to the patient, the system is flushed with 2 L of normal saline solution to eliminate many of the charcoal impurities associated with emboli.[21,22] Prerinsing of the charcoal with dextrose just prior to its use prevents hypoglycemia by allowing glucose equilibration during hemoperfusion.[23]

Anticoagulation with heparin is achieved by an increase in the clotting times to 2½ to 3 times the normal value. Blood is withdrawn from the patient via an arteriovenous or venovenous shunt and passed through the cartridge with a roller pump in an antigravity direction at rates varying from 100 to 300 ml/min.[24] Pressure devices used to detect rises in pressure across the column help detect thrombosis inside the device. The charcoal system cartridges are used for approximately 3 hours before replacement of the cartridge.[23] Periodic blood level monitoring, with calculation of extraction efficiency, can aid in the determination of when the column should be changed. The resin cartridge has been used for up to 10 hours in some cases.[23]

Efficacy. Charcoal hemoperfusion is a useful therapeutic modality for a variety of intoxicants that are poorly removed by hemodialysis or peritoneal dialysis. Comparison of the efficiency of extraction of various intoxicants with hemoperfusion and hemodialysis shows plasma extraction ratios to be significantly greater for both charcoal and resin hemoperfusion when compared to hemodialysis (Table 3–2).

Complications. The problems of severe thrombocytopenia and microembolization have largely been eliminated with the newer hemoperfusion systems. However, thrombocytopenia is still the most common problem with both charcoal and resin hemoperfusion, but the reduction in platelet count is not usually associated with bleeding. Clinical studies report platelet losses of approximately 40% during a hemoperfusion procedure. A return to pretreatment values can be expected in 24 to 48 hours after the completion of hemoperfusion.[21]

Other side effects, such as hypocalcemia, hypoglycemia, hypothermia, and leukopenia have been reported, but are generally mild. Hypotension has also occurred in some clinical trials of hemoperfusion in patients with hepatic coma.[25] If it is necessary for the clinician to administer vasopressors, they should be adminis-

Table 3–2. Plasma extraction ratios for drugs frequently involved in poisoning incidents. (From Winchester JF, et al: Present and future uses of hemoperfusion with sorbents. *Artif Organs,* 2[4]:353, 1978.)

DRUG	HEMODIALYSIS	CHARCOAL HEMOPERFUSION	RESIN HEMOPERFUSION
Phenobarbital	0.27	0.5	0.8–0.9
Amobarbital	0.26	0.3	0.9
Carbromal	0.25–0.4	0.5–0.6	1.0
Glutethimide	0.16	0.6–0.7	0.8
Tricyclic antidepressants	0.2–0.5	0.2–0.5	0.7–0.9
Acetaminophen	0.4	0.5	—
Paraquat	0.5	0.6	0.9
Salicylates	0.5	0.5	—
Digoxin	0.15	0.3–0.6	0.4

$$\text{Extraction ratio} = \frac{\text{inlet concentration} - \text{outlet concentration}}{\text{inlet concentration}}$$

tered distal to the charcoal column, as they are adsorbed by the column. There is also some evidence that substances such as catecholamines, cortisol, aldosterone, and thyroxine may be adsorbed by the charcoal, but the clinical significance of this is unknown.[26]

CHOICE OF DIALYTIC PROCEDURE

The decision as to whether or not to remove an intoxicant by the use of a dialytic procedure should be based primarily on the clinical status of the patient and secondarily on the type and quantity of the intoxicant that has been ingested. The choice of the particular procedure, however, should be based on both the properties of the intoxicant and the patient's clinical status. Both peritoneal dialysis and hemodialysis are limited to intoxications involving drugs that are water soluble, exhibit low protein binding, and are of a size that allows them to pass through the peritoneal or dialysis membrane. Charcoal hemoperfusion, on the other hand, can be used for drugs that are not easily removed by HD or PD because of their lipophilic nature or strong protein-binding properties. However, this also may be a potential limitation, since hemoperfusion does not correct fluid status, electrolytes, or acid-base balance abnormalities.

PATIENT CRITERIA

The implementation of a dialytic procedure should be considered for intoxicated patients who have one or more of the following conditions:[27] (1) severe intoxication manifested by abnormal vital signs and acid-base, fluid, and electrolyte abnormalities, (2) prolonged coma with its potential complications, (3) compromised excretory routes in the presence of renal failure, liver disease, or cardiac insufficiency, (4) progressive clinical deterioration despite intensive care and therapeutic interventions, (5) ingestion of a potentially lethal dose of an intoxicant, and (6) a blood level that is in the potentially lethal range.

DRUG CRITERIA

A thorough knowledge and understanding of the physical characteristics and pharmacokinetic parameters of the ingested intoxicant can be extremely helpful to the clinician in the assessment of the need for implementation of a dialytic procedure. These include particle size, protein-binding characteristics, volume of distribution, distribution phase, and fraction excreted unchanged by the kidney

Size. The particle size of the intoxicant should be small enough to allow diffusion through the pores of the artificial membrane during HD. Since CHP and RHP are not limited by a dialysis membrane, the particle size is not a limiting factor.[28,29]

Protein binding. The intoxicant must not be highly bound to plasma proteins, because proteins are too large to be filtered through a dialysis membrane. Only the free fraction, or the fraction of the intoxicant in the plasma that is not protein bound, is dialyzable. However, in severe intoxications, because the protein-binding sites can become saturated, the free fraction of the ingested intoxicant may be increased, and hence dialysis may become a useful therapeutic modality.[29,30] The relative importance of the degree of protein binding during CHP remains to be investigated; however, it has been postulated that increasing the percentage of unbound drug increases the rate of drug uptake.[31]

Volume of distribution. The intoxicant ideally should have a small volume of distribution. Intoxicants that are highly lipid soluble have large volumes of distribution, and only a small fraction of the intoxicant is present in the plasma. Only the intoxicant that is in plasma is available for removal by a dialytic procedure.[29]

Distribution phase. Distribution of an intoxicant from tissue stores to plasma may be the rate-limiting step in a dialytic procedure. For example, when equilibration of an intoxicant from tissues to the plasma lags behind dialytic removal from plasma, the plasma concentration may decrease rapidly, suggesting therapeutic success. However, when the intoxicant redistributes from tissue to plasma, a secondary rebound increase in the plasma concentration may occur, resulting in a recurrence of toxic manifestations.[28,29,32]

Fraction excreted unchanged by the kidney. As a general guide, intoxicants that are largely excreted unchanged in the urine are expected to be effectively removed by the implementation of a dialytic procedure because of their hydrophilic nature.[28]

ASSESSING THE EFFECTIVENESS OF DIALYTIC PROCEDURES

Presently, it is difficult for the clinician to assess the effectiveness of a dialytic procedure, because of the inherent problems that have been associated with the various parameters used to evaluate the contribution of these procedures to the total therapeutic outcome of the intoxicated patient. The commonly used parameters are clinical status of the patient, pharmacokinetic parameters, amount of drug eliminated, dialysis clearance, and extraction ratio.

CLINICAL STATUS

When an intoxicated comatose patient awakens subsequent to the initiation of a dialytic procedure, the method is usually considered successful. However, initiation of the dialytic procedure is only one of several factors that may have been responsible for the clinical improvement. For example, good supportive care may have contributed to the therapeutic outcome of the patient. Furthermore, when such a case is reported, a comparison is commonly made with the existing literature concerning intoxications treated without implementation of a dialytic procedure. However, it is important for the clinician to ascertain whether or not the comparisons are made with the appropriate patient population, e.g., age, sex, weight, prior disease states, quantity ingested, degree of intoxication, interval elapsing between ingestion and initial treatment, and types of initial treatment.[28]

PHARMACOKINTEIC PARAMETERS

There are several factors associated with the intoxicated state that could affect the pharmacokinetics of an intoxicant, making it difficult to assess changes caused by the dialytic procedure. For example, absorption could be affected by GI paralysis. If the absorption rate constant becomes larger than the elimination rate constant, the terminal part of the log-drug-concentration-time curve does not accurately reflect elimination. Correction of unstable vital functions, e.g., anoxia, hypotension, and hypothermia, could enhance elimination of the intoxicant, which could be attributed to the dialytic procedure. Saturation phenomena may occur in enzyme-catalyzed metabolism, active renal tubular secretion, and protein- and tissue-binding sites, resulting in concentration-dependent elimination kinetics in the intoxicated patient. Distribution characteristics of the substance must also be taken into account. When half-life data are given, it is often not known whether the drug is still equilibrating with body tissues or whether elimination has reached the beta or slow phase for drug elimination.[33,34]

AMOUNT OF DRUG ELIMINATED

Quantitation of the amount of drug eliminated is important in the assessment of dialytic efficacy. However, this is a difficult task. Although the amount eliminated by a dialytic procedure is often given in the literature, the total drug ingested is usually unknown, and it may be difficult to calculate the fraction of the body burden eliminated. For agents such as the tricyclic antidepressants, for example, that have large volumes of distribution and correspondingly low concentrations in the plasma, an insignificant amount of the total tissue load is expected to be removed.[33]

DIALYSIS CLEARANCE

Dialysis clearance is frequently used as a measure of dialyzability of intoxicants. The clearance of any intoxicant can be defined as the ability of an organ to irreversibly remove an intoxicant from perfusing blood. Clearance can be described as the volume of plasma cleared of a drug in a given time, and can be calculated using the following equation.

$$Cl_D = \frac{Q_b \cdot (C_{bi} - C_{bo})}{C_{bi}}$$

Cl_D is the dialysis clearance, Q_b is the blood flow through the dialysis machine, and C_{bi} and C_{bo} are the concentrations of the intoxicant in the blood entering and leaving the dialysis machine, respectively. This equation assumes that the intoxicant concentration of the dialysate approaches zero, which is usually accomplished by the use of large volumes of dialysate, by frequent replacement of the dialysate, or by inclusion of substances that will bind the intoxicant in the dialysate.[35]

Another method used to calculate clearance is independent of blood flow and can

also be used for peritoneal dialysis. It is expressed by the following equation.

$$Cl_D = \frac{R}{t\ C_p\ MID}$$

R is the total amount of intoxicant removed in the dialysate, t is the length of dialysis, and C_p MID is the arterial plasma level at the midpoint of dialysis.[29]

Dialysis clearance, however, is not a reliable indicator of the efficiency of a dialytic procedure, as shown in Figure 3–4, owing to the fact that dialysis clearance is partly a function of volume of distribution.[35] If the drug, e.g., digoxin, has a large volume of distribution, the amount of plasma cleared of the drug represents only a small percentage of its total body burden. However, clearance calculations may assist the clinician in comparing various dialytic procedures for a given intoxicant.

EXTRACTION RATIO

The extraction ratio can be used to evaluate the efficacy of removal of an intoxi-

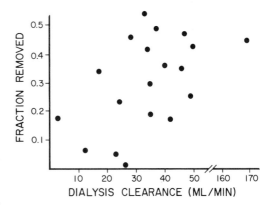

Fig. 3–4. A plot of the fraction of drug in the body (immediately prior to hemodialysis) removed by a 6-hour hemodialysis versus dialysis clearance. (From Gwilt PR, and Perrier D: Plasma protein binding and distribution characteristics of drugs as indices of their hemodialysis. *Clin Pharmacol Ther*, 24 [2]:154, 1978.)

Table 3–3.   Dialyzability of Common Intoxicants.

SUBSTANCE	PHARMACOKINETIC PARAMETERS[a]				CLEARANCE DURING DIALYTIC PROCEDURES (ML/MIN)[b]				COMMENTS[c]
	T½ (HR)	VD (L/KG)	PB (%)	FE (%)	PD	HD	CHP	RHP	
ALCOHOLS									
Ethanol		0.7				110[38]	59–78[39]		Although rarely necessary in uncomplicated alcohol excess, HD may be useful if blood levels exceed 400 mg/dl.
Ethylene glycol						174[40]			HD has been reported to be effective.[41]
Isopropanol									PD and HD have been reported to cause clinical improvement.[42–44]
Methanol						150[45]			Dialysis is recommended when visual impairment, severe acidosis or blood levels over 50 mg/dl occur. PD removes 3× and HD 25× as much as renal excretion.[46–50]
ANALGESICS									
Acetaminophen	2.75–3.25[e]			2–3	3[51]	120[52]	190[24]		Acetaminophen and its metabolites may be removed by HD or CHP. However, efficacy in preventing or reducing the severity of liver damage is poor, possibly owing to late initiation of therapy.[53–55]
Acetylsalicylic acid	2–19[d]	0.1–0.2	50–90	5–85	45–90[56]	35–100[57]	100[58]	27–74[39]	PD, HD, CHP, and RHP are all effective. HD has the advantage of reversing acidosis. PD may be enhanced by dialysis solutions containing 5% albumin. Ingestion of 500 mg/kg, severe acidosis, or blood levels greater than 80 mg/dl may be considerations for dialysis.[24,59,60]

Drug									Comments
Propoxyphene	11.8			1.5	8[61]	138[61]	124[62]		Both HD and PD remove only small amounts of the drug. Clinical improvement has not been demonstrated.
ANTITUBERCULAR DRUGS									
Isoniazid	1–3.6	0.6	0	57–66		24–59[63]			Anecdotal reports suggest HD may be effective, and it is recommended if there is ingestion of more than 5 g or renal failure.
BRONCHODILATORS									
Theophylline	3–7	0.33–0.74	15			38[64]	110[65]	225[66]	CHP or RHP recommended in serious overdosage and may be considered at blood levels greater than 70 μg/ml.[67–69]
CARDIOVASCULAR DRUGS									
Digoxin	36	5.2	23	59	8[70]	10–40[71]	25–90[72]	82–143[73]	PD and HD are not effective, owing to drug's large Vd and tissue binding. HD may be used to treat hyperkalemia unresponsive to other methods. Data on CHP and RHP are inconclusive. Although case reports suggest improvement, pharmacokinetic analysis shows removal of only a small fraction of drug.[74]
Phenytoin	8–60[d]	0.6–0.8	90	1–5			10[75]	79–189[22]	Data on therapeutic levels suggest HD is not useful. Data on CHP are inadequate.
Procainamide	2.2–4.7[e]	1.5	15	40–60			33–37[76]		HD may be valuable in patients with toxicity severe enough to cause life-threatening arrhythmias and hypotension.[77]
Propranolol	4	3.6–4.6	90–96	1			18.6[78]		HD does not appear to remove a significant amount of drug. Cases have been reported; however, further study is needed.[80]
Quinidine	6–7	3	80	10–50		11.3–42.5[79]			

Table 3–3. Dialyzability of Common Intoxicants. (Continued)

SUBSTANCE	PHARMACOKINETIC PARAMETERS[a]				CLEARANCE DURING DIALYTIC PROCEDURES (ML/MIN)[b]				COMMENTS[c]
	T½ (HR)	VD (L/KG)	PB (%)	FE (%)	PD	HD	CHP	RHP	
METALS									
Arsenic							87[81]		Although the arsenic-hemoglobin complex is not thought to be dialyzable, in the presence of renal failure, dialysis will remove the BAL-arsine complex.
Bromide									Dialysis may be indicated for blood levels above 20 mEq/L, intolerance to salt loading, or presence of renal failure.[82–84]
Iron					0.4[85]				Dialysis recommended in the presence of renal failure. In dogs with normal renal function, desferoxamine promoted greater renal excretion than hemodialysis.[86,87]
Lead									Although clinical results have been poor, the use of PD and HD in the presence of renal failure has been suggested.[88–90]
Lithium	7–20	0.6		97	15–25	13–15[91]	30–50[92]		Dialysis lowers blood levels and improves clinical status. It has been recommended for lithium levels greater than 3.5 mEq/L or renal failure. However, owing to slow equilibration between intra- and extracellular compartments, rebound increases frequently occur.
Mercury					1–5[93]	5[94]			Dialysis is useful in treating uremia, but its value in removing mercury remains to be demonstrated.[95,96]

								Comments
PSYCHOTHERAPEUTIC AGENTS								
Phenothiazines	16–36	20	91–99	1		0.5[97]		Owing to high tissue binding, phenothiazines are poorly dialyzable.
Tricyclic antidepressants	8–90	20–59	75–94	1–5			240[98]	Owing to rapid tissue binding and large Vd, it seems unlikely that HD, CHP will be of benefit unless performed within a few hours of ingestion.[99–100]
SEDATIVES/ HYPNOTICS								
Barbiturates (short-acting)	12–28	0.1–1.1	40–65	5–20	10[101–102]	25–55[103]	80[104]	PD, HD, CHP, and RHP have been reported to remove barbiturates. Ingestion of 3 g or blood levels of 50 μg/ml may be consideration for extracorporeal removal. However, clinical improvement has not been documented.[98]
Barbiturates (long-acting)	48–144	0.7	20–45	27–50	10[101–102]	60[103]	80[104]	PD, HD, CHP, and RHP have been reported to remove barbiturates. Ingestion of 5 g or blood levels of 100 μg/ml may be considerations for extracorporeal removal. Case reports suggest clinical improvement.[98]
Chloral hydrate (see Trichlorethanol)								
Ethchlorvynol	5.6–25[e]	4	35–50	10	18.5[105]	64[105]		Although PD, HD, and CHP have been suggested for ingestion of greater than 10 g or blood levels greater than 150 μg/ml, these procedures have not been shown to remove significant amounts of drug.[62,106]
Glutethimide	5–22[e]	2	54	2	5.3[107]	30[107]	150[108]	Although data are limited, CHP or RHP may be beneficial at blood levels above 40 μg/ml or ingestion of 10 g. A rebound rise in levels may occur following termination of hemoperfusion.[109–110]

Table 3–3. Dialyzability of Common Intoxicants. (Continued)

SUBSTANCE	PHARMACOKINETIC PARAMETERS[a]				CLEARANCE DURING DIALYTIC PROCEDURES (ML/MIN)[b]				COMMENTS[c]
	T½ (HR)	VD (L/KG)	PB (%)	FE (%)	PD	HD	CHP	RHP	
Meprobamate	6–17	0.75	20	8–20	11[110]	20[111]	40–221[112]	208[112]	CHP and RHP have been reported to be effective and may be considered at blood levels of 120 µg/ml.[113]
Methaqualone	20–60	6		80	7.5[114]	23[114]	56[62]		HD has not been shown to prevent or shorten coma. CHP or RHP may be considered at blood levels of 40 µg/ml, but adequate data on efficacy are not available.
Methyprylon	4[e]			3			80[115]	160–210[116]	HD and CHP have been reported to remove drug and cause clinical improvement and may be considered after ingestion of 6 g or blood levels greater than 40 µg/ml.[117,118]
Primidone	5–10	1	0	1					Clinical improvement has been reported with HD (see also its metabolite, phenobarbital).[119]
Trichlorethanol	8[e]	1	35–51				162[120]		HD has been reported effective and may be considered at blood levels of 50 µg/ml.[121]

MISCELLANEOUS

			Comments
Amanita phalloides			Case reports have suggested the use of CHP, but data are inconclusive.[122–124]
Camphor	1		Case reports have suggested use of RHP. Lethal doses range from 50–500 mg/kg.[125,126]
Organophosphates	53–59[27]	59–83[127]	Case reports have suggested use of CHP.[128,129]
Paraquat	10[130]	72[130]	HD does not appear to be effective. CHP has not been shown to cause clinical improvement, although some drug is removed. The toxic dose is 4 mg/kg.[131–134]

Key to Table 3–3.
ABBREVIATIONS:
t½   = Half-life
VD   = Volume of distribution
PB   = Protein binding
FE   = Fraction excreted unchanged
PD   = Peritoneal dialysis
HD   = Hemodialysis
CHP = Charcoal hemoperfusion
RHP = Resin hemoperfusion
FOOTNOTES:
[a] Values take from references 136–139.
[b] Individual references cited in table.
[c] Blood level guidelines from references 1, 134, 135.
[d] Intoxicant exhibits dose-dependent kinetics at therapeutic levels.
[e] Literature suggests kinetics are altered in overdose patients.

cant and is calculated by the following formula:

$$\text{Extraction ratio} = \frac{\text{inlet concentration} - \text{outlet concentration}}{\text{inlet concentration}}$$

Several examples utilizing the extraction ratio principle are shown in Table 3–2. It appears that resin hemoperfusion is more effective than charcoal hemoperfusion, which is more effective than hemodialysis. Although the application of this concept is useful in comparing various dialytic procedures, it does not help the clinician to assess the fraction of total body burden removed during a dialytic procedure, because the distribution volume is not taken into account.[25,36]

PREDICTING THE EFFECTIVENESS OF DIALYTIC DEVICES

Pharmacokinetic principles may be used by the clinician to determine the effectiveness of dialytic procedures in removing drugs from intoxicated patients. The following two parameters should be considered: (1) volume of distribution and (2) clearance of the intoxicant.

VOLUME OF DISTRIBUTION

The larger the volume of distribution of the intoxicant, the smaller the fraction of body burden cleared per unit of time by the use of a dialytic device. Also, the efficacy of a dialytic procedure is expected to increase as the percentage of the unbound intoxicant in the plasma is increased. As a result, the ratio of percentage of unbound intoxicant to volume of distribution of the intoxicant can be used as an index of dialyzability. A mathematical model based on this concept has been developed specifically for HD to assist the clinician in estimating the fraction of the intoxicant that will be removed from the body in a given time period, using the volume of distribution and percentage of unbound intoxicant in the plasma.[35] This can be expressed as: % unbound/Vd(L/kg). Values for volume of distribution and percentage bound to plasma proteins of

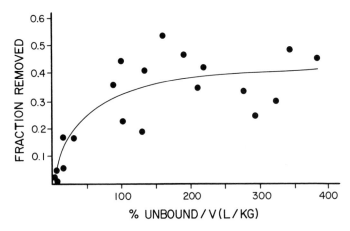

Fig. 3–5. A plot of the fraction of drug in the body (immediately prior to hemodialysis) removed by a 6-hour hemodialysis versus the ratio of the percent of drug (unbound to plasma proteins) in the plasma to the volume of distribution (V) of the drug. (From Gwilt PR, and Perrier D: Plasma protein binding and distribution characteristics of drugs as indices of their hemodialysis. *Clin Pharmacol Ther,* 24 [2]:164, 1978.)

common intoxicants are provided in Table 3–3.

Generally, it has been reported that when the percentage of unbound intoxicant in the plasma is divided by the apparent volume of distribution of that intoxicant, and the ratio obtained is greater than 80, a significant amount (20 to 50%) of the intoxicant ingested will be removed with 6 hours of HD. However, if the ratio obtained is under 20, an insignificant amount of the intoxicant (less than 10%) will be removed during 6 hours of HD (Figure 3–5).

This mathematical model, however, has several limitations. Presently, the pharmacokinetic parameters (e.g., volume of distribution and percentage unbound) of an intoxicant are often derived from normal individuals, and are generally unavailable for acutely and/or chronically intoxicated patients. In addition, the particle size of the intoxicant is not considered. For example, vancomycin, which is 90% unbound and which has a volume of distribution of 0.6 L/kg, would be expected to be dialyzable. However, due to its large particle size (1800 daltons), it is poorly dialyzable.

DIALYSIS CLEARANCE RELATIVE TO TOTAL BODY CLEARANCE

A mathematical model has been developed that can be used to assess the contributions of both HD and CHP or RHP to the total amount of an intoxicant that can be eliminated from the body during a given period (T).[33] The first step is to calculate the total body clearance, which can be defined as the sum of the clearances by the liver, kidney, and other eliminating organs of the body, and can be most simply expressed as $Cl_T = Vd \times K$, where Vd is the volume of distribution, and K is the elimination rate constant $\left(K = \dfrac{0.693}{t^{1/2}} \right)$ of an intoxicant. The $t^{1/2}$ and

Vd values of common intoxicants are listed in Table 3–3. The results obtained should be added to the reported clearances by the dialytic procedures (Cl_D), in order to calculate the total clearance (Cl_{TD}) of an intoxicant by both the eliminating body organ systems and the dialytic procedure: $Cl_{TD} = Cl_T + Cl_D$.

After the total clearance has been calculated, the fraction of the total amount of the ingested intoxicant that can be removed by the dialytic procedure can be calculated with the following equation.

$$\frac{Cl_D}{Cl_{TD}} \left(1 - e^{-Cl TD^{t}/VD} \right)$$

If the fraction removed in 6 hours is greater than 50%, the intoxicant is considered highly dialyzable. If the fraction removed is between 20% and 50%, the intoxicant is considered moderately dialyzable. If the fraction is less than 20%, it is unlikely that dialysis will contribute significantly to the removal of the intoxicant.

This model assumes that (1) the elimination of all intoxicants, including the dialytic procedures, follows first-order kinetics, (2) the dialytic procedure is initiated in the postabsorptive, postdistributive phase, and (3) in intoxicated patients, the intoxicant has a normal volume of distribution. However, because pharmacokinetic parameters are altered in intoxicated patients and may not follow these assumptions, this model may also have a limited predictive value in assessing the dialyzability of different intoxicants.[33,35,37]

The indications and efficacy of different dialytic procedures for common intoxicants are listed in Table 3–3. The dose and blood level at which to initiate a dialytic procedure, also listed, serve only as guidelines. The clinical condition of the patient should be the primary consideration.

Clearances are given as an aid to the clinician in comparing various dialytic procedures. The clearances provided, however, are only representative and can vary with the apparatus, blood flow, and individual patient characteristics. Furthermore, since the literature is often inadequate regarding the use of dialytic procedures in the removal of different intoxicants, various pharmacokinetic properties that influence their dialyzability are also provided. Their significance is discussed in the section on drug criteria. It should also be noted that the pharmacokinetic properties are reported for normal patients and may be significantly different for intoxicated patients.

Removal of intoxicants by the use of different dialytic procedures has been shown to benefit some acutely or chronically intoxicated patients. The criteria for selection of these patients should be stringent, however, since most patients can be treated by supportive and symptomatic care alone. The assessment of the efficacy of the different dialytic devices for a particular intoxicant is difficult at the present time in the majority of cases because, in published reports, the methodology and quantitative analysis used to assess the removal of intoxicants from intoxicated patients have been poor. However, some basic pharmacokinetic principles are provided to help the clinician to assess the literature and at the same time to predict the usefulness of the different dialytic procedures in the removal of intoxicants from intoxicated patients.

REFERENCES

1. Winchester JF, et al: Dialysis and hemoperfusion of poisons and drugs—update. *Trans Am Soc Artif Organs*, 23:762–842, 1977
2. Clemmesen C, and Nilson E: Therapeutic trends in management of barbiturate poisoning. The Scandinavian methods. *Clin Pharmacol Ther*, 2(2):220–229, 1961.
3. Young RK, et al: Respiratory intensive care: A 10 year survey. *Br Med J*, 1:307–310, 1974.
4. Arieff AI, and Friedman EA: Coma following non-narcotic drug overdosage: Management of 208 adult patients. *Am J Med Sci*, 266:405–426, 1973.
5. Sargen JA, and Gotch FA: Principles and biophysics of dialysis. In *Replacement of Renal Function by Dialysis*. 2nd Ed. Edited by W Brukker, FM Parsons and JF Maher. Boston, Martinus Nijhoff Publishers, 1979, pp. 38–68.
6. Hampers CL, Schupak E, Lowrie EG, and Lazarus JM (eds): *Long-Term Hemodialysis*. 2nd Ed. New York, Grune and Stratton, 1973, pp. 1–31.
7. Brukker W: Haemodialysis: A historical review. In *Replacement of Renal Function by Dialysis*, 2nd Ed. Edited by W Brukker, FM Parsons, and JF Maher. Boston, Martinus Nijhoff Publishers, 1979, pp. 3–37.
8. Hoenich NA, Frost TH, and Kerr DNS: Dialyzers. In *Replacement of Renal Function by Dialysis*. 2nd Ed. Edited by W Brukker, FM Parsons, and JF Maher. Boston, Martinus Nijhoff Publishers, 1979, pp. 80–124.
9. Maher JF: Selective dialysis for removal of large solutes: A reappraisal. *Kidney Int*, 3(Suppl): 361–364, 1975.
10. Maher JF, and Nolph KD: Resistance to diffusion in dialyzers. *Clin Nephrol*, 1:333–335, 1973.
11. Maeda K, et al: Dialysate regeneration: 30 liter dialysate supply system with sorbents. *Kidney Int*, 10:S289–295, 1976.
12. Wing AJ and Magowan M (eds): *The Renal Unit*. 1st Ed. Philadelphia, JB Lippincott, 1975, pp. 151–160.
13. Dunea G: Peritoneal dialysis and hemodialysis. *Med Clin North Am*, 55:155–175, 1971.
14. Nolph KD: Peritoneal dialysis. In *Replacement of Renal Function by Dialysis*. 2nd ed. Edited by W Brukker, FM Parsons and JF Maher. Boston, Martinus Nijhoff Publishers, 1979, pp. 277–321.
15. Maxwell MH, Rokney RE, and Kleeman CR: Peritoneal dialysis: 1. Technique and applications. *JAMA*, 170:917–924, 1959.
16. Jones HJ: Peritoneal dialysis. *Br Med Bull*, 27:165–169, 1971.
17. Gault HM, et al: Fluid and electrolyte complications of peritoneal dialysis. *Ann Intern Med*, 75:253–262, 1971.
18. Boen ST: Kinetics of peritoneal dialysis. *Medicine*, 40:243–287, 1961.
19. Simon NM, and Krumlovsky FA: The role of dialysis in the treatment of poisonings. *Ration Drug Ther*, 3:1–7, 1971.
20. Raja RM, Kramer MS, and Rosenbaum JL: Recirculation peritoneal dialysis with sorbent redy cartridge. *Nephron*, 16:134–142, 1976.
21. Vale JA, et al: Use of charcoal hemoperfusion in the management of severely poisoned patients. *Br Med J*, 1:5–19, 1975.
22. DeGroot G, Maes RAA, and Van Heyst AN: The use of hemoperfusion in the elimination of absorbed drug mixtures in acute intoxications. *Neth J Med*, 20:142–148, 1977.
23. Passer JA: Hemoperfusion: A new treatment for severe drug overdose. *Nebr Med J*, 63:116–119, 1978.
24. Gelfand MC, et al: Treatment of severe drug overdosage with charcoal hemoperfusion. *Trans Am Soc Artif Intern Organs*, 23:599–605, 1977.
25. Winchester JF, Gelfand MC, and Tilstone WJ: Hemoperfusion in drug intoxication: Clinical

and laboratory aspects. *Drug Metab Rev* (FJ Di Carlo, ed), 8(1):69–104, Marcel Dekker, Inc., N.Y., 1978.

26. Leber HW, Geissler RH, and Post D: Carbromal intoxication—hemodialysis or hemoperfusion? *Acta Pharmacol Toxicol (Copenh) (Suppl),* 41(2):78–84, 1977.

27. Schreiner GE: The role of hemodialysis (artificial kidney) in acute poisoning. *Arch Intern Med,* 102:896–913, 1958.

28. Maher JF: Principles of dialysis and dialysis of drugs. *Am J Med,* 62:475–481, 1977.

29. Gibson TP, and Neson HA: Drug kinetics and artificial kidneys. *Clin Pharmacokinetics* 2:403–426, 1977.

30. Malizia E, Signore L, and Crimi G: Chlorpromazine plus thioridazine poisoning and treatment with extracorporeal dialysis. *Acta Pharmacol Toxicol (Copenh) (Suppl),* 41(1):163–170, 1977.

31. Chang TMS: A 1978 perspective of hemoperfusion. *Artif Organs,* 2:359–366, 1978.

32. Gibson TP, Nelson HA, and Ivanovich P: Digoxin removal from an anephric patient by hemoperfusion over XAD-4. *Artif Organs,* 2(4) 398–401, 1978.

33. Takki S, et al: Pharmacokinetic evaluation of hemodialysis in acute drug overdose. *J Pharmacokinet Biopharm,* 6(5): 427–442, 1978.

34. Tilstone WS, Reavey PC, and Winchester JF: Clearance models to assess the efficacy of procedures enhancing drug removal in self-poisoning. *Acta Pharmacol Toxicol (Copenh) (Suppl),* 41(2): 102–106, 1977.

35. Gwilt PR, and Perrier D: Plasma protein binding and distribution characteristics of drugs as indices of their hemodialysis. *Clin Pharmacol Ther,* 24(2):154–161, 1978.

36. Winchester JF, et al: Present and future uses of hemoperfusion with sorbents. *Artif Organs,* 2(4):353–358, 1978.

37. Watanabe AS: Pharmacokinetic aspects of the dialysis of drugs. *Drug Int Clin Pharm,* 11:407–416, 1977.

38. Elliott RW, and Hunter PR: Acute ethanol poisoning treated by haemodialysis. *Postgrad Med J,* 50:515–517, 1974.

39. Widdop B, et al.: Experimental drug intoxication: Treatment with charcoal hemoperfusion. *Arch Toxicol,* 34:27–36, 1975.

40. Underwood F, and Bennett WM: Ethylene glycol intoxication. Prevention of renal failure by aggressive management. *JAMA,* 226:1453–1454, 1973.

41. Hagstam KL, et al: Ethylene-glycol poisoning treated by haemodialysis. *Acta Med Scand,* 178:599–606, 1965.

42. Freireich AW, et al: Hemodialysis for isopropanol poisoning. *N Engl J Med,* 277:699–700, 1967.

43. King LH, Bradley KP, and Shires DL: Hemodialysis for isopropyl alcohol poisoning. *JAMA,* 211:1855, 1970.

44. Dua SL (Letter): Peritoneal dialysis for isopropyl alcohol poisoning. *JAMA,* 230:35, 1974.

45. Setter JG, et al: Studies on the dialysis of methanol. *Trans Am Soc Artif Intern Organs,* 13:178–182, 1967.

46. McCoy HG, et al: Severe methanol poisoning. *Am J Med,* 67:804–810, 1979.

47. Gonda A, et al: Hemodialysis for methanol intoxication. *Am J Med,* 64:749–757, 1978.

48. Keyvan–Larijarni H, and Tannenberg AM: Methanol intoxication: Comparison of peritoneal dialysis and hemodialysis treatment. *Arch Intern Med,* 134:293–296, 1974.

49. Wenzl JE, Mills SD, and McCall JT: Methanol poisoning in an infant. Successful treatment with peritoneal dialysis. *Am J Dis Child,* 116:445–447, 1968.

50. Humphrey TJ: Methanol poisoning: Management of acidosis with combined haemodialysis and peritoneal dialysis. *Med J Aust,* 1:833–835, 1974.

51. Maclean D, et al: Treatment of acute paracetamol poisoning. *Lancet,* 2:849–852, 1968.

52. Proudfoot AT, and Wright N: Acute paracetamol poisoning. *Br Med J,* 3:557–558, 1972.

53. Farid NR, Glynn JP, and Kerr DNS: Hemodialysis in paracetamol self-poisoning. *Lancet,* 2:396–398, 1972.

54. Rigby RJ, et al: The treatment of paracetamol overdose with charcoal haemoperfusion and cysteamine. *Med J Aust,* 1:396–399, 1978.

55. Penn RG: A theoretical approach to the management of paracetamol overdosage. *J Int Med Res* (Suppl) 4:98–104, 1976.

56. Fischer RL: Intermittent peritoneal dialysis using 5% albumin in the treatment of salicylate intoxication in children. *J Pediatr,* 58:226–236, 1961.

57. Kallen RJ, Zaltman S, Coe FL, and Metcoff J: Hemodialysis in children: Technique, kinetic aspects related to varying body size and application to salicylate intoxication, acute renal failure and some other disorders. *Medicine,* 45:1–50, 1966.

58. Rosenbaum JL, et al: Resin hemoperfusion in the treatment of drug intoxications. *Trans Am Soc Artif Intern Organs,* 16:134–140, 1970.

59. Etteldorf JN, et al: Intermittent peritoneal dialysis in the treatment of experimental salicylate intoxication. *J Pediatr,* 56:1–10, 1960.

60. Schlegel RJ, et al: Peritoneal dialysis for severe salicylism: An evaluation of indications and results. *J Pediatr,* 69:553–552, 1966.

61. Gary NE, et al: Acute propoxyphene hydrochloride intoxication. *Arch Intern Med,* 121:453–457, 1968.

62. Torrente A, et al: Fixed bed uncoated charcoal hemoperfusion in treatment of intoxications: Animal and patient studies. *Nephron,* 24:71–77, 1979.

63. Schneider E, Jungbluth H, and Oppermann F: Acute isoniazid intoxication: A neurological electroencephalographic and toxicological follow-up study. *Klin Wochenschr,* 49:904–910, 1971.

64. Levy G, et al: Hemodialysis clearance of theophylline. *JAMA,* 237:1466–1467, 1977.

65. Russo ME: Management of theophylline intoxication with charcoal column hemoperfusion. *N Engl J Med*, 300(1):24–26, 1979.

66. Lawyer C, et al: Treatment of theophylline neurotoxicity with resin hemoperfusion. *Ann Intern Med*, 88:516–517, 1978.

67. Zwillich CW, et al: Theophylline-induced seizures in adults: Correlation with serum concentrations. *Ann Intern Med*, 82:784–787, 1975.

68. Ehlers SM, Zaske DE, and Sawchuck RJ: Massive theophylline overdose. *JAMA*, 240:474–475, 1975.

69. Muir KT, and Pond SM (Correspondence): Removal of theophylline from the body by hemoperfusion. *Clin Pharmacokinet*, 4:320–321, 1979.

70. Ackerman GL, Doherty JE, and Flanigan WJ: Peritoneal dialysis and hemodialysis of tritiated digoxin. *Ann Intern Med*, 67:718–729, 1967.

71. Holt, DW, Trail TA, and Brown CB: The treatment of digoxin overdosage. *Clin Nephrol*, 3:119–122, 1975.

72. Tobin M, Cerra F, Steinbach J, and Moorkerjee B: Hemoperfusion in digitalis intoxication: A comparative study of coated vs uncoated charcoal. *Trans Am Soc Artif Intern Organs*, 23:730–731, 1977.

73. Smiley JW, March NM, and Del Guercio ET: Hemoperfusion in the management of digoxin toxicity. *JAMA*, 240:2736–2737, 1978.

74. Slattery JT, and Koup JR: Hemoperfusion in the management of digoxin toxicity: Is it warranted? *Clin Pharmacokinet*, 4:395–399, 1979.

75. Martin E, et al: Removal of phenytoin by hemodialysis in uremic patients. *JAMA*, 238:1750–1753, 1977.

76. Gibson TP, et al: Artificial kidneys and clearance calculations. *Clin Pharmacol Ther*, 20:720–726, 1976.

77. Atkinson AJ, et al: Hemodialysis for severe procainamide toxicity: Clinical and pharmacokinetic observations. *Clin Pharmacol Ther*, 20(5):585–592, 1976.

78. Lowenthal DT, et al: Pharmacokinetics of oral propranolol in chronic renal disease. *Clin Pharmacol Ther*, 16:761–769, 1974.

79. Reimold EW, et al: Use of hemodialysis in the treatment of quinidine poisoning. *Pediatrics*, 52:95–99, 1973.

80. Woie L, and Oyri A: Quinidine intoxication treated with hemodialysis. *Acta Med Scand*, 195:237–239, 1974.

81. Gilberson A, et al: Hemodialysis of acute arsenic intoxication with transient renal failure. *Arch Intern Med*, 136:1303–1304, 1976.

82. Butte W, Meyer GJ, and Vollnberg W: Detoxification methods for bromureide poisoning: Comparison of haemodialysis, haemofiltration and haemoperfusion on bastard dogs. *Arch Toxicol*, 41:61–67, 1978.

83. Trump, DL, and Hochberg MC: Bromide intoxication. *Johns Hopkins Med J*, 138:119–123, 1976.

84. Collins J: A case of self-poisoning with carbrital. *Postgrad Med J*, 46:584–586, 1970.

85. Covey TV: Ferrous sulphate poisoning. *J Pediatr*, 64:218–226, 1964.

86. Whitten CF, Chen YC, and Gibson GW: Studies in acute iron poisoning. II. Further observations of desferoxamines in the treatment of acute experimental iron poisoning. *Pediatrics*, 38:102–110, 1966.

87. Greengard J: Iron poisoning in children. *Clin Toxicol*, 8(6):575–597, 1975.

88. Smith HD, King LR, and Margolin EG: Treatment of lead encephalopathy: The combined use of EDTA and hemodialysis. *Am J Dis Child*, 109:322–324, 1965.

89. Mehbod J: Treatment of lead intoxication. Combined use of peritoneal dialysis and edetate calcium disodium. *JAMA*, 201:972–974, 1967.

90. Pederson RS: Lead poisoning treated with haemodialysis. *Scand J Urol Nephrol*, 12:189–190, 1978.

91. Wilson JH, et al: Peritoneal dialysis for lithium poisoning. *Br Med J*, 2:749–750, 1971.

92. Amdisen A, and Skjoldborg H: Hemodialysis for lithium poisoning. *Lancet*, 2:213, 1969.

93. Lowenthal DT, Chardo F, and Reidenberg MM: Removal of mercury by peritoneal dialysis. *Arch Intern Med*, 134:139–141, 1974.

94. Maher JF, and Schreiner GE: The dialysis of mercury and mercury-BAL complex. *Clin Res*, 1:298, 1959.

95. Kahn A, Denis R, and Blun D: Accidental ingestion of mercuric sulphate in a 4-year old child. *Clin Pediatr*, 16:956–958, 1977.

96. Leumann EP, and Brandenberger H: Hemodialysis in a patient with acute mercuric cyanide intoxication. Concentrations of mercury in blood, dialysate, urine, vomitus and feces. *Clin Toxicol*, 11(3):301–307, 1977.

97. Avram MM, and McGinn JT: Extracorporeal hemodialysis in phenothiazine overdosage. *JAMA*, 97:142–143, 1966.

98. Trafford JAP, et al: Haemoperfusion with R–004 amberlite resin for treating acute poisoning. *Br Med J*, 2:1453–1456, 1977.

99. Wright N, and Cooke D (letter): Hemodialysis and forced diuresis for tricyclic antidepressant poisoning. *Br Med J*, 4:407, 1974.

100. Iverson BM, Willassen YW, and Bakke OM (letter): Charcoal hemoperfusion in nortriptyline poisoning. *Lancet*, 1(8060):388–389, 1978.

101. Berman LB, and Vogelsang P: Removal rates for barbiturates using two types of peritoneal dialysis. *N Engl J Med*, 270:77–80, 1964.

102. Knochel JP, and Barry KG: THAM dialysis: An experimental method to study diffusion of certain weak acids in vivo. II. Secobarbital. *J Lab Clin Med*, 65:361–369, 1965.

103. Henderson LW, and Merrill JP: Treatment of barbiturate intoxication with a report of recent experiences at Peter Bent Brigham Hospital. *Ann Intern Med*, 64:876–891, 1966.

104. Rosenbaum JL, Kramer MS, and Raja R: Resin hemoperfusion for acute drug intoxication. *Ann Intern Med*, 136:263–266, 1976.

105. Teehan BP, et al: Acute ethchlorvynol (Placidyl) intoxication. *Ann Intern Med*, 72:875–881, 1975.

106. Lynn RI, et al: Resin hemoperfusion for treatment of ethchlorvynol overdose. *Ann Intern Med*, 91:549–553, 1979.

107. Von Hartitzch B, et al: Treatment of glutethimide intoxication: An in vivo comparison of lipid, aqueous and peritoneal dialysis with albumin. *Proc Clin Dial Transplant Forum,* 3:102, 1973.

108. Ambre JJ, and Fischer LJ: Identification and activity of the hydroxy metabolite that accumulates in the plasma of humans intoxicated with glutethimide. *Drug Metab Dispos,* 2:151–158, 1974.

109. Koffler A, et al: Fixed bed charcoal hemoperfusion. Treatment of drug overdose. *Arch Intern Med,* 138(11):1691–1694, 1978.

110. Martin AM, et al: Charcoal haemoperfusion in the management of severe poisoning. *Br Med J,* 1:392, 1975.

111. Lubo PI, et al: Use of hemodialysis in meprobamate overdosage. *Clin Nephrol,* 7:73–75, 1977.

112. Hoy W, Schwab G, and Freeman RB: Clearance of meprobamate by hemoperfusion over columns of charcoal and amberlite resin. *Artif Organs,* 2:395–397, 1978.

113. Graae J, and Ladetoged J: Severe meprobamate poisoning treated by hemodialysis and peritoneal dialysis. *Nord Med,* 81:601–603, 1969.

114. Proudfoot AT, et al: Peritoneal dialysis and hemodialysis in methaqualone (Mandrax) poisoning. *Scott Med J,* 13:232–236, 1968.

115. Mandelbaum JM, and Simon NM: Severe methyprylon (Noludar) intoxication treated by hemodialysis. *JAMA,* 216:139–140, 1971.

116. Chang TMS, et al: The efficiency of the ACAC microcapsule artificial kidney for the removal of glutethimide, methyprylon and methaqualone in patients with acute intoxication. *Trans Am Soc Artif Intern Organs,* 19:87–91, 1973.

117. Yudis M, et al: Hemodialysis for methyprylon (Noludar) poisoning. *Ann Intern Med,* 68:1301–1304, 1968.

118. Pancorbo AS, et al: Hemodialysis in methyprylon overdose. Some pharmacokinetic considerations. *JAMA,* 237:470–471, 1977.

119. Blair AA, Hallpike JF, and Lascelles PT: Acute diphenylhydantoin and primidone poisoning treated by peritoneal dialysis. *J Neurol Neurosurg Psychiatry,* 31:520–523, 1968.

120. Vaziri ND, et al: Hemodialysis in treatment of acute chloral hydrate poisoning. *South Med J,* 70:377–378, 1977.

121. Stalker NE, et al: Acute massive chloral hydrate intoxication treated with hemodialysis: A clinical pharmacokinetic analysis. *J Clin Pharmacol,* 18: 136–142, 1978.

122. Rockel A, et al: Hemodialysis and cross-dialysis treatment of phalloidin intoxication in the unanesthetized rat. *Res Exp Med,* 165:101–109, 1975.

123. Gazzard BG, et al: Charcoal hemoperfusion in the treatment of fulminant hepatic failure. *Lancet,* 1:1301–1307, 1974.

124. Wauters JP, Rossel C, and Farquet JJ (letter): Amanita phalloides poisoning treated by early

charcoal hemoperfusion. *Br Med J,* 2(6150):1465, 1978.

125. Kopelman R, et al: Camphor intoxication treated by resin hemoperfusion. *JAMA,* 241:727–728, 1979.

126. Antman E, et al: Camphor overdosage. Therapeutic considerations. *NY State J Med,* 78:896–897, 1978.

127. Okonek S. Probable progress in the therapy of organophosphate poisoning. Extracorporeal hemodialysis and hemoperfusion. *Arch Toxicol,* 35:221–227, 1976.

128. Luzhnikov EA, et al (letter): Plasma perfusion through charcoal in methylparathion poisoning. *Lancet,* 1:38–39, 1977.

129. Okonek S: Hemoperfusion with coated activated charcoal in the treatment of organophosphate poisoning. *Acta Pharmacol Toxicol (Copenh) (Suppl)* 41:85–90, 1977.

130. Okonek S, Hofmann A, and Henningsen B: Efficacy of gut lavage, hemodialysis and hemoperfusion in the therapy of paraquat or diquat intoxication. *Arch Toxicol,* 36:43–51, 1976.

131. Vale JA, et al: The treatment of paraquat poisoning using oral solvents and charcoal hemoperfusion. *Acta Pharmacol Toxicol (Copenh) (Suppl),* 41(2):109–117, 1977.

132. Solfrank G, et al: Hemoperfusion through activated charcoal in paraquat intoxication. *Acta Pharmacol Toxicol (Copenh) (Suppl),* 41(2):91–101, 1977.

133. Spector D, et al: Fatal paraquat poisoning: Tissue concentrations and implications for treatment. *Johns Hopkins Med J,* 142:110–113, 1978.

134. Goulding R: Experience with hemoperfusion in drug abuse. *Kidney Int,* 10:S338–S340, 1976.

135. Basett H, Wright JA, and Cravey RH: Therapeutic and toxic concentrations of more than 100 toxicologically significant drugs in blood, plasma or serum: a tabulation. *Clin Chem,* 21(1):44–62, 1975.

136. Ritschel WA: *Handbook of Basic Pharmacokinetics.* Hamilton, IL., Drug Intelligence Publications, 1976.

137. Pagliaro LA, and Benet LZ: Pharmacokinetic data. Critical compilation of terminal half-lives, percent excreted unchanged, and changes of half-life in renal and hepatic dysfunction for studies in humans with references. *J Pharmacokinet Biopharm,* 3(5):333–383, 1975.

138. Knoben JE, Anderson PO, and Watanabe AS: *Handbook of Clinical Drug Data.* 4th Ed. Hamilton, IL, Drug Intelligence Publications, 1976.

139. Anderson RJ, Gambertoglio JG, and Schrier RW: *Clinical Use of Drugs in Renal Failure.* Springfield, IL, Charles C Thomas, 1976.

140. Avery GS (ed): *Drug Treatment.* 1st Ed. Acton, MA, Publishing Sciences Group, 1976, pp. 890–896, 970–975.

Section II

Management of Common Drug Overdosages

Chapter 4

Barbiturates

Vasilios A. Skoutakis
Sergio R. Acchiardo

Intentional and accidental ingestion of barbiturates still remains one of the most common types of intoxication in all developed countries. In Britain, for example, acute barbiturate intoxication accounts for about 70% of the total hospital admissions due to acute poisonings. This contributes to 2,000 adult deaths each year.[1] In the United States, the consumption of barbiturates is close to 1,000,000 pounds per week, or about 4,500,000 doses. This enormous usage continues to result in some 3,000 barbiturate deaths a year.[2]

In contrast to many forms of poisoning, acute barbiturate intoxication is (1) more often purposeful than accidental, (2) more common in adults than children, and (3) more frequent among members of the health care team. Intoxication also may be a pharmacologic accident, especially in the elderly, due to "automatism." The prescribed tablet or capsule produces not sleep but an amnesic state. Aware of the need for medication but forgetful that is has been taken, the patient continues to repeat the dose at intervals until the supply has been exhausted and intoxication becomes evident.[3]

Acute barbiturate poisoning, therefore, remains a continuing problem in all developed societies, and one that every health care team member will encounter during his professional life. An understanding of the clinical diagnostic considerations, the causes of the toxicologic manifestations, the appropriate laboratory tests, and available therapeutic measures is a requisite for the optimal management of the patient who is intoxicated by barbiturate agents.

CASE REPORT

A 26-year-old white female was admitted to the emergency room in coma at 5:00 PM. A discussion with the patient's husband revealed that the patient had been moody and depressed for the previous 5 weeks, but was not taking any prescription drugs and had no known allergies. At 3:30 PM of the day of admission, he found his wife lying unresponsive near the bedside, without any evidence (empty medicine bottles, pills, or syringes) of drug overdosage.

On admission to the ER, the patient was noted to be cyanotic and to have moderate respiratory distress. The vital signs at this time were blood pressure, 110/55 mm Hg; temperature, 35.0°C; pulse, 90/min and regular; and respirations, 12/min. The patient was not responsive to either verbal or painful stimuli. The gag reflex was absent. Deep tendon reflexes were diminished. The pupils were dilated 5 mm bilaterally and responded slowly to light. No alcoholic odor was present on the patient's breath. Auscultation of the chest revealed bilateral rales and rhonchi throughout the lungs. Abdominal examination showed diminished bowel sounds. Examination of the skin failed to show any pathologic abnormalities. The electrocardiogram revealed nonspecific ST-segment and T-wave changes.

CLINICAL ASSESSMENT AND MANAGEMENT OF THE PATIENT

The initial assessment of the patient is of paramount importance, not only to gain a baseline knowledge of the patient's condition from which his progress can be judged, but also to decide upon the therapeutic measures to preserve life. Assessment should include consideration of the following: (1) major clinical diagnostic considerations, (2) immediate therapeutic and diagnostic measures indicated, (3) significance of the toxicology laboratory results, (4) causes of the toxicologic manifestations, (5) indicated therapeutic measures, (6) possible complications, (7) determinants of successful therapy, and (8) prognosis.

MAJOR CLINICAL DIAGNOSTIC CONSIDERATIONS

In this case, we were presented with a patient in coma. The patient did not have historical evidence of pre-existing diseases such as hypertension, cirrhosis, chronic pulmonary disease, renal insufficiency, or diabetes mellitus. She had, however, a history of depression and a possible drug overdose, but there was no information to confirm that suspicion. The initial physical examination revealed signs of (1) respiratory depression, (2) impaired level of consciousness, (3) bilaterally dilated pupils that responded slowly to light, (4) hypotension, and (5) hypothermia.

However, the differential diagnosis as to the cause of the patient's current status could not be made clinically at the time, because the history was doubtful and because many substances and/or conditions are capable of producing these signs and symptoms (e.g., sedative-hypnotics, opiates, alcohol, ether, or other liquid hydrocarbons, diabetic and hyperosmolar coma, and carbon monoxide intoxication.

IMMEDIATE THERAPEUTIC AND DIAGNOSTIC MEASURES

As with all patients in coma, immediate measures must be instituted to support life. In the patient presented, the oropharynx was suctioned, a sample for arterial blood gas (ABG) determination was promptly drawn, and a cuffed endotracheal tube was inserted and connected to 95% oxygen. At the same time, access to the patient's circulation was established via an intravenous line, and blood was obtained for hematologic (Hemo-10 with differentials), biochemical (SMA-12), and basic toxicologic (alcohol, barbiturates, opiates) determinations. In addition, the patient was catheterized and 450 ml of urine were collected for urinalysis and drug screening.

Subsequently, a solution of 50 ml of 50% dextrose in water was administered to counteract any possible effects of hypoglycemia, but this resulted in no response from the patient. This was followed by the administration of four doses of naloxone hydrochloride (Narcan), 0.4 mg each at 5-minute intervals, but again no response was elicited. If the patient's respiratory depression had been solely due to a narcotic analgesic, an immediate improvement in respiratory rate would have been noted. Respiratory depression induced by barbiturates or other CNS depressants would not have been reversed following the administration of naloxone hydrochloride.

In doubtful cases in which the history, clinical manifestations, and initial diagnostic measures are not helpful, confirmation of the diagnosis is made possible by chemical analysis either of plasma or urine. In the present case, the results from the laboratory revealed a positive EMIT urinary drug screen for barbiturates, and a serum phenobarbital and secobarbital level of 11.8 mg/dl and 2.8 mg/dl, respectively. Other pertinent laboratory values on admission and during hospitalization are shown in Table 4–1.

CAUSES OF THE TOXICOLOGIC MANIFESTATIONS

The causes of the CNS depression, respiratory depression, hypotension, hypothermia, and decreased bowel sounds,

Table 4–1. Laboratory Findings During Hospitalization for Barbiturate Intoxication.

STUDIES	12/10/77[a]	12/11/77[b]	12/12/77[c]	12/15/77[d]
BUN (mg/100 ml)	16	15	14	15
Creatinine (mg/100 ml)	1.0	1.0	1.1	1.0
Calcium (mg/100 ml)	9.0	—	—	9.1
Phosphorus (mg/100 ml)	3.1	—	—	3.1
Sodium (mEq/L)	138	140	142	142
Chloride (mEq/L)	96	98	102	102
Potassium	5.4	5.3	5.0	4.5
Bicarbonate (mEq/L)	10	21	26	24
Blood glucose (mg/100 ml)	110	124	118	105
Hematocrit (%)	41	41	41	41.5
WBC (no/mm^3)	15,000	13,000	8,000	6,000
Urinary pH	5.0	8.0	7.8	6.0
Specific gravity	1.018	1.020	1.021	1.018
Arterial blood gases				
pH	7.15	7.41	7.45	7.41
P$_{CO_2}$ (mm Hg)	60	38	40	40
P$_{O_2}$ (mm Hg)	40	92	93	95
Intake (ml/24 hours)	2,300	9,000	7,000	2,950
Output (ml/24 hours)	2,700	9,400	7,600	3,140
Serum drug levels (mg/100 ml)				
Secobarbital	2.8	1.1	0.5	0
Phenobarbital	11.8	4.1	2.1	0
Stage of coma	4	2	1	
Blood pressure	110/55	120/70	120/80	128/85
Temperature (°C)	36.0	36.5	37.0	36.8

[a] Admission.
[b] Supportive care, forced diuresis, and alkalinization of urine started.
[c] Forced diuresis, alkalinization of urine, and artificial support of respiration stopped (48 hours post-admission).
[d] Patient's biochemical, hematologic, and clinical status prior to discharge.

which were manifested in the present case, can be related to the sedative-hypnotic actions of the barbiturate agents.

Central Nervous System Effects

In acute barbiturate intoxication, the degrees of depression of the central nervous system may vary from mild incoordination, with slurred speech and disorientation, to profound coma, with absence of deep tendon, pupillary, pharyngeal, laryngeal and even cranial reflexes. Any of these effects can be achieved deliberately or accidentally by any barbiturate given in sufficient dosage. The exact way in which barbiturates cause these effects is not known, but depression of the ascending reticular activating system (RAS), which is located in the central core of the brain stem, is thought to be the mechanism of action.[7]

Respiratory Effects

Barbiturates are respiratory depressants, affecting both the respiratory drive and the mechanism for the rhythmic character of respiratory movement. Initially, the neurogenic drive is most sensitive to depression by the barbiturate agents. As the dose of barbiturates is increased, the sensitivity of the medullary center to P_{CO_2} and pH changes becomes diminished. Eventually, as intoxication becomes more severe, there is a shift in the control of respiration from the P_{CO_2}-sensitive areas of the medulla to the more primitive receptors of the carotid and aortic bodies. With further accumulation of the parent compound or the production of active metabolites, the powerful hypoxic drive also fails, subjecting the patient to dangerous respiratory depression.[8] This then contributes to the severe acid-base problems, as seen in the initial evaluation of blood gases in the patient under consideration.

Cardiovascular Effects

In high drug concentrations or acute intoxications, the barbiturates have a direct suppressant effect on the myocardium and vascular musculature. The effect on the myocardium results in a reduction of the contractile force of the heart muscle and a decrease in the cardiac output.[9,10] The effect on the tone of the musculature of the peripheral vessels results in an excessive capillary exudation and venous pooling. This contributes to a subsequent diminution in venous return to the heart, further decreasing cardiac output, and a consequent fall in blood pressure and electrocardiogram abnormalities,[9,10] as seen in the patient presented.

Hypothermia

Significant hypothermia, with average temperature readings at 34 to 35°C, is frequently found in patients intoxicated with barbiturate drugs. In the case presented, the initial temperature on admission was recorded to be 35°C. Hypothermia present in these patients results from the direct suppressant effect of the barbiturates in the thermoregulatory centers in the hypothalamus.[8]

Gastrointestinal Effects

Reduction in gastrointestinal tone and motility following barbiturate intoxication again reflects the CNS depression. Patients who are unconscious and lack bowel sounds may be regarded as severely intoxicated. In addition, the clinician should remember that restoration of GI function during recovery from acute barbiturate intoxication, with resumption of peristalsis and absorption of retained drug residue, may result in relapse of symptoms.

SIGNIFICANCE OF THE TOXICOLOGY LABORATORY RESULTS

An important factor that must be considered by the clinician when using serum barbiturate drug levels to assess the clinical condition of the intoxicated patient and severity of the intoxication is drug tolerance. Patients on long-term barbiturate therapy or those abusing these drugs may have high blood barbiturate levels and yet show no toxic signs or symptoms.[4] In general, however, the therapeutic range for short-acting barbiturates is below 2 mg/dl. Toxicity and coma are usually noted when the serum drug level exceeds 3 mg/dl. For long-acting barbiturates, levels as high as 5 mg/dl may be considered therapeutic. Toxicity and coma are usually noted when the serum drug level is in excess of 8 mg/dl.[5]

In the case discussed here, the results from the laboratory assisted the clinician in (1) confirming the suspected diagnosis, (2) identifying the specific agents responsible, (3) assessing the severity of the intoxication, (4) distinguishing symptoms caused by the drug from those caused by other disorders, (5) initiating appropriate treatment based on the kinetics of the drugs, and (6) using the initial results as a baseline in monitoring the patient's progress.

However, when a patient is admitted to a hospital following the ingestion of a known barbiturate agent, and the appropriate laboratory facilities are not available, evaluation of the depth and severity of coma can be used by the clinician to assess the severity of the intoxication. Table 4–2 shows the four grades of coma that are based on Reed's work and that are currently used to assess the depth of coma at The University of Tennessee Center for the Health Sciences.[6] If this classification is applied to the case presented, the patient can be categorized as being in Grade 4 coma.

INDICATED THERAPEUTIC MEASURES

The treatment of barbiturate-intoxicated patients has changed dramatically over the past 40 years. These changes have resulted in a marked improvement in patients' survival rates.

In the 1930s and early 1940s, the mainstays of treatment were massive gastric lavage with fluids and the administra-

Table 4–2. Evaluation of Depth and Severity of Coma.

GRADE OF COMA	SYMPTOMS
Grade 1	Patient responds to painful stimuli. Deep tendon reflexes are present. Gag reflex is present. Blood pressure is normal and stable. Respirations are of an adequate rate and depth.
Grade 2	Patient does not respond to painful stimuli. Deep tendon reflexes are present. Gag reflex is present. Blood pressure is normal and stable. Respirations are adequate but may be slow.
Grade 3	Patient does not respond to painful stimuli. Deep tendon reflexes are absent. Gag reflex is present or absent. Blood pressure is stable but may be low. Respirations are adequate but may be slow.
Grade 4	Patient does not respond to painful stimuli. Deep tendon reflexes are absent. Gag reflex is absent. Blood pressure is unstable and needs support. Respirations are unstable and need support.

tion of powdered charcoal. However, in 1942, Harstad and associates showed that only small quantities of barbiturates could be removed by this technique, and that delayed utilization of lavage and charcoal was ineffective.[11] They also pointed out that pulmonary aspiration frequently associated with barbiturate intoxication, which resulted from an unprotected airway, often produced fatal pneumonias.

During the late 1940s and early 1950s, the administration of CNS stimulants such as picrotoxin, bemegride (Tegimide), ethamivan (Emivan), and Megimide nikethamide (Coramine) was extensively employed by clinicians. However, despite this aggressive treatment, the duration of coma was not shortened, and the morbidity and mortality rates remained high (40%). This was because of increased oxygen demand, convulsions, psychotic reactions, hyperpyrexia and cardiac arrhythmias produced by the analeptic agents.[12]

Although analeptic therapy continued in most countries, Scandinavian physicians showed that supportive therapy of the vital functions produced more favorable results than did vigorous attempts at arousal of these patients. Their recommendation for supportive therapy without the use of analeptics has become known as the "Scandinavian Method" and has been widely accepted. The widespread implementation of this technique has resulted in a decrease in the morbidity and mortality rate from 40% to 1%.[13]

Presently, the treatment procedures for the management of the barbiturate-intoxicated patient are (1) correction of life-threatening symptoms, (2) prevention of further absorption of the drug from the GI tract, (3) facilitation of removal of the absorbed drug, and (4) symptomatic and supportive care as indicated. A practical approach to the management of the barbiturate-intoxicated patient is illustrated in Figure 4–1.

Correction of Life-Threatening Symptoms

Since the major complications and deaths in acute barbiturate intoxications are due to respiratory and cardiovascular causes, maintenance of effective pulmonary gas exchange and circulating blood volume is the key to successful management of these patients.

If the patient is deeply unconscious, as in the present case, a cuffed endotracheal

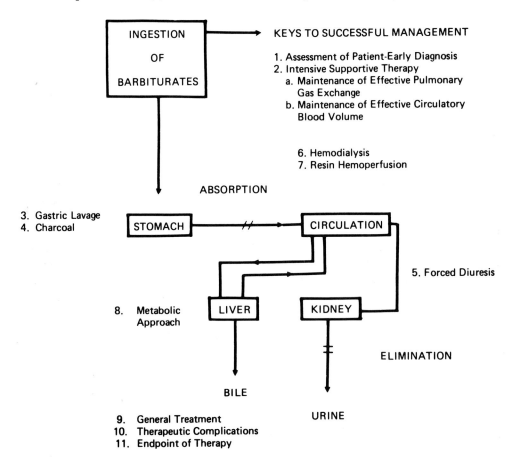

Fig. 4–1. Approach to the management of barbiturate overdosage.

tube should be inserted and room air administered. Higher concentrations of oxygen should be avoided when possible, since carbon dioxide provides a major stimulus for breathing. Overcorrection of hypoxia may be followed by prolonged apnea when the intermittent positive pressure breathing is discontinued. Therefore, the partial pressure of carbon dioxide should be kept as close to 40 mm Hg as possible. If assisted ventilation is required for longer than 48 to 72 hours, tracheostomy should be considered.

In the present case, after an adequate airway was secured, the next step was to determine whether ventilation was sufficient. This was accomplished by the measurement of arterial blood gases (pH, P_{CO_2}, P_{O_2}, HCO_3^-) at 45-minute intervals for the initial 6 hours and once a day for the next 4 days. (For laboratory results, see Table 4–1.) Hypoxic patients who are adequately ventilated may revert to a lesser grade of coma. This presumably occurs because hypoxia lowers the serum pH, thus favoring the presence of the nonionized form of the barbiturates. Since the nonionized form of the drug is the active component, lowering of the pH deepens the coma.

Hypotension, which also was present in this patient, is frequently associated with barbiturate overdosages. The mechanism of hypotension is a drug-induced dilation of the capacitance vessels (venous circulation), with a consequent pooling of blood and reduction in effective vascular volume. This hemodynamic defect accounts for the effective reduction in cardiac output and the consequent fall in blood pressure. Therefore, fluid replacement therapy, rather than the once-recommended vasopressor therapy, should be administered. The administration of a vasopressor agent can worsen the situation by further reducing effective vascular volume and by decreasing cardiac output.

If hypotension persists in the face of a normal central venous pressure (CVP),

dopamine, 2 to 4 μg/kg/min, appears to be the drug of choice, because it increases cardic output and preserves renal blood flow.[14] In the case presented, the elevation of the foot of the bed and the intravenous infusion of 1 L of 0.45% saline solution in 5% glucose solution (300 mg/hr) resulted in an increase in the patient's blood pressure from 110/55 to 120/70 mm Hg.

Prevention of Further Absorption

The techniques involved in the prevention of absorption of the barbiturate still remaining in the GI tract are (1) lavage or emesis, and (2) administration of activated charcoal and a saline cathartic.

Lavage and/or emesis. If the barbiturate has produced coma, the patient should be intubated with a cuffed endotracheal tube, and lavage should be performed. However, if the patient is alert, gastric evacuation can be performed by the use of an emetic. In those cases where more than 6 to 8 hours have elapsed prior to admission, and the patient is still in coma, gastric lavage usually produces negligible results. This phenomenon is due to the fact that the acidic environment favors the nonionized form of the barbiturates and hence absorption.[15] Therefore, the decision as to when emesis or lavage is indicated depends on (1) the accuracy of initial history, (2) the interval between when the patient is seen and the time that the drug was ingested, (3) the quantity of the drug ingested, and (4) overall clinical condition of the patient.

The use of emetics (syrup of ipecac) to remove unabsorbed barbiturate from the GI tract should be discouraged in lethargic patients. Syrup of ipecac has a lag time of 20 to 30 minutes before vomiting is initiated. During this time, the patient may become comatose, which would greatly increase the possibility of pulmonary aspiration if vomiting occurs.

Administration of apomorphine to induce emesis overcomes the problem of delayed onset encountered with syrup of ipecac. The onset of emesis with apomorphine occurs in 2 to 3 minutes and the effects can be terminated with any of the available narcotic antagonists such as naloxone (Narcan). However, the potentially serious side effects of apomorphine, such as CNS depression, cardiac arrhythmias, convulsions, and cardiovascular collapse, tend to overshadow the potential benefits it might have.[16] Therefore, apomorphine is not a rational alternative to syrup of ipecac.

In the case presented, the patient was intubated with a cuffed endotracheal tube, and a large-bore (28-French) nasogastric tube was inserted into the stomach. Lavage was performed with isotonic saline solution used as a lavage fluid. During lavage, the patient was placed in a modified Trendelenburg position on his left side, with the foot of the bed slightly elevated. The purpose of this technique was to avoid aspiration while the gastric contents were being emptied. Lavage of this patient resulted in the removal of capsule particles. The endpoint of lavage was the continuous appearance of 2 L of clear gastric aspirate.

Activated charcoal and cathartics. Mann and associates have shown that 1 g of activated charcoal is capable of binding 300 to 350 mg of barbiturate.[17] The dose that has been recommended is 1 g/kg mixed with enough water to produce a fine slurry with the consistency of thick soup.[17] However, since the amount ingested in many intoxications is not reliably known, a practical dose would be approximately 50 to 100 g. In addition, activated charcoal should not be administered concomitantly with syrup of ipecac, because its nonspecific adsorbent properties would inactivate the actions of syrup of ipecac.

The purpose of the administration of saline cathartics is to facilitate the intestinal transit of unabsorbed barbiturate, and thus to reduce the amount absorbed.

In the case presented, activated charcoal was administered after lavage, as a 25% w/v (25 g of charcoal powder in a total volume of 100 ml) tap water suspension. In addition, sodium sulfate (250 mg/kg of body weight) also was administered, to facilitate removal of the charcoal-barbiturate complex from the gastrointestinal tract.

Magnesium sulfate and magnesium citrate also can be used (250 mg/kg of body weight). However, in case of impending or manifest renal failure, magnesium-containing cathartics should be avoided because hypermagnesemia may develop and contribute to CNS depression, cardiac arrhythmias, and death.[18] Many patients require additional doses of a saline cathartic to achieve results. The endpoint of saline cathartic administration in this patient was the passage of a charcoal-laden stool.

Facilitation of the Removal of the Absorbed Barbiturate

Before the methods available to remove absorbed barbiturate from the body are discussed, a brief review of the pharmacologic and pharmacokinetic properties of these drugs is necessary, because they both suggest and impose limitations on the treatment of barbiturate intoxications.

All barbiturates are chemical derivatives of barbituric acid (Figure 4–2), and are classified as sedative-hypnotic drugs. The pharmacologic and pharmacokinetic char-

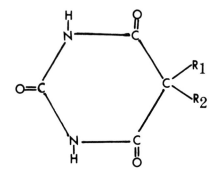

Fig. 4–2. Chemical structure for derivatives of barbituric acid.

Table 4–3. Barbiturates: Relation Between Physiochemical Factors,
Distribution, Fate, Duration of Action, and Toxicity.

OFFICIAL NAME	TRADE NAME	CLASSIFICATION	PARTITION COEFFICIENT*	PLASMA PROTEIN BINDING†	BRAIN PROTEIN BINDING‡	DELAY IN ONSET OF ACTIVITY	% EXCRETED UNCHANGED BY KIDNEYS§	DEGRADATION BY LIVER SLICES‖	pKa**	DURATION (HRS) OF ACTION IN THERAPEUTIC DOSES	SERUM LEVELS ASSOCIATED WITH TOXICITY (MG/DL)	SIGNIFICANT DIALYSIS OF DRUG***
Barbital	Veronal	Long-acting	1	0.05	0.06	22	65–90	—	7.8	12–24	8 or more	H (yes)
Phenobarbital	Luminal		3	0.20	0.19	12	27–50	—	7.3	12–24		P (yes)
Amobarbital	Amytal	Intermediate-acting	—	—	—	—	1	—	7.7	8–10		H (minimally effective)
Butabarbital	Butisol		—	—	—	—	2	—	7.7	8–10	5 or more	
Allobarbital	Diadol		—	—	—	—	—	—	—	8–10		P (no)
Secobarbital	Seconal	Short-acting	52	0.44	0.39	0.1	5	0.28	7.9	4–6	3 or more	H (no)
Pentobarbital	Nembutal		39	0.35	0.29	0.1	1	0.21	8.0	6–8		P (no)
Hexobarbital	Evipal	Ultra-short-acting	580	0.65	0.50	—	1	0.38	7.4	3–4	1.5 or more	H (no)
Thiopental	Pentothal									3–4		P (no)

* (Concentration in methylene chloride): (concentration in aqueous phase) of the nonionized form at approximately 25°C. Binding of 0.001 M barbituric acids by 1% bovine serum in M/15 phosphate buffer at pH 7.4; fraction bound.

† Minutes until anesthesia after intravenous injection in mice.

‡ Fraction of barbiturate bound by rabbit brain homogenates.

§ Approximate percentage of total dose excreted unchanged in urine of man.

‖ Fraction degraded in vitro by liver slices in 3 hours.

** Ionization exponent at 25°C.

*** H = Hemodialysis

   P = Peritoneal Dialysis

acteristics of each drug are largely determined by the chemical nature of the sidechains at the R_1 and R_2 positions (Figure 4–2). In general, those agents with long sidechains possess a short duration of action and high degrees of potency, lipid solubility, protein binding, and ionization (pKa). Furthermore, they are primarily inactivated by hepatic biotransformation (e.g., ultrashort- and short-acting barbiturates).

In contrast, those agents with shorter sidechains exhibit a longer duration of action and lower degrees of potency, lipid solubility, protein binding, and ionization. The primary route of elimination from the body is by the kidneys (e.g., long-acting barbiturates). The pharmacologic and pharmacokinetic properties of greatest importance to therapy for each class of barbiturates have been listed in Table 4–3.[19]

The three methods currently used to facilitate the removal of absorbed barbiturate from the body are (1) forced diuresis, (2) urinary alkalinization, (3) peritoneal dialysis, hemodialysis, and hemoperfusion.

Forced diuresis. Forced diuresis increases the excretion of barbiturate by increasing the volume and flow of urine in the renal tubules, thereby reducing the concentration of the barbiturate and the time it has to undergo passive reabsorption. Although the elimination of all barbiturates is increased during forced diuresis, the elimination of short-acting and intermediate-acting barbiturates is not increased sufficiently to justify this procedure in most cases.[21] The greatest effect is seen with long-acting barbiturate ingestions.[21] Mann and associates have reported that the half-life of phenobarbital can be reduced with forced diuresis by 61%, from a normal half-life of 96 hours to 37 hours.[17]

Before forced diuresis can be initiated, however, the adequacy of the patient's urinary flow and renal function must be established. Furthermore, constant monitoring of the patient and replacement of urinary losses of fluid and electrolytes, once treatment has been initiated, are essential. In case presented, furosemide (Lasix), in a dose of 1 mg/kg of body weight every 6 hours, and 5% dextrose in normal saline solution, infused at 350 to 400 ml/hr, were administered intravenously to enhance the urinary excretion of phenobarbital (initial levels of 11.8 mg/dl). The aim of forced diuresis was to produce a urine output of 300 to 400 ml/hr or 8 to 10 L/day.

Alkalinization of urine. As previously discussed, barbiturates are weak acids, whose pKa values (pH at which 50% of the drug is ionized and 50% is nonionized) range from 7.2 to 8.0 (see Table 4–3). The greater the value of pH as compared to pKa, the greater the extent of ionization. This is clinically important because the lipid membranes of the body permit rapid transit only to nonionized forms. Therefore, alkalinization of the urine, with the administration of such agents as sodium bicarbonate, sodium lactate, or acetazolamide (Diamox), would enhance the renal excretion of barbiturates, because in the presence of an alkaline urine, nonionized intratubular barbiturate would be converted to the ionized, relatively impermeable form.[22] As a result, the passive back-diffusion of barbiturate across the tubule would be reduced.[23]

The mild systemic alkalosis produced by the administration of alkalinizing agents also produces a favorable pH gradient between the blood and tissues. This promotes a shift of barbiturate out of the tissue and CNS into the systemic circulation, thus further enhancing excretion.[24]

Alkalinization of the urine is of little or no value in the treatment of short-acting and intermediate-acting barbiturates, since their principal means of elimination is by hepatic degradation.[19] In the treatment of toxicity due to long-acting barbiturates, alkalinization of the urine would increase their excretion 5- to 10-fold. For example, at pH 7.2, phenobarbital is 50% ionized, and at pH 8.0, it is 85% ionized. This is in contrast to secobarbital, which is 17% ionized at pH 7.2 and only 56% ionized at pH 8.0.[25]

In the case presented, sodium bicarbonate was administered in an initial intravenous dose of 44.3 mEq, followed by a constant infusion in D$_5$NS (5% dextrose in normal saline solution). The rate of infusion was determined by serial measurements of the urinary pH. The endpoint of therapy was the maintenance of a urinary pH of 8 or greater. During the first 24 hours of therapy with forced diuresis and alkalinization of the urine, the patient's serum phenobarbital and secobarbital levels decreased from 11.8 mg/dl and 2.8 mg/dl to 4.1 mg/dl and 1.1 mg/dl, respectively. In addition, the patient's overall condition reverted from a Grade 4 to a Grade 2 coma (see Table 4–2).

Peritoneal dialysis, hemodialysis, and hemoperfusion. An increased rate of barbiturate removal from the body is the objective when peritoneal dialysis, hemodialysis, or hemoperfusion is initiated. In general, intermediate-acting and long-acting barbiturates can be extracted in greater quantity than the short-acting barbiturates. This observation can be attributed to the fact that short-acting barbiturates exhibit a greater degree of binding to plasma proteins, are more lipid soluble, and have low plasma-to-tissue concentration ratios as compared to the intermediate-acting and long-acting barbiturates. As a result, the short-acting barbiturates are less dialyzable.[19,26]

Peritoneal dialysis is an effective way to facilitate the removal of long-acting barbiturates; it is somewhat effective with the intermediate-acting class, and its clinical value with short-acting barbiturates is questionable.[27] Overall, a standard PD will double the total elimination (renal and hepatic) of phenobarbital, and will produce a rate of drug removal that approximates the removal rate obtained during forced alkaline diuresis. However, the removal of short-acting drugs may be enhanced by no more than 35%.[28]

Based on the pharmacokinetic properties of the barbiturate agents, two clever maneuvers have been used to facilitate the peritoneal removal of barbiturates: (1) addition of albumin to the dialysate and (2) alkalinization of the dialysate solution. Berman and associates used a 5% albumin solution for dialysis and noted that the peritoneal concentrations of secobarbital, pentobarbital, and phenobarbital after 60 minutes of equilibrium were twice as high as the concentrations reached in protein-free dialysate.[29] Knochel and associates have also reported that when the dialysate is buffered with tris(hydroxymethyl) aminomethane (THAM) and the pH of peritoneal fluid is maintained at 8.2 or greater, the peritoneal removal rates of short-acting and long-acting barbiturates were remarkably increased.[30] However, THAM is no longer available in this country.

Schreiner and associates have reported that HD is nine times more effective than forced diuresis and regular PD for long-acting agents, and six times more effective for short-acting agents.[31] However, despite this fact, the mortality rate of patients undergoing dialysis for barbiturate intoxication has been reported to be between 12.5% and 35%.[32] This unexplained high mortality rate, therefore, precludes the use of HD for routine treatment of barbiturate intoxications, and only patients with Grade 4 coma not responding to standard therapeutic approaches should be considered.

Newer methods of HD are being developed that alter the mortality rate by reducing the time needed for dialysis. Yatsidis was the first to demonstrate activated charcoal hemoperfusion as a means of removing barbiturates in intoxicated patients.[32] In two cases of self-administered overdose, a mean reduction of 71% and 76% in plasma levels of phenobarbital and barbital, respectively, was achieved during the charcoal treatment. Rosenbaum and associates have also reported that by using RHP, they were able to treat patients acutely intoxicated with short-acting and long-acting barbiturates.[34] However, more research is necessary before this therapy can be recommended on a routine basis.

Currently, intensive supportive therapy is the recommended treatment of choice for patients acutely intoxicated with barbiturate agents. However, in some cases when (1) standard therapy is ineffective and the patient's condition is deteriorating, (2) renal and/or hepatic impairment precludes enhanced excretion of the barbiturate by conventional means, and (3) the serum barbiturate level is extremely high and the patient's condition is critical, any of the previously discussed dialytic procedures should be considered.

The choice of which dialytic procedure to use depends on (1) the dialyzability of the agent ingested (see Table 4–3), (2) age of the patient, and (3) availability of adequate facilities and trained personnel. Generally, HD is the most commonly used method in our institution for patients intoxicated with long-acting barbiturates and who are not responding to standard therapeutic regimens. None of these procedures were used in the case presented.

Symptomatic and Supportive Care

Subsequent to the initial intensive therapeutic interventions (e.g., securing of airway, provision of ventilation assistance, stabilization of blood pressure, initiation of gastric lavage, administration of activated charcoal and a cathartic, and forced diuresis), supportive measures constitute the cornerstone of therapy for the barbiturate-intoxicated patient. Supplemental measures such as alkalinization of urine should be reserved for those patients who have ingested long-acting barbiturates, and treatment with dialysis

(e.g., PD, HD, or hemoperfusion) should be implemented when routine measures are ineffective and the patient's condition is deteriorating.

The importance of good nursing care for these patients cannot be overemphasized. Patients should be placed on alternating-pressure-type mattresses and turned frequently to prevent tissue damage due to drying. Vital signs should be monitored frequently, and close observation of fluid intake and output is mandatory.

POSSIBLE COMPLICATIONS

The most commonly observed complications due to acute barbiturate intoxications are shock, pneumonia, renal shutdown, skin blisters, hypothermia, thrombophlebitis and pulmonary embolisms, and withdrawal symptoms.

Shock. The mechanism of shock is a disproportion between blood volume and capacity of the vascular bed. This hemodynamic defect accounts for the reduction in cardiac output and consequent fall in blood pressure.[35] Other factors attributable to the development of shock are severe impairment of respiration and the direct depressant effect of the barbiturates on the myocardium and the vasomotor center in the central nervous system.[35]

The use of vasopressor drugs should be avoided in the treatment of hypovolemic shock in these patients, because these agents would lead to an increased workload of the heart, arterial and venous constriction, a decrease in venous return of blood to the heart, and a consequent decrease in cardiac output. Hence, they potentiate hypovolemia, which is a major intrinsic mechanism in the initiation of the shock state.[36]

Treatment of shock is directed primarily towards restoration of the effective plasma volume. Large volumes of fluid should be administered, guided by central venous pressure measurements, to prevent fluid imbalances. The fluid challenge is beneficial, not only in reversing the hemodynamic defect, but in promoting diuresis and excretion of barbiturate. If a vasopressor is needed, dopamine is the drug of choice because in appropriate dosage it enhances cardiac output and preserves renal blood flow without increased peripheral resistance.[14]

Pneumonitis. Aspiration pneumonitis often complicates barbiturate intoxication and is a major cause of death.[37] It should be treated aggressively with early administration of parenteral steroids, intubation with assisted ventilation, meticulous and aseptic care of the airway, and bronchoscopy if necessary. Prophylactic antibiotics are unnecessary and can result in superinfection. If the patient becomes febrile, gram staining of the sputum should dictate the antibiotic of choice.

Renal shutdown. Acute tubular necrosis secondary to shock and hypoxia may result in renal shutdown. Therefore, forced diuresis should never be initiated until adequate urine flow and renal function have been established.

Skin blisters. Blisters of the skin occur in approximately 6% of acute barbiturate intoxications, because of capillary damage by the reduced blood flow and perhaps by a direct toxic action of the barbiturates.[38] Although they are not specific for barbiturate overdose, they can suggest the diagnosis of barbiturate poisoning in the unconscious patient. These blisters should be treated like second-degree burns.

Hypothermia. Severe hypothermia is frequently found in patients with acute barbiturate intoxication, and should be treated gradually with warming blankets. During the recovery phase, however, pyrexia will almost invariably occur. This fever does not necessarily mean the presence of an infection and should not be viewed with undue concern. Return to normality occurs spontaneously after a period of some hours or possibly days.

Thrombophebitis and pulmonary embolism. Deep-vein thrombosis and thromboembolism can occur in patients with prolonged coma, and can be a late cause of death. Elastic stockings, inflatable cuffs, and foot boards can be used. Low-dose heparinization should be considered in those patients likely to be comatose for several days.[32]

Withdrawal symptoms. Every patient recovering from acute barbiturate intoxication should be watched closely for withdrawal symptoms. These symptoms (e.g., excitement, sleeplessness, convulsions, delirium, and toxic psychosis) may occur during diminution of drug levels in addicted individuals. These withdrawal symptoms should be treated with phenobarbital (Luminal).[39] The initial dosage should be 30 mg of phenobarbital for each 100 mg of intermediate-acting and short-acting barbiturates previously used, divided into four 6-hour doses per day.

If, after administration of the initial phenobarbital dose, withdrawal symptoms continue, the dosage may be raised until the patient is comfortable. Once a stabilizing dosage has been obtained, gradual reduction in phenobarbital dosage over 3 to 4 weeks may then be instituted.[39] Seizures occurring in the withdrawal state may be treated with diazepam (Valium), 0.1 to 0.3 mg/kg/dose, to a maximum of 10 mg/dose IV, over 2 to 3 minutes.[39] In the case presented, no complications were encountered, and the patient was discharged 5 days postadmission.

DETERMINANTS OF SUCCESSFUL THERAPY

Excellent results in the treatment of even the most severe barbiturate overdose can be expected with the following simple techniques: (1) maintenance of the airway with the use of endotracheal or tracheostomy intubation, and mechanical assistance in order to provide adequate ventilation as measured by blood gases, (2) changes in vital signs, depth of coma, and fluid and electrolyte balance, (3) strict avoidance of CNS stimulants, (4) prevention of further absorption of the drug from the stomach by gastric lavage and administration of activated charcoal, (5) facilitation of drug removal from the body by forced diuresis and/or alkalinization of urine, (6) management of hypotension with a central venous pressure catheter, and electrolyte solution replacement to maintain the systolic blood pressure above 95 mm Hg, (7) prevention of respiratory infection with frequent turning and suctioning to remove secretions, and (8) attention to detail of eye care, skin blisters, maintenance of sterile indwelling catheter, and management of withdrawal symptoms.

PROGNOSIS

Prognosis in barbiturate intoxication is determined chiefly by the age of the patient, the dose, the nature of barbiturate swallowed, and the time interval between ingestion and discovery. Factors that may give rise to an unfavorable course are severe hypothermia, shock, aspiration pneumonitis, acute renal failure or pre-existing cardiovascular disorders. However, if the patient can be kept alive for the first 12 to 24 hours after ingestion, survival is likely. If coma persists over several days despite the fall in blood barbiturate level, lumbar puncture should be performed. Severe changes in the spinal fluid (increase in total protein) indicates serious, mostly irreversible central damage, and thus an unfavorable prognosis.

REFERENCES

1. Matthew H, and Lawson AAH (eds): *Treatment of Common Acute Poisonings.* 3rd Ed. Edinburgh, Churchill Livingstone, 1975, pp. 4–9.
2. Murphee HB: The continuing problem of barbiturate poisoning. *Am Fam Physician, 8*:108–109, 1973.
3. Richards R: A symptom of poisoning by hypnotics of the barbituric acid group. *Br Med J, 1*:331, 1934.
4. Conney AH: Pharmacological implications of microsomal enzyme induction. *Pharmacol Rev, 19*:317–366, 1967.
5. Schreiner GE: The role of hemodialysis (artificial kidney) in acute poisoning. *Arch Intern Med, 102*:896–913, 1958.
6. Reed CE, Driggs MF, and Goote CC: Acute barbiturate intoxication: A study of 300 cases based on a physiologic system of classification of the severity of the intoxication. *Ann Intern Med, 37*:303, 1952.
7. French JD, Verzeano M, and Magoun HW: A neural basis of the anesthetic state. *Arch Neurol Psychiatry, 69*:519–529, 1953.
8. Ngai SH: General anesthetics: Effects upon physiological systems. In *Physiological Pharmacology.* Vol. I, Chap. A2. Edited by WW Root and FG Hofmann. New York, Academic Press, 1963.
9. Price HL: General anesthesia and circulatory homeostasis. *Physiol Rev, 40*:189–218, 1960.
10. Marck LC: *Acute Barbiturate Poisoning.* Edited by H Matthew. Amsterdam, Excerpta Medica, 1971, pp. 85–92.
11. Harstad E, Meiler KO, and Simeson MH: Uber din Wert Der Magens pulung bei der Behandlung con Akuten Vergiftungen. *Acta Med Scand, 112*:478–514, 1942.
12. Clemmesen C: The treatment of poisoning during the past twenty-five years: A retrospective review. *Dan Med Bull, 6*:209–213, 1959.
13. Matthew H, and Lawson AH: Acute barbiturate poisoning: A review of two years experience. *Q J Med, 35*:539–552, 1966.
14. Golberg LI and Useih YY: Clinical use of dopamine. *Ration Drug Ther, 11*:1, 1977.
15. Shapiro FL, and Smith HT: The treatment of barbiturate intoxication. *Mod Med, 37*:104–110, 1969.
16. Okum R: Therapy of barbiturate overdose. *Geriatrics, 26*:113–118, 1971.
17. Mann JB, and Sandberg DH: Therapy of sedative overdosage. *Pediatr Clin North Am, 17*:617–628, 1970.
18. Alfrey AC, et al: Hypermagnesemia after renal homotransplantation. *Ann Intern Med, 73*:367–371, 1970.
19. Sharpless SK: Hypnotics and sedatives: The barbiturates. In *The Pharmacological Basis of Therapeutics.* 4th Ed. Edited by LS Goodman and A Gilman. New York, Macmillan, 1970, pp. 98–120.
20. Linton AL, Luke RG, and Briggs JD: Methods of forced diuresis and its application in barbiturate poisoning. *Lancet, 2*:377–379, 1967.
21. Bunn HF, and Lubash GD: A controlled study of induced diuresis in barbiturate intoxication. *Ann Intern Med, 62*:246–251, 1965.
22. Waddell WJ, and Butler TC: The distribution and excretion of phenobarbital. *J Clin Invest, 36*:1217–1226, 1957.
23. Giotti A, and Maynert EW: Renal clearance of barbital and the mechanism of its reabsorption. *J Pharmacol Exp Ther, 101*:296–309, 1951.
24. Golberg MA, Barlow CE, and Roth LJ: The effects of carbon dioxide on the entry and accumulation

of drugs in the central nervous system. *J Pharmacol Exp Ther, 131*:308–318, 1961.

25. Robinson RR, Gunnells JC, and Clapp JR: Treatment of acute barbiturate intoxication. *Mod Treatment, 8*:561–579, 1971.

26. Setter JG, Maher JF, and Schreiner GE: Barbiturate intoxication: Evaluation of therapy including dialysis in a large series selectively referred because of severity. *Arch Intern Med, 117*:224–236, 1966.

27. Mattocks AM, and El-Bassiouni, EA: Peritoneal dialysis: A review: *J Pharm Sci, 60*:1767–1782, 1971.

28. Henderson LW, and Merrill JP: Treatment of barbiturate intoxication. *Ann Intern Med, 64*:876–891, 1966.

29. Berman LB, and Vogelsang P: Removal rates of barbiturates using two types of peritoneal dialysis. *N Engl J Med, 270*:77–80, 1964.

30. Knochel JP, et al: Intraperitoneal Tham: An effective method to enhance phenobarbital removal during peritoneal dialysis. *J Lab Clin Med, 64*:257–268, 1964.

31. Schreiner GE, and Teehan BP: Dialysis of poisons and drugs: Annual review. *Am Soc Artif Intern Organs, 18*:563–599, 1972.

32. Hadden J, et al: Acute barbiturate intoxication: Concepts of management. *JAMA, 209*:893–900, 1969.

33. Yatsidis H, et al: Treatment of severe barbiturate poisoning. *Lancet, 2*:216–217, 1965.

34. Rosenbaum JL, Kramer MS, and Raja R: Resin hemoperfusion for acute drug intoxication. *Arch Intern Med, 136*:263–266, 1976.

35. Shubin H, and Weil MH: The mechanism of shock following suicidal doses of barbiturates, narcotics and tranquilizer drugs with observations of the effects of treatment. *Am J Med, 38*:853–863, 1965.

36. Weil MH, and Shubin H: The "VIP" approach to the bedside management of shock. *JAMA, 207*:337–340, 1969.

37. Goodman JM, et al: Barbiturate intoxication: Morbidity and mortality. *West J Med, 124*:179–186, 1976.

38. Beveridge GW, and Lawson HB: Occurrence of bullous lesions in acute barbiturate intoxication. *Br Med J, 1*:835–837, 1965.

39. Rumack BH (ed): Barbiturate management. In *Poisindex*. Denver, Colorado, Micromedex, Inc., May, 1978.

Chapter 5

Nonbarbiturates

Vasilios A. Skoutakis
Sergio R. Acchiardo

There is a constant endeavor on the part of the pharmaceutical, scientific, and medical communities to produce new nonbarbiturate sedative-hypnotic drugs as satisfactory alternatives to barbiturates. However, like the barbiturates, the nonbarbiturates have disadvantages and side effects; they are popular in self-intoxication or poisoning and are frequently chosen by those abusing or taking drugs for "kicks." National statistics from the Drug Abuse Warning Network (DAWN) indicate that during the months of July, August, and September of 1976, 2496 drug-related deaths (cited by medical examiners), and 46,321 drug-related injuries (cited by emergency departments) were reported in 24 of the largest metropolitan areas in the United States. During this period, 4.5% of the deaths and 8.5% of the injuries were due to nonbarbiturate sedative-hypnotic drugs.[1] Additional published reports also attest to the problem of abuse and/or overdosages with these drugs.[2-11]

Because of the widespread use, abuse, and frequently occurring drug overdosages and deaths, clinicians should become familiar with the potential toxic and lethal consequences as well as the management of patients who have been intoxicated with nonbarbiturate sedative-hypnotic drugs. This chapter therefore will discuss the clinical manifestations and mechanisms of nonbarbiturate-induced toxicities and the therapeutic interventions necessary for the successful management of patients acutely intoxicated with nonbarbiturate drugs.

77

CASE REPORT

A 24-year-old female had made several previous suicide attempts with drug ingestions. At this time, following another suicide attempt, she was brought to the emergency room in a coma resulting from an ingestion of 15 g of glutethimide (Doriden), which occurred approximately 3½ hours prior to admission. Upon initial examination, vital signs were blood pressure, 140/65 mm Hg; pulse, 82 beats/min; respirations, 11 to 13/min, shallow, and spontaneous; and temperature, 36.8°C. The pupils were widely dilated and reacted sluggishly to light. Corneal, doll's eye, and tendon reflexes were not elicited, and there was no response to deep pain. No abnormal reflexes were noted, and bowel sounds were absent. Results of an x-ray examination of the chest were negative, and other routine laboratory test results, such as serum electrolyte determination, urinalysis, hematologic indices, and EKG, were within normal limits.

Blood gases on admission were Po_2, 57 mm Hg; Pco_2, 48 mm Hg; serum pH, 7.4; and serum bicarbonate (HCO_3^-), 16 mEq/L. Results of analyses of serum and urine samples were negative for all drugs, with the exception of glutethimide. The serum glutethimide level was reported to be 4.2 mg/dl. Because the patient had a diminishing respiratory effort and was progressing to apnea, assisted ventilation with an Ohio respirator was instituted 6 hours postadmission. Arterial blood gas values 2 hours later were Po_2, 96 mm Hg; Pco_2, 40 mm Hg; and serum pH, 7.41.

Thereafter, arterial blood gases, blood pressure, central venous pressure and urine output were monitored and maintained adequately. Gastric lavage was performed, and activated charcoal and a saline cathartic were administered. No forced diuresis or hemodialysis was performed, although the glutethimide serum level was increased to 5.2 mg/dl, approximately 9 hours postadmission. Supportive and symptomatic care constituted the cornerstone of therapy. At 22 hours postadmission, deep tendon reflexes had returned. At 26 hours postadmission, shallow spontaneous respirations and deep pain responses were evident. Thereafter, although some fluctuations in the clinical condition were noted, the patient could respond to verbal stimuli 36 hours postadmission. The patient regained consciousness about 48 hours after drug ingestion, and further recovery was uneventful. The patient was discharged from the hospital 5 days postadmission.

CLINICAL ASSESSMENT AND MANAGEMENT OF THE PATIENT

In order for the clinician to successfully assess and treat patients who have been intoxicated with sedative-hypnotic drugs of the nonbarbiturate type, the following should be considered: (1) identification of drugs classified as nonbarbiturates, (2) manifestations and mechanisms of nonbarbiturate-induced toxicities, (3) the role and significance of the toxicology laboratory results, (4) indicated therapeutic measures, (5) general prognosis.

DRUGS CLASSIFIED AS NONBARBITURATES

Hypnotics, sedatives, depressants, tranquilizers, relaxants, psychotropics, soporifics, and nonbarbiturates are only a few of the terms commonly used to characterize a large, heterogeneous group of compounds that possess CNS-depressant properties. These terms have so often been applied interchangeably that many clinicians consider them synonymous. However, since in acute intoxications, all these compounds, with otherwise diverse chemical structures and pharmacologic properties, have in common the ability, like barbiturate drugs, to produce a depression of the CNS, the term nonbar-

Table 5–1. Chemical Classes, Representative Examples, Trade Names, Sedative-Hypnotic Doses, and Half-Lives of Commonly Ingested Nonbarbiturates.

Chemical Class	Representative Examples	Trade Names	Adult Oral Dose — Sedative	Adult Oral Dose — Hypnotic	Half-Life (hrs)
Benzodiazepines	Chlordiazepoxide, U.S.P.	Libritabs	5–10 mg, 2–3× daily	25 mg	6–28
	Chlordiazepoxide hydrochloride, U.S.P.	Librium, A-Poxide, SK-Lygen	5–20 mg, 3–4× daily	25 mg	6–28
	Clorazepate dipotassium	Tranxene	5–10 mg, 2–3× daily	15–20 mg	—
	Clorazepate monopotassium	Azene		20–25 mg	—
	Diazepam	Valium	10–15 mg, 3–4× daily	10 mg	20–70
	Flurazepam	Dalmane	2–10 mg, 2–4× daily	15–30 mg	51–100
	Lorazepam	Ativan	0.5–1 mg, 2–3× daily	2–4 mg	10–15
	Oxazepam	Serax	10–15 mg, 3–4× daily	10–30 mg	4–13
	Prazepam	Verstran	10–20 mg, 2–3× daily	10–20 mg	24–500
Carbonic acid esters of alcohols	Ethinamate	Valmid		500–1000 mg	2–3
Carbamic acid esters of glycols	Meprobamate	Equanil, Miltown	400 mg, 3–4× daily	800 mg	10–11
Tertiary acetylenic alcohols	Ethchlorvynol	Placidyl	100–200 mg, 2–3× daily	500–1000 mg	5–25
Chloral derivatives	Chloral hydrate	Noctec, Felsules	250 mg, 3× daily	500–2000 mg	4–9.5
	Chloral betaine	Beta-Chlor			
	Triclofos	Triclos		870–1000 mg	4–9.5
Cyclic ether	Paraldehyde	Paraldehyde	5–10 ml	10–30 ml	0.5–1
Inorganic salts	Bromides		500–1000 mg, 3–4× daily	3000–4000 mg	288
Piperidione derivatives	Methyprylon	Noludar	50–100 mg, 3–4× daily	200–400 mg	3–6
	Glutethimide	Doriden	125–250 mg, 1–3× daily	250–500 mg	5–22
2,3-Disubstituted quinazolines	Methaqualone	Quaalude, Sopor, Parest	100 mg, 4× daily	200–400 mg	0.5–16

biturates is more advisable and the one that will be used in this chapter. Table 5–1 summarizes the chemical classes, generic and trade names, and therapeutic dosages and half-lives of the most commonly used, abused, or ingested nonbarbiturate drugs.

MANIFESTATIONS AND MECHANISMS OF NONBARBITURATE-INDUCED TOXICITIES

Taken as prescribed by a clinician, the nonbarbiturate agents may be beneficial for the symptomatic relief of anxiety, irritability, tension, and the symptomatic treatment of insomnia. When prescribed in such low doses, most of these agents produce a state of drowsiness and are referred to as *sedatives.* In higher doses, they produce a state of CNS depression that resembles normal sleep and are referred to as *hypnotics.* When taken chronically and in excessive amounts or when abused, the nonbarbiturates not only have a high potential for the development of tolerance and physical and psychological dependence,[12,13] but can also depress a wide range of physiologic and cellular functions in many vital organ systems, resulting in many undesirable effects. These progressive dose-related effects can be summarized as follows:

biogenic monoamines). Therefore, during a poisoning or an acute overdosage, there is a progressive CNS depression characterized by drowsiness, which is followed by ataxia, nystagmus, vertigo, slurred speech, headache, paresthesia, and subjective visual disturbances. A brief period of confusion, excitement, delirium, and hallucinations may also occur.

As more of the drug is absorbed and distributed throughout body tissues, in addition to the depression of RAS, the cerebral cortex, limbic system, and hypothalamus are also depressed. As a result, the depth of coma increases, the hypothalamic thermoregulatory and medullary vasomotor centers do not function properly, and the peripheral autonomic ganglionic transmission is impaired. Therefore, the intoxicated patient will exhibit severe respiratory depression, a shock syndrome, progressive inhibition of superficial and deep tendon reflexes, and no response to painful stimuli. The Babinski sign may become positive, the skin and mucous membranes will be cyanotic, pupils may be somewhat constricted and may or may not respond to light, GI motility may be decreased, and body temperature may be reduced. Urinary volume may also be decreased as a result of hemodynamic changes and an

$$\text{Sedation} \rightleftharpoons \text{Hypnosis} \rightleftharpoons \text{Anesthesia} \rightleftharpoons \text{Coma} \rightarrow \text{Death}$$

The CNS is particularly sensitive to nonbarbiturate agents. It is believed that the nonbarbiturate agents, like the barbiturates, block multineuronal conduction at the ascending reticular activating system (RAS) of the brain stem.[14] This system is thought to maintain a background of wakefulness under normal conditions. It is believed that inhibition of central synaptic transmission results from interference with the release of one or more of the central neurotransmitters (e.g., acetylcholine, gamma-aminobutyric acid, or

increased secretion of the antidiuretic hormone from the posterior pituitary. If death occurs, it is usually the result of either respiratory failure, cardiovascular collapse, kidney failure, or a combination of any of these.[2–11]

The majority of the toxicologic manifestations presented and discussed in this section were also manifested in the patient described in the case report (e.g., coma, decreased respirations, hypotension, hypothermia, widely dilated pupils, decreased bowel sounds, absence of deep tendon reflexes, and nonresponsiveness to painful stimuli).

ROLE AND SIGNIFICANCE OF THE TOXICOLOGY LABORATORY RESULTS

The patient intoxicated with CNS-depressant drugs usually has respiratory and cardiovascular depression. The non-barbiturate sedative-hypnotic drugs produce no distinguishing clinical symptoms. Therefore, definite diagnosis of a patient acutely intoxicated with CNS depressants is often difficult. Furthermore, as with any disease state or overdosage with other CNS-depressant drugs, the reaction of intoxicated patients to a nonbarbiturate drug depends upon a number of variables, including (1) the type and quantity of drug used, (2) time elapsed since ingestion, (3) underlying medical or psychological problems, (4) the degree of tolerance, if any, which the patient has developed toward that drug, (5) the ingestion of multiple drugs, and (6) the history obtained from the intoxicated patient, which sometimes may be helpful, other times unreliable or misleading, and most of the time unobtainable because of the CNS-depressant effects of the nonbarbiturate drugs.

Table 5–2. Toxic Doses and Blood Levels of Commonly Ingested Nonbarbiturates in Adults.*

DRUG	TOXIC DOSE	TOXIC LEVELS
Benzodiazepines	0.5–1.5 g	5–30 μg/ml
Ethinamate	5–10 g	10–20 μg/ml
Meprobamate	5–8 g	50–100 μg/ml
Etchlorvynol	4–6 g	20 μg/ml
Chloral hydrate	4–10 g	100 μg/ml
Paraldehyde	60–90 ml†	500 μg/ml
Bromides	15–20 g	50 μg/ml
Methyprylon	3–6 g	30–60 μg/ml
Glutethimide	5–8 g	10–80 μg/ml
Methaqualone	3–7.5 g	20–80 μg/ml

* For specific clinical signs and symptoms and therapeutic interventions, consult discussion section in text.
† Equivalent to 59.6–89.5 g paraldehyde.

In the overall assessment of the patient, therefore, the etiologic diagnosis is often impossible to establish without laboratory analysis of a drug sample or body fluids. As with the barbiturates, however, it must be remembered that all nonbarbiturate drugs are capable of producing tolerance and physical and psychological dependence.[12,13] Therefore, patients on long-term nonbarbiturate therapy or those abusing these drugs may have high blood nonbarbiturate levels and yet show no toxic signs and symptoms. Table 5–2 summarizes the toxic doses and toxic blood levels of the commonly ingested nonbarbiturate drugs, to assist the clinician in assessing the etiologic diagnosis and severity of the nonbarbiturate intoxication.

INDICATED THERAPEUTIC MEASURES

Treatment of the patient acutely intoxicated with nonbarbiturate drugs is primarily directed toward maintenance of normal body homeostasis while the drug is being metabolized. In a few instances, acceleration of normal excretory pathways may be induced by the implementation of special measures. Therefore, treatment can be conveniently divided into three areas: (1) emergency supportive measures and symptomatic treatment, (2) nonspecific therapy, and (3) specific therapeutic interventions based on the pharmacologic, pharmacokinetic, and toxicologic properties of the nonbarbiturate drug.

General Supportive Measures and Symptomatic Treatment

The implementation of the basic physiologic principles of management of toxic emergencies presented and discussed in Chapter 1 are still valid and applicable in the treatment of the nonbarbiturate-intoxicated patient. These general emergency supportive measures and symptomatic treatment include (a) assessment of the patient's clinical condition, adequacy of ventilation, and maintenance of the airway, (b) maintenance of adequate cardiovascular stability, (c) avoidance of the administration of analeptics (CNS stimulants) and avoidance of the prophylactic use of antibiotics, (d) frequent and careful monitoring of vital signs, depth of coma, and prevention of sequelae of shock and hypoxia, fluid and electrolyte abnormalities, and pulmonary, renal, and cardiovascular complications; (e) attention to detail of eye care and skin blisters if present, frequent positional changes and suctioning of oropharyngeal secretions, and maintenance of sterile indwelling and intravenous catheters.

Nonspecific Therapy

Prevention of further absorption of the ingested nonbarbiturate drug is the clinician's major goal when implementing nonspecific therapeutic procedures. Therefore, all patients who have ingested nonbarbiturate drugs should receive syrup of ipecac (10 ml orally for children under 1 year old, 15 ml orally for children 1 to 5 years old, and 15 to 30 ml for children over 5 years old; 30 ml orally for adults), with copious amounts of fluid to evacuate the stomach. Because of its CNS- and respiratory-depressant effects, the administration of apomorphine in place of syrup of ipecac is not recommended. If contraindications to emesis are present (e.g., coma, seizures, or absence of the gag reflex), gastric lavage with the largest tolerable tube should be performed. Following gastric evacuation, activated charcoal (30 to 50 g) and a saline cathartic (250 mg/kg) should be administered to these patients, since neither emesis or gastric lavage empties the stomach completely. Activated charcoal adsorbs the ingested nonbarbiturate present within the GI tract and prevents its absorption into the blood. The saline cathartic promotes intestinal evacuation of the nonbarbiturate-charcoal complex, further decreasing the potential toxic effects of the ingested nonbarbiturate drug.

Specific Therapeutic Interventions

Further treatment of nonbarbiturate intoxication involves specific therapeutic interventions based on the pharmacologic, pharmacokinetic, and toxicologic properties of the ingested nonbarbiturate drug.

Benzodiazepine derivatives. This group of drugs includes chlordiazepoxide, chlorazepam, diazepam, flurazepam, lorazepam, nitrazepam, oxazepam, prazepam, clorazepate dipotassium and chlorazepate monopotassium (see Fig. 5–1 and Table 5–3). Acute overdosage with these particular nonbarbiturates is common, but fortunately they do not produce severe toxic symptoms even when ingested in high doses. Ingestions of 500 to 1500 mg, for example, have been reported with only minor toxicity.[2] Furthermore, no fatalities have yet been documented as solely due to one of these agents, although poorly documented deaths related to diazepam,[2,15] and one case of cardiac arrest caused by oral diazepam intoxication in a child, have been reported.[16]

The intravenous use of these agents, however, has been reported to result in

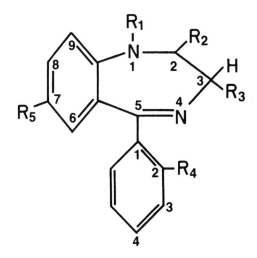

Fig. 5–1. Structure of 1,4-benzodiazepine. See Table 5–3 for substitution salts.

Table 5–3. Substitution Salts for Commonly Used 1,4-Benzodiazepines.

DRUG	TRADE NAME	R_1	R_2	R_3	R_4	R_5
Chlordiazepoxide hydrochloride	Librium	—H	$-N{<}^{H}_{CH_3}$	—H	—H	—Cl
Chlordiazepoxide	Libritabs					
Chlorazepate dipotassium	Tranxene Tranxene-SD	—H	$=O \leftrightarrow {<}^{OH}_{OK}$	—COOK	—H	—Cl
Diazepam	Valium	—CH$_3$	=O	—H	—H	—Cl
Flurazepam	Dalmane	$-CH_2-CH_2-N{<}^{C_2H_5}_{C_2H_5}$	=O	—H	—H	—Cl
Lorazepam	Ativan	—H	=O	—OH	—Cl	—Cl
Oxazepam	Serax	—H	=O	—OH	—H	—Cl
Prazepam	Verstran	—CH$_2$◁	=O	—H	—H	—Cl

respiratory depression and death.[2,15–18] Benzodiazepine overdosage usually produces no other symptoms besides sleepiness and Grade 0 to Grade 1 coma, even following large overdosages. During the initial phase of the intoxication, minor extrapyramidal signs with some excitement may be present, as well as symptoms such as dry mouth, tachycardia, dilated pupils, and absent bowel sounds (anticholinergic effects). Coma unresponsive to stimulation such as sternal pressure is quite uncommon. Deep coma, marked hypotension, or severe respiratory or cardiovascular depression in an intoxicated patient indicate that perhaps other CNS-depressant drugs have been ingested as well.[2,15,19]

In therapeutic doses, all benzodiazepines are rapidly and almost completely absorbed after oral administration. Maximum absorption occurs within 30 to 180 minutes, the duration of the process varying in different studies and with different compounds.[20] Furthermore, at physiologic pH, all benzodiazepines are highly lipid soluble and are readily distributed in body tissues. These drugs are metabolized in the liver, and the metabolites are then excreted in the urine.[20,21]

Regarding the metabolism and elimination half-lives, two kinetic properties define the clinical profile of the various benzodiazepines: (1) the formation of pharmacologically active metabolites and (2) the length of elimination half-lives of the adminstered drug and its active metabolite(s). Table 5–4 summarizes the peak times and peak plasma levels, volume of distribution, binding, principal active metabolites, elimination half-lives, and maximum therapeutic levels of the commonly used benzodiazepines.[20] There are no data available for the pharmacokinetic parameters of these agents during intoxication, but it is expected that those parameters will be prolonged and/or increased in such cases.

Presently, there is no specific treatment regarding the management of patients acutely intoxicated with any of the benzodiazepine agents, and successful recovery usually results form the implementation of only emergency supportive measures and symptomatic treatment. Respiratory depression, if it occurs, should be treated with assisted ventilation. Forced diuresis and hemodialysis are ineffective and therefore not recommended.[2,19,22]

Hypotension, if present, should be treated initially with fluids, and vasopressor agents should be used only in unresponsive cases. In addition, although the

Table 5-4. Pharmacokinetic Parameters of Commonly Used 1,4-Benzodiazepines.

DRUG	ORAL DOSE (mg)	PEAK TIME (hrs)	PEAK LEVEL (ng/ml)	VOLUME DISTRIBUTION (V_d [L/kg])	BINDING (%)	ELIMINATION HALF-LIVES ($t\frac{1}{2}$, in hrs)	PRINCIPAL ACTIVE METABOLITE(S)
Chlordiazepoxide	25	0.5–4.0	370–2050	0.26–0.58	94–97	6–28[s]	Norchlordiazepoxide Demoxepam Nordiazepam Oxazepam
Diazepam	10	1.5–2.0	177–400	0.95–2.0	96.8–98.6	20–70[m]	Nordiazepam Oxazepam Temazepam
Flurazepam	90	1.0	40–80	3.4	NA	51–100[ml]	N-Desalkylflurazepam 3-hydroxy-N-desalkylflurazepam
Lorazepam	2	1.0–2.0	17	0.70–1.0	85	12.6[s,m]	Unknown
Oxazepam	15	1.4	119–190	0.6	87–90	4–13[s]	Unknown

[s]   After single oral dose
[m]   After multiple oral dose
[ml]   Data refer to N-desalkylflurazepam
NA not available in humans.

successful use of physostigmine salicylate and naloxone hydrochloride as antidotes in accidental diazepam overdosages has been reported,[23,24] the routine use of these two agents in the treatment of benzodiazepine overdosages is not recommended, because the potential risks associated with their administration outweigh the benefits.

Addiction resulting from the extensive use or abuse of the benzodiazepines has been reported.[12,13] It is possible, therefore, that acute overdosage with any of the benzodiazepine agents or any of the other nonbarbiturate drugs can be superimposed on a state of chronic addiction to the same or other sedative-hypnotic agents. In such cases, the patient may be successfully treated for the acute intoxication, only to enter a withdrawal syndrome. With diazepam, withdrawal will usually occur if the daily ingested dose has reached 80 to 120 mg and if abuse has occurred for 40 to 50 days,[25] whereas with chlordiazepoxide, withdrawal symptoms will be present if the daily ingested dose has reached 300 to 600 mg and if abuse has occurred for 2 to 6 months.[26]

For the newer benzodiazepines, although the necessary dosage and duration of abuse have not been established with certainty, withdrawal symptoms should be expected and the clinician should follow such patients closely. The withdrawal symptoms reported to have occurred with the benzodiazepines include apprehension, anorexia, nausea, vomiting, tremulousness, insomnia, confusion, seizures, and hallucinations.[2,12,13,15,19,25,26]

Treatment of the withdrawal syndrome must be carried out in the hospital and requires barbiturate substitution (e.g., 30 mg of phenobarbital is equivalent to 5 mg of diazepam or 25 mg of chlordiazepoxide) or the administration of one of the benzodiazepines. If phenobarbital is to be used, one fourth of the calculated dose should be administered and increased as necessary to relieve abstinence symptoms.

Thereafter, a gradual tapering off of phenobarbital can be instituted as soon as the patient has become stable for at least 48 hours. If one of the benzodiazepine drugs is to be administered, a sufficient dose should be given initially, based on the patient's prior history of daily dosage and duration of abuse of the specific agent, in order to control or relieve the abstinence symptoms. The dosage then should be decreased by 10% per day for the next 10 to 14 days.[27–29]

Ethinamate. Ethinamate is part of a group of compounds that are carbamic acid esters of alcohol. Patients intoxicated with ethinamate have symptoms similar to those of barbiturate overdosage, which may include hypotension, respiratory depression, and coma.[3,30,31] In contrast to most other nonbarbiturate and barbiturate agents, the CNS depression produced by ethinamate overdosage is often of short duration. Death may result from respiratory failure and/or cardiovascular collapse. Ingestion of 15 g of ethinamate has caused death, although some patients have survived the ingestion of as much as 28 g of the drug.[3,30]

In therapeutic doses, ethinamate is readily absorbed from the gastrointestinal tract and distributed in body fat, liver, and brain tissue. The half-life is reported to be 2¼ hours, and ethinamate is almost completely cleared from the plasma within 10 to 15 hours. It is extensively metabolized in humans, as reflected in its short duration of action. Only a small amount is excreted in the urine.[32,33] There are no data available regarding the pharmacokinetic parameters of ethinamate during acute intoxication, but it is expected that the above-reported values are prolonged and/or increased in such cases.

Treatment of patients acutely intoxicated with ethinamate consists of general supportive measures, prevention of further absorption of the drug, and continuous symptomatic care. Enhancement of the excretion of ethinamate by forced diuresis in severely intoxicated patients is not recommneded because of the pharmacokinetic parameters of the drug. Hemodialysis has been shown to be somewhat effective in the removal of ethinamate from the body, and may be considered in those patients unresponsive to standard therapeutic measures.[3,31]

Prolonged use of high doses of ethinamate may lead to tolerance and physical and psychological dependence. Withdrawal of ethinamate has been followed by agitation, syncopal episodes, tremulousness, hyperactive reflexes, convulsions, disorientation, delusions, and hallucinations.[34]

Treatment of physical dependence upon ethinamate consists of cautious and gradual withdrawal of the drug. The patient should be hospitalized, and the daily dose of ethinamate should be reduced by 500 mg to 1 g every 2 to 3 days until administration of the drug has been discontinued. Alternatively, phenobarbital can be used, with an initial dose of 100 mg administered every 6 hours and increased as necessary until the symptoms subside. Thereafter, once the patient's condition has been stabilized for at least 48 hours, the dosage of phenobarbital should be gradually reduced over a period of 10 to 14 days.[27-29]

Meprobamate. Meprobamate is included in a group of compounds that are the carbamic acid esters of glycols. Overdosage with meprobamate can result in drowsiness, lethargy, stupor, coma, convulsions, hypotension, shock, and circulatory and respiratory collapse.[4,35-41] Death may result from respiratory failure or hypotension.[4,36-38,40,41] It is difficult to describe the amount of meprobamate necessary for toxicity, since there is variability among patients with regard to the metabolism (e.g., slow or fast acetylation), and hence detoxication of the drug. Ingestion of 12 g of meprobamate has resulted in death,[37] although some patients have survived the ingestion of up to 40 g.[4,39,42]

Usually, blood concentrations of 100 to 200 μg/ml are associated with deep coma, requiring intensive treatment. Concentrations above 200 μg/ml are often fatal. Deaths have also been reported to occur, however, at lower concentrations.[38,40,43]

In therapeutic doses, meprobamate is readily absorbed from the GI tract, and peak concentrations in the plasma occur after 1 to 2 hours. The plasma half-life of meprobamate averages about 10 to 11 hours.[44] Meprobamate is widely distributed throughout the body. It diffuses across the placenta and appears in the milk of nursing mothers at concentrations of up to four times those in the maternal plasma. About 90% or more of a dose is excreted in the urine, mainly as a hydroxylated metabolite and its glucuronide conjugate. The remaining portion of the drug is excreted unchanged in the urine.[44,45] There are no data available regarding the pharmacokinetic properties of meprobamate in acute overdosages, but it is expected that the above values are prolonged and/or increased in such cases.

The treatment of meprobamate-intoxicated patients consists of decreased absorption of the drug, promotion of excretion, and symptomatic care as indicated. When gastric lavage is indicated, it must be thorough, since death has resulted after initial recovery and has been attributed to incomplete gastric emptying and delayed absorption of meprobamate.[40-41] The combination of the physiochemical properties of meprobamate (low solubility in water and stability in gastric or intestinal juices), the decreased motility of the gut, and the hypotension commonly present in these patients, allows delayed absorption and the formation of drug-containing mass concentrations.

Jenis and associates have reported a case in which 25 g of meprobamate was found in the stomach of a patient at autopsy.[40] Schwartz reported a case in which gastrotomy of a meprobamate-intoxicated patient resulted in the recovery of 24 g of meprobamate, even after gastric lavage with 10 L of normal saline solution was performed.[41] If the patient is not comatose or convulsing, or if the gag reflex is present, emesis should be initiated. In addition, following lavage and/or emesis, activated charcoal should be administered to adsorb any remaining drug, and a saline cathartic should be administered to facilitate the removal of the drug-charcoal complex.

If the patient is severely poisoned and is in Grade 3 or Grade 4 coma, forced alkaline diuresis may be indicated to promote or enhance the excretion of meprobamate.[38,46,47] A solution of 5% dextrose in water with ½-normal saline solution and a diuretic such as furosemide (1 mg/kg of body weight) in a single dose should be administered to obtain a urine flow of 3 to 6 ml/kg/hr. After good urinary flow is obtained, a solution of 5% dextrose, with sodium bicarbonate added to produce 0.2% to 0.45% isotonicity, and 40 mEq of potassium chloride per liter of solution should be administered to the patient to produce alkalinization. The goal should be a urinary pH greater than 7.0, and pH should be monitored hourly.

Hemodialysis or charcoal hemoperfusion have been reported effective in the removal of meprobamate from the body, whereas peritoneal dialysis is apparently not as effective.[48,49] However, HD or CHP should be considered only in patients unresponsive to forced alkaline diuresis or who have pulmonary edema or severe acid-base problems.

Hypotension due to meprobamate overdosage is seen commonly and is thought to be the result either of a direct effect of the drug on the arterial musculature or an indirect consequence of generalized skeletal muscle relaxation, with reduction in muscular tone. As a result, administration of fluids or plasma expanders to correct the hypotension may lead to severe pulmonary edema, as has often been reported in the literature. The best way to correct the hypotension in these patients is to increase cardiac contractility by the use of inotropic drugs.[50]

Tolerance and physical and psychological dependence have been reported to occur following prolonged use of high doses of meprobamate.[12,13] Withdrawal symptoms reported after the abrupt withdrawal of such high doses include insomnia, vomiting, tremors, muscle twitches, anxiety, headaches, ataxia, convulsions, and psychotic behavior, at times resembling delirium tremens.[51] Death has been reported to occur following withdrawal of meprobamate.[52]

Treatment of physical dependence on meprobamate consists of cautious and gradual withdrawal of the drug over a period of 1 or 2 weeks. Alternatively, the patient may be stabilized on phenobarbital, which is then withdrawn over 10 to 14 days. Phenobarbital is administered orally, 30 mg for each 400 to 800 mg of meprobamate the patient has been taking daily. The total daily dose of phenobarbital is usually divided into three or four doses and is administered every 6 hours. As soon as the patient has been stabilized and has been without symptoms for 48 hours, the dose of phenobarbital is decreased by 30 mg/day. The patient should be closely monitored and preferably hospitalized, and general supportive and symptomatic care should be given as needed.[27-29]

Ethchlorvynol. Acute intoxication with ethchlorvynol, a tertiary acetylenic alcohol, produces symptoms similar to barbiturate overdosage. These may include coma, which can be of several days' duration, hypotension, hypothermia, respiratory depression, and apnea. Mydriasis, areflexia, and bradycardia may also occur.[5,53-56] A diagnostic sign helpful in ethchlorvynol intoxications is the characteristic pungent aromatic odor of the breath and/or materials removed by gastric lavage from intoxicated patients, present because ethchlorvynol is a tertiary alcohol.

The various complications that have been reported to occur in ethchlorvynol-intoxicated patients are pulmonary edema, severe infections, cardiopulmonary arrest, peripheral neuropathy, severe pancytopenia, thrombocytopenia and renal failure, and hemolysis.[5,53–56,57–60] Death may result from respiratory failure, hypotension, or complications of prolonged coma. The exact dose of ethchlorvynol necessary to produce toxic effects is not clear. Patients have recovered after ingesting doses of from 10 to 25 g, following a period of coma lasting from 5 to 7 days.[60] Death has resulted in persons with blood levels of approximately 14 mg/100 ml, which is 10 times the maximum level attained after the ingestion of 1 g.[60] Toxic blood levels have been reported to be greater than 2 mg/dl.[61]

In therapeutic doses, ethchlorvynol is readily absorbed from the GI tract. The onset action of the drug is rapid, and CNS depression occurs within 30 minutes following usual oral hypnotic doses.[60] A single dose of 500 mg of ethchlorvynol given to nine normal subjects produced a rapid rise in plasma ethchlorvynol concentration to about 4.2 μg/ml in 2 hours, followed by a fall to about 2.4 and 1.6 μg/ml at 4 and 6 hours respectively.[62] The decline of serum levels of ethchlorvynol is biphasic and fits a two-compartment open model. The half-life for the first (distribution) phase is 5 to 6 hours. The half-life for the second (elimination) phase has been reported to be 25 hours[63] and, following ethchlorvynol overdosage, greater than 100 hours.[64] Studies of ethchlorvynol distribution indicate that there is extensive tissue localization of the drug, particularly in adipose tissue.[63,65] Ethchlorvynol is metabolized in the liver, and about 10% has been reported to be excreted unchanged in the urine.[62,63,65]

In the treatment of patients acutely intoxicated with ethchlorvynol, intensive supportive therapy, with emphasis on the respiratory and cardiovascular functions, is essential. Hypotension should be treated initially with fluids. If the patient does not respond to fluid administration, vasopressor agents should be used. Hypothermia, which is commonly present, should be treated carefully with blankets or temperature-controlled water blankets. Forced diuresis is not effective and may complicate the pulmonary problems seen in these patients. Dialytic procedures (e.g., PD, HD, CHP, or RHP) have been reported to be somewhat effective.[5,53,56,66] However, they should be reserved for patients who do not respond to standard therapeutic approaches or who have severe acid-base and electrolyte imbalances.

Tolerance and physcial and psychological dependence have been reported to occur with ethchlorvynol.[12,13] Withdrawal symptoms are best treated with either reinstitution of ethchlorvynol and a gradual tapering off, or with substitution of phenobarbital. The initial dose of phenobarbital should be 100 to 200 mg. If, within the first hour, signs of withdrawal have not subsided, a second dose of 100 to 200 mg of phenobarbital should be administered. This dose should be continued every 1 to 2 hours until the patient is comfortable. Thereafter, administration of phenobarbital should be scheduled at 6-hour intervals. After the patient has been stabilized, a gradual withdrawal schedule for phenobarbital should be implemented.[27–29]

Withdrawal has been reported to occur also in neonates, following maternal ingestion of an amount appropriate for nighttime sedation. Withdrawal symptoms in a neonate should be treated with a short course of 3 to 5 mg/kg of phenobarbital.[67]

Chloral derivatives. Chloral derivatives such as chloral hydrate, chloral betaine, and triclofos are widely used, and cases of severe intoxication, either through intentional or accidental overdosage, have been reported.[6,68-72] Acute intoxication with these preparations also takes place when chloral is mixed with alcohol to provide "knock-out drops," popularly known as "Mickey Finn." Although only chloral hydrate intoxication will be discussed here in detail, the toxic effects and treatment of chloral betaine and triclofos are similar.

Acute chloral hydrate intoxications produce symptoms similar to barbiturate overdosage; these may include coma, hypotension, hypothermia, respiratory depression and cardiac arrhythmias, miosis, vomiting, areflexia, and muscle flaccidity.[6,68,71,72] Esophageal stricture, gastric necrosis and perforation, and GI hemorrhage have also been reported.[69,70] During the recovery phase after an acute intoxication, hepatic and renal function may be impaired, and this may result in transient jaundice and/or albuminuria. If death occurs, it is usually the result of respiratory failure or hypotension. The toxic oral dose of chloral hydrate for adults is approximately 10 g, although death has been reported with as little as 4 g, and individuals have survived after ingesting as much as 30 g.[73,74]

In therapeutic doses, chloral hydrate is rapidly absorbed from the stomach and starts to act within 30 minutes. It is widely distributed throughout the body, and is metabolized by the liver and erythrocytes to form trichloroethanol (an active metabolite) and trichloroacetic acid (an inactive metabolite).[75,76] The reduction of chloral hydrate to trichloroethanol is catalyzed by alcohol dehydrogenase and other enzymes. Trichloroethanol may also be conjugated with glucuronic acid to form trichloroethanol glucuronide (urochloralic acid), an inactive metabolite, or it may be further metabolized to trichloroacetic acid.

About 16% to 35% of a dose may be excreted in the urine in 24 hours as glucuronide and about 5% as free trichloroethanol. A small portion of glucuronide is excreted in the bile. Trichloroacetic acid is slowly excreted over 24 to 48 hours. Chloral hydrate is not excreted unchanged in the urine.[75,76] Trichloroethanol is also an active hypnotic, and with chloral hydrate it passes to the cerebrospinal fluid, into milk, and through the placenta to the fetus.[77]

Treatment of patients intoxicated with chloral hydrate consists of general supportive measures and frequent monitoring of cardiac arrhythmias, especially in children. Because chloral hydrate is a halogenated hydrocarbon, in large doses it depresses the contractility of the myocardium and shortens the refractory period, as do many hydrocarbon anesthetics. In symptomatic overdose cases, liver and renal studies should be obtained early as baselines and should be followed throughout the patient's hospitalization, since toxicity in these two organ systems is not unusual.

Forced diuresis is also recommended because of the pharmacokinetic parameters of chloral hydrate. Mannitol, in a dose of 2 g/kg for children or to a maximum of 100 g/dose for adults, or furosemide, 1 mg/kg for children or to a maximum of 40 to 80 mg for adults, should be administered. Hemodialysis has also been advocated and may be useful in patients unresponsive to normal supportive care, or in patients in whom acid-base or fluid and electrolyte problems may become uncontrollable.[71,78]

Prolonged use of chloral hydrate may lead to tolerance and dependence, and the symptoms include apprehension and weakness, anxiety, headache, dizziness, tremors, nausea, vomiting, abdominal cramps, insomnia, and convulsions similar to those experienced by alcoholics.[73,79] Withdrawal symptoms are best treated with either reinstitution of chloral hydrate if hepatic, renal, or other abnormalities are not present, or substitution of phenobarbital. Once the patient has been stabilized in a specific dosage regimen for at least 48 hours, a gradual withdrawal schedule for chloral hydrate or phenobarbital should be implemented over a period of 7 to 10 days.[27-29]

Paraldehyde. Patients acutely intoxicated with paraldehyde, a cyclic ether, have symptoms similar to those of chloral hydrate intoxication, which may include coma, severe hypotension, respiratory depression, pulmonary edema, renal complications, oliguria, azotemia, albuminuria, liver toxicity, and cardiac failure.[7,80-82] Diagnosis of paraldehyde intoxication is facilitated by the characteristic odor of the drug on the patient's breath. Although fatalities are not common, administration of 25 ml of paraldehyde orally or 12 ml rectally has caused death. The minimum lethal blood level is reported to be about 50 mg/dl.[7,80,82,83] Death is usually the result of respiratory failure. However, several fatalities have also been attributed to pulmonary edema and right-sided heart failure or metabolic acidosis.[7,80,82,83]

In therapeutic doses, paraldehyde is readily absorbed when given orally, rectally, or intramuscularly, and is distributed throughout the tissues. About 30 minutes are required for paraldehyde to reach maximum concentrations in the brain after oral administration, and 80% of a given dose is metabolized to acid metabolites in the liver and excreted in the urine.[84] A significant portion (7%) is excreted unchanged through the lungs, giving the breath the characteristic odor.[85] Paraldehyde diffuses across the placenta and may cause respiratory depression in neonates.[86]

General supportive measures constitute the cornerstone of management. Clinical improvement has occurred following dialysis for paraldehyde intoxication, but removal of the drug has not been documented.[87] In addition, correction of metabolic acidosis was achieved in two patients who underwent hemodialysis,[7,88] and in one patient who underwent peritoneal dialysis.[80]

Chronic paraldehyde intoxication results in tolerance and dependence. The paraldehyde addict may become acquainted with the drug when it is used for the treament of alcoholism and then may prefer it to alcohol. Paraldehyde addiction resembles alcoholism and withdrawal may result in delirium tremens and vivid hallucinations.[89] The treatment of paraldehyde withdrawal symptoms is similar to that of alcohol withdrawal symptoms, e.g., administration of sedatives, anticonvulsants, and antibiotics based on the patient's clinical status, as well as frequent monitoring of the patient for the prevention, detection, and/or treatment of fluid and electrolyte abnormalities and carbohydrate metabolism aberrations.[90,91]

Bromides. The bromides are inorganic salts that have been widely used in the past for their sedative and anticonvulsant effects. However, because the blood concentration necessary to produce a therapeutic effect is usually close to that at which toxic effects become evident, bromide salts have largely been replaced by more effective, less toxic agents. The bromide salts are still used occasionally in the treatment of grand mal and focal epilepsy, and they are often found in nostrums, nerve tonics, and headache remedies.

Acute bromide intoxication occurs rarely. Because the drug tends to be irritating to the GI tract, it is difficult for a patient or individual to ingest and retain without vomiting a sufficient amount to elevate plasma bromide to a toxic level. If taken daily, however, a toxic level may be attained over a period of weeks, and overdosages have been reported.[8,92-94] Bromides replace chloride in extracellular body fluids and have a half-life in the body of about 12 days.[95] They may be detected in the milk of nursing mothers and in the fetus.[96]

Most patients show signs of intoxication with serum bromide levels of 12 to 25 mEq/L, or greater than 5 mg/dl.[8,93] The symptoms of bromide intoxication, or "bromism," include mental dullness, slurred speech, weakened memory, apathy, anorexia, constipation, drowsiness, and loss of sensitivity to touch and pain. These symptoms disappear when the drug is discontinued, but continued use leads to more serious symptoms, including restlessness, disorientation, ocular disturbances, ataxia, hallucinations, delirium, stupor, and coma.[8,92,97-100] Cerebral spinal fluid pressure may be raised, and in cases of severe intoxication, papilledema may be present. The "bromism" syndrome has been mistaken for acute alcoholic intoxication, general paresis, encephalitis, cerebral tumor, multiple sclerosis, uremia, and other disease entities.[73,97] Bromide rash, of an acneiform, nodular, or sometimes erythematous type, is also of fairly common occurrence in bromide-intoxicated patients.[101]

Standard supportive measures are indicated in the treatment of the patient intoxicated with bromide salts. In addition, 1 L of sodium chloride injection should be given every 3 to 4 hours by intravenous infusion. A rapidly acting diuretic such as furosemide (Lasix) (1 mg/kg of body weight) should also be given to promote the excretion of bromide.[8,92,102-104] In chronic intoxications, bromide administration should be stopped, and sodium chloride, 2 to 3 g three or four times daily, should be given by mouth with at least 4 L of fluid per day.

Ammonium chloride, 2 to 3 g three or four times daily, may be substituted for sodium chloride if desired, to avoid a positive balance of sodium and if there is no danger of uncompensated acidosis. Psychosis, if present, can be controlled by the administration of 300 mg of chlorpromazine (Thorazine) daily.[105] Recovery usually requires from 1 to 3 weeks. In severe cases of bromide intoxication, or when the usual treatment cannot be used,

hemodialysis can be used to remove bromide from the body.[106,107]

Methyprylon. Methyprylon, along with glutethimide (see next section), is a piperidione derivative. The main symptoms of methyprylon overdosage are coma lasting anywhere from 5 to 30 hours, respiratory depression, hypotension (the most dangerous complication), tachycardia, and hyper- or hypothermia.[9,108-110] Paradoxical excitability, e.g., hyperactivity and convulsions, have also been reported.[108,110,111] Methyprylon is absorbed rapidly from the GI tract. In therapeutic doses, approximately 60% of a dose is excreted in the urine as metabolites, together with 3% of unchanged methyprylon.

The therapeutic half-life of methyprylon has been reported to be 3 to 6 hours.[112] Information regarding the pharmacokinetic parameters of methyprylon in acute overdosages in not available, and the range of toxicity is not clearly defined. One fatal case has been reported after the ingestion of 6 g,[9] whereas other patients have ingested up to 30 g and have survived.[111] The therapeutic blood level of methyprylon is less than 1 mg/dl. Toxic manifestations are usually present with blood levels of 3 to 6 mg/dl, and blood levels of 10 mg/dl or greater are potentially lethal.[108]

Supportive therapy constitutes the mainstay of treatment of methyprylon-intoxicated patients.[103] CNS stimulants should be avoided, as they are of no proven benefit and may cause convulsions. Phases of excitation or convulsions may be controlled by the cautious administration of diazepam, 1 mg/kg of body weight. Fluids and electrolytes should be monitored closely and replaced as necessary. Hypotension is usually resistant to the administration of fluids, and vasopressor drugs may be needed to prevent shock.

The use of forced diuresis or alkalinization of the urine is not recommended, since only a small percentage of methypry-lon is excreted unchanged in the urine. In addition, there is no evidence that dialysis alters the outcome of the intoxication or the length of coma. However, in cases of severe intoxication, where standard therapeutic measures are ineffective and the clinical condition of the patient is deteriorating, hemodialysis or charcoal hemoperfusion may be of value.[112-115]

Prolonged use or abuse of methyprylon may lead to tolerance and physical and psychological dependence.[12,13] Methypry-lon withdrawal has been reported to cause confusion, restlessness, excitement, sweating, polyuria, generalized convulsions, and auditory and visual hallucinations.[116] Psychotic behavior was precipitated in a patient who had discontinued the daily use of 4.8 g of methyprylon, and death has been reported after withdrawal of methyprylon in a patient who had been taking 7.5 to 12 g daily for about 18 months.[117]

Withdrawal resulting from addiction can be treated with resubstitution of methyprylon in a decreasing dosage scale, or with substitution of phenobarbital. The initial dose of phenobarbital should be 100 to 200 mg administered every 6 hours and increased as needed until withdrawal symptoms are controlled. When the patient's clinical condition has been stable for at least 48 hours, the dosage of phenobarbital should be gradually reduced over a period of 10 to 14 days.[27-29]

Glutethimide. Overdosage with glutethimide, another piperidione derivative, produces symptoms similar to those of barbiturate overdosage, but with considerable fluctuations in the depth of coma and wakefulness. Sudden apnea and convulsions may occur, with signs of raised intracranial pressure and severe hypotension, and persistent acidosis may develop. Anticholinergic effects such as mydriasis, dryness of the mouth, paralytic ileus, and urinary bladder atony often occur.[10,118-125]

In therapeutic doses, glutethimide is absorbed slowly and irregularly from the GI tract, with peak plasma concentrations reached in 1 to 6 hours. The range of the elimination half-life has been reported to be between 5 and 22 hours, with an average value of 11.6 hours.[126,127] The erratic absorption of glutethimide may be due to the fact that the drug is poorly soluble in water. Whole tablets of glutethimide were recovered from the stomach of a patient who died 3 days after ingesting a fatal dose, in spite of the fact that the patient had undergone gastric lavage shortly after admission to the hospital.[123] The ingestion of alcohol along with the tablets greatly facilitates absorption from the stomach. Glutethimide is widely distributed in body tissues and fat and passes diffusion barriers. It is hydroxylated to water-soluble derivatives and conjugated in the liver. Some metabolites, and possibly glutethimide itself, are excreted in the bile and reabsorbed in the intestine. Therafter, they are excreted in the urine after more than 48 hours. Therefore, excretion of the metabolites in the urine is slow.[126,127]

Although enterohepatic circulation was once suggested as being responsible for the cyclical coma and fluctuations in the level of consciousness seen in glutethimide-intoxicated patients,[120,122] it is now believed that the probable cause is the accumulation of the active metabolite of glutethimide, 4-hydroxy-2-ethyl-2-phenyl-glutaramide.[121] Cyclic coma may also occur as a result of continued absorption of glutethimide from the gut. The anticholinergic effects of glutethimide decrease bowel motility until the glutethimide has been metabolized, at which time bowel motility returns, more glutethimide is absorbed, and coma once again ensues, completing the circular pattern. This phenomenon also explains why plasma levels of glutethimide do not correlate with the clinical course of intoxicated patients.

Autopsy findings commonly include cerebral and pulmonary edema, visceral hemorrhage, and pneumonia.[10,118,119,123,124] A dose of 5 g is sufficient to produce severe intoxication. The lethal dose is between 10 and 20 g.[118,119,123,124] Toxic manifestations are usually present with blood levels of glutethimide greater than 3 mg/dl, whereas severe symptoms are present with blood levels of greater than 10 mg/dl, unless the patient has a tolerance for glutethimide.[119,123] After ingestion of 1 g of glutethimide, the blood concentration of glutethimide has been reported to be 7 mg/dl.[119]

Intensive supportive therapy is indicated in all glutethimide-intoxicated patients.[123,128–131] Acidosis should be corrected with the intravenous administration of sodium bicarbonate. Sudden episodes of apnea and raised intracranial pressure can be treated with the intravenous administration of 500 ml of 20% mannitol over a 20-minute period, followed by the intravenous administration of 5% dextrose over the next 4 hours. Fluids should be used initially to correct hypotension, and vasopressors should be reserved for refractory hypotension. Convulsions should be treated by the cautious intravenous administration of diazepam, 1 mg/kg of body weight.

The use of CNS stimulants, gastric lavage with castor oil, and the administration of physostigmine salicylate to counteract the anticholinergic effects of gluthethimide are of no value and should be avoided. The potential risks associated with the administration of these agents outweigh the possible benefits. Methods to enhance excretion of glutethimide, such as forced diuresis, also are not likely to be effective, as suggested by the pharmacokinetic parameters of glutethimide, and therefore are not recommended. Hemodialysis, however, can be of assistance to the clinician where uncontrollable acid-base and fluid and electrolyte prob-

lems are present.[132] In addition, although lipid dialysis has been recommended by some investigators,[133] it appears to be of questionable value.

Careful supportive and symptomatic care results in the survival of more than 95% of patients intoxicated with glutethimide. In cases where standard supportive measures are ineffective and the clinical condition of the patient is deteriorating, charcoal and resin hemoperfusion are effective techniques available to the clinician for the successful treatment of these patients.[115,134]

Prolonged use or abuse of glutethimide can lead to tolerance and physical and psychological dependence.[12,13] Manifestations of glutethimide withdrawal have been reported to include nausea, vomiting, abdominal cramping, tachycardia, sweating fever, agitation, and tremulousness. Major reactions include convulsions, delirium, or both, characterized by confusion, disorientation, and hallucinations.[135–138] The lowest dosages reported to have been followed by abstinence convulsions were 2.5 g and 5 g daily in two patients who had taken the drug for 3 months and several weeks, respectively.[138]

Withdrawal symptoms due to addiction can be treated with resubstitution of glutethimide in a decreasing dosage scale, or with substitution of phenobarbital. Phenobarbital may be started at 100 to 200 mg every 6 hours, and increased as necessary until withdrawal symptoms subside. After a stabilization period of from 1 to 2 days, the dosage of phenobarbital should be gradually tapered off.[27–29]

Methaqualone. The symptoms produced by mild intoxication with methaqualone, a 2,3-disubstituted quinazoline, are the same as those produced by the barbiturates and most other nonbarbiturates. In severe methaqualone overdosage, however, the coma is accompanied by pyramidal signs such as hypertonia, hyperreflexia, myoclonia, and/or convulsions.[10,139-145] Cardiac and respiratory depression occurs less frequently than with barbiturate overdosage. Pupillary dilation is commonly present. Pulmonary and cutaneous edema, hepatic damage, renal insufficiency, and bleeding may occur. Spontaneous vomiting and increased secretions are common and may lead to pneumonitis or respiratory obstruction. Reflexes are usually active, and the patients react to painful stimuli.[140,142,146,147] Ingestion of 2.4 g of methaqualone usually produces coma in adults. Ingestion of 8 g has caused death, although one patient survived the ingestion of 22 g.[148]

Methaqualone is rapidly absorbed from the GI tract when administered in therapeutic doses. After a single oral dose of 300 mg given to seven healthy subjects, the maximum blood concentration occurred after an average of 3 hours, and the concentration diminished in a biphasic manner. The biologic half-life was calculated to be about 50 minutes for the first component and 16 hours for the second. Distribution studies indicate that there is extensive tissue localization of the drug, particularly in adipose tissue. The major route of metabolism in humans involves nonspecific hydroxylation, and glucuronide and sulfate derivatives are excreted in the urine. About 2% is excreted unchanged in the urine.[149,150]

In methaqualone-intoxicated patients, the half-life is not known. Peak plasma levels are reached erratically, suggesting that the drug remaining in the gut is absorbed continuously. Methaqualone levels between 2 and 8 mg/dl are consistent with significant intoxication in the majority of patients. In severe overdosages manifested by coma, hypertonicity, hyperreflexia, and myoclonia, the serum methaqualone level is generally higher than 8 mg/dl.[141,142,150,151]

Treatment of the methaqualone-intoxicated patient consists of general supportive measures, prevention of further absorption of the drug, and symptomatic care as indicated.[142] Convulsions, if present, may be treated with the intravenous administration of diazepam, 0.1 to 0.3 mg/kg in a child and up to 10 mg in an adult. Forced diuresis is not indicated, since less than 2% of active methaqualone is excreted in the urine. Furthermore, because pulmonary edema is a relatively common finding in the majority of patients intoxicated with this drug, forced diuresis should be contraindicated.

Hemodialysis and charcoal hemoperfusion have been shown to be somewhat effective in removing large amounts of methaqualone in severely intoxicated patients.[115,144,146,147] The cornerstone of treatment, however, should be conservative therapy, and HD and CHP should be reserved for patients unresponsive to standard therapeutic and supportive measures, those who have fluid and electrolyte and acid-base abnormalities, or those with methaqualone levels in excess of 10 mg/dl. In addition, during hospitalization, frequent monitoring of biochemical and hematologic indices, periodic x-ray examinations, and electrocardiograms are indicated, since liver, renal, cardiovascular, respiratory, and hematologic abnormalities have been reported to occur in severely intoxicated patients.[139-147]

Prolonged use of methaqualone leads to the development of tolerance and psychological and physical dependence.[152-155] Abrupt cessation of methaqualone, in persons with a history of daily ingestion of 1.5 to 2 g for several months, has been reported to cause withdrawal symptoms.[155] Usually, symptoms appear 24 hours after termination of drug intake and include restlessness, mental confusion, visual hallucination, brisk reflexes, tremor, hyperthermia, generalized convulsions, and delirium.[152-155]

Withdrawal resulting from addiction can be treated with resubstitution of the drug in a decreasing dosage scale, or with substitution of phenobarbital. The initial dose of phenobarbital should be 100 mg (3 to 6 mg/kg) every 6 hours, increased as necessary until withdrawal symptoms subside. After stabilization for 48 hours, the dosage of phenobarbital should be gradually reduced over a period of days or 1 or 2 weeks.[27-29] The withdrawal symptoms of one of our patients showed dramatic improvement following the oral administration of thioridazine (Mellaril) in a dosage of 800 mg/day. Patients being withdrawn from methaqualone should be closely monitored, preferably hospitalized, and supportive and symptomatic care should be given as needed.

GENERAL PROGNOSIS

The prognosis for patients intoxicated with nonbarbiturate drugs depends upon several factors: (1) type and quantity of drug(s) ingested or intravenously administered, (2) time elapsed between ingestion and initiation of treatment, (3) underlying medical or psychological problems, (4) degree of tolerance, if any, (5) ingestion or intravenous administration of multiple drugs with synergistic actions, and (6) accuracy of historical facts or evidence regarding the drugs ingested or intravenously administered.

In the majority of patients, however, and even in those severely intoxicated with nonbarbiturate drugs, recovery is usually successful when careful standard therapeutic approaches are applied. Forced diuresis, hemodialysis, and charcoal hemoperfusion are infrequently necessary, and they are indicated only in those patients in whom the implementation of standard therapeutic approaches is unsatisfactory.

REFERENCES

1. Anon: Drug related deaths and injuries. U.S. Government Printing Office, 720–12611, Drug Enforcement Administration, United States Department of Justice, Washington D.C., 1977.
2. Greenblatt DJ, et al: Acute overdosages with benzodiazepine derivatives. *Clin Pharmacol Ther*, 21:497–514, 1977.
3. Davis RP, et al: Treatment of intoxication with ethinyl cyclohexyl carbamate (Valmid) by extracorporeal hemodialysis: Case report, Yale. *J Biol Med*, 32:192–196, 1959.
4. Allen MD, Greenblatt DJ, and Noel BJ: Meprobamate overdosage: A continuing problem. *Clin Toxicol*, 11:501–515, 1977.
5. Teehan BP, et al: Acute ethchlorvynol (Placidy®) intoxication. *Ann Intern Med*, 72:875–882, 1970.
6. Lansky LL: An unusual case of childhood chloral hydrate poisoning. *Am J Dis Child*, 127:275–276, 1974.
7. Hayward JN, and Boshell BR: Paraldehyde intoxication with metabolic acidosis: Report of two cases, experimental data and a critical review of the literature. *Am J Med*, 23:965–976, 1957.
8. Trump DL, and Hochberg MC: Bromide intoxication. *Johns Hopkins Med J*, 138:119–123, 1976.
9. Reidt WU: Fatal poisoning with methyprylon (Noludar®), a nonbarbiturate sedative. *N Engl J Med*, 255:231–232, 1956.
10. Wright N, and Roscoe P: Acute glutethimide poisoning. Conservative management of 31 patients. *JAMA*, 214:1704–1706, 1970.
11. Inaba DS, et al: Methaqualone abuse. *JAMA*, 244:1505–1509, 1973.
12. Essig CF: Newer sedative drugs that can cause states of intoxication and dependence of barbiturate type. *JAMA*, 196:126–129, 1966.
13. Essig CF: Addiction to nonbarbiturate sedative and tranquilizing drugs. *Clin Pharmacol Ther*, 5:334–343, 1964.
14. Harvey SC: Hypnotics and sedatives. In *The Pharmacological Basis of Therapeutics*. 6th Ed. Edited by AG Gilman, LS Goodman, and A. Gilman. New York, Macmillan, 1980.
15. Palmer GC: Use, overuse, misuse, and abuse of benzodiazepines. *Ala J Med Sci*, 15:383–392, 1978.
16. Berger R, Green G, and Melneck A: Cardiac arrest caused by oral diazepam intoxication. *Clin Pediatr*, 14:842–844, 1975.
17. Baker AB: Induction of anesthesia with diazepam. *Anaesthesia*, 24:388–394, 1969.
18. Prensky AM, et al: Intravenous diazepam in the treatment of prolonged seizure activity. *N Engl J Med*, 276:779–784, 1967.
19. Rumack BH (ed): Management of benzodiazepines. In *Poisindex*. Denver, Colorado, Micromedex, Inc., August, 1980.
20. Bellantuono C, et al: Benzodiazepines. *Drugs*, 19:195–219, 1980.
21. Breimer DD: Clinical pharmacokinetics of hypnotics. *Clin Pharmacokinet*, 2:93–109, 1977.
22. Ruedy J: Acute drug poisoning in the adult. *Can Med Assoc J*, 109:603–608, 1973.
23. DiLiberti J, O'Brien ML, and Turner T: The use of physostigmine as an antidote in accidental diazepam intoxication. *J Pediatr*, 86:106–107, 1975.
24. Bell EF: The use of naloxone in the treatment of

diazepam poisoning. *J Pediatr,* 87:803–804, 1975.

25. Hollister LE, et al: Diazepam in newly admitted schizophrenics. *Dis Nerv Syst,* 24:746–750, 1963.

26. Hollister LE, Motzenbecker FP, and Degan RO: Withdrawal reactions from chlordiazepoxide (Librium). *Psychopharmacologia,* 4:235–246, 1963.

27. Wilker A: Diagnosis and treatment of drug dependence of the barbiturate type. *Am J Psychiatry,* 125:758–765, 1968.

28. Smith DE, and Wesson DR: A new method for treatment of barbiturate dependence. *JAMA,* 213:294–295, 1970.

29. Gay GR, et al: A new method of outpatient treatment of barbiturate withdrawal. *J Psychedelic Drugs,* 3:81–88, 1971.

30. Editorial note: Current concepts in therapy of sedative hypnotic drugs. V. Nonbarbiturates. *N Engl J Med,* 256:314–316, 1957.

31. Langecker H, et al: Ein Suicid-Versuch mit Valamin mit einem Bertrag zur elimination und therapie. *Arch Toxicol,* 19:293-301, 1962.

32. Clifford JM, Cookson JH, and Wickham PE: Absorption and clearance of secobarbital, heptabarbital, methaqualone and ethinamate. *Clin Pharmacol Ther,* 16:376–389, 1974.

33. Murata T: Metabolic fate of 1-ethynylcyclohexyl carbamate. II. Studies on the glucuronide excreted in the urine of humans receiving 1-ethynylcyclohexyl carbamate. *Chem Pharm Bull (Tokyo),* 9:146, 1961.

34. Ellinwood EH, Ewing JA, and Hoaken PCS: Habituation to ethinamate. *N Engl J Med,* 266:185–186, 1962.

35. Bedson HS: Coma due to meprobamate intoxication: Report of a case confirmed by chemical analysis. *Lancet,* 1:288–290, 1959.

36. Kamin I, and Shaskan DA: Death due to massive overdose of meprobamate. *Am J Psychiatry,* 115:1123–1124, 1959.

37. Powell LW Jr, Mann GT, and Kaye S: Acute meprobamate poisoning. *N Engl J Med,* 259:716–718, 1958.

38. Maddock RK Jr, and Bloomer HA: Meprobamate overdosage: Evaluation of its severity and methods of treatment. *JAMA,* 201:999–1003, 1967.

39. Hiestand EC: Overdosage with meprobamate. Presentation of a case. *Ohio State Med J,* 52:1306–1307, 1956.

40. Jenis EH, Payne RJ, and Goldbaum LR: Acute meprobamate poisoning: A fatal case following a lucid interval. *JAMA,* 207:361–362, 1969.

41. Schwartz HS: Acute meprobamate poisoning with gastrotomy and removal of a drug-containing mass. *N Engl J Med,* 295:1177–1178, 1976.

42. Woodward MG: Attempted suicide with meprobamate. *Northwest Med,* 56:321–322, 1957.

43. Felby S: Concentrations of meprobamate in the blood and liver following fatal meprobamate poisoning. *Acta Pharmacol Toxicol,* 28:334–337, 1970.

44. Walkenstein SS, et al: The excretion and distribution of meprobamate and its metabolites. *J Pharmacol Exp Ther,* 123:254–258, 1958.

45. Meyer MC, and Straughn AB: Meprobamate: Bioavailability monograph. *J Am Pharm Assoc,* 17:173–176, 1977.

46. Rumack BH: Management of meprobamate. In *Poisindex.* Denver, Colorado, Micromedex, August, 1980.

47. Gibson TP, et al: Enhanced renal tubular secretion of meprobamate: Role of saline-furosemide diuresis. *Clin Toxicol,* 7:29–35, 1974.

48. Winchester JF, et al: Dialysis and hemoperfusion of poisons and drugs—update. *Trans Am Soc Artif Intern Organs,* 23:762–842, 1977.

49. Crome P, and Higgenbottom T: Severe meprobamate poisoning: Successful treatment with hemoperfusion. *Postgrad Med J,* 53:698–699, 1977.

50. Lhoste F, Lemaire F, and Rapin M: Treatment of hypotension in meprobamate poisoning. *N Engl J Med,* 296:1004, 1977.

51. Haizlip TM, and Ewing JA: Meprobamate habituation: A controlled clinical study. *N Engl J Med,* 258:1181–1186, 1958.

52. Swanson LA, and Okada T: Death after withdrawal of meprobamate. *JAMA,* 184:780–781, 1963.

53. Westervelt FB Jr: Ethchlorvynol (Placidyl) intoxication, experience with five patients, including treatment with hemodialysis. *Ann Intern Med,* 64:1229–1236, 1966.

54. Glauser FL, et al: Ethchlorvynol (Placidyl®) induced pulmonary edema. *Ann Intern Med,* 84:46–48, 1976.

55. Westerfield BT, and Blovin RA: Ethchlorvynol intoxication. *South Med J,* 70:1019–1020, 1977.

56. Hyde JS, Lawrence AG, and Males JB: Ethchlorvynol intoxication: Successful treatment by exchange transfusion and peritoneal dialysis. *Clin Pediatr,* 7:739–741, 1968.

57. Klock JC: Hemolysis and pancytopenia in ethchlorvynol overdose. *Ann Intern Med,* 81:131–132, 1974.

58. Kuenssberg EV: Side-effects of ethchlorvynol. *Br Med J,* 2:1610, 1962.

59. Schultz JC, Crowder DG, and Medart WS: Excretion studies in ethchlorvynol (Placidyl®) intoxication. *Arch Intern Med,* 117:409–411, 1966.

60. Algeir EJ, Katsas GS, and Luongo MA: Determination of ethchlorvynol in biologic mediums, and report of two fatal cases. *Am J Clin Pathol,* 38:125–130, 1962.

61. Done AK: The toxic emergency. *Emergency Med,* 7:193–201, 1975.

62. Dawborn JK, Turner A, and Pattison G: Ethchlorvynol as a sedative in patients with renal failure. *Med J Aust,* 2:702–704, 1972.

63. Cummins LM, Martin YC, and Scherfling EE: Serum and urine levels of ethchlorvynol in man. *J Pharm Sci,* 60:261–263, 1971.

64. Rumack BH: Management of ethchlorvynol poisoning. In *Poisindex:* Denver, Colorado, Micromedex, Inc., August, 1980.

65. Cravey RH, and Baselt RC: Studies of the body

distribution of ethchlorvynol. *J Forensic Sci,* 13:532–536, 1968.

66. Rosenbaum JL, Kramer MS, and Raja R: Resin hemoperfusion for acute drug intoxication. *Arch Intern Med, 136:*263–266, 1976.
67. Rumack BH, and Walrowens PA: Neonatal withdrawal following maternal ingestion of ethchlorvynol (Placidyl®). *Pediatrics, 52:*714–716, 1973.
68. Marshall AJ: Cardiac arrhythmias caused by chloral hydrate. *Br Med J,* 2:994, 1977.
69. Vellar IDA, et al: Gastric necrosia—a rare complication of chloral hydrate intoxication. *Br J Surg,* 59:317–319, 1972.
70. Gleich GJ, Mongan ES, and Vaules DW: Esophageal strictures following chloral hydrate poisoning. *JAMA, 201:*266–267, 1967.
71. Stalker NE, et al: Acute massive chloral hydrate intoxication treated with hemodialysis. A clinical pharmacokinetic analysis. *J Clin Pharmacol, 18:*136–142, 1978.
72. Gustafson A, Svensson SE, and Ugander L: Cardiac arrhythmias in chloral hydrate poisoning. *Acta Med Scand, 201:*227–230, 1977.
73. Sharpless SK: Hypnotics and sedatives. II. Miscellaneous agents. In *The Pharmacological Basis of Therapeutics.* 4th Ed. Edited by LS Goodman and A Gilman. New York, Macmillan, 1970, pp. 121–124.
74. Hawes AJ: Safety of chloral. *Br Med J,* 2:627, 1968.
75. Owens AH Jr, and Marshall EK Jr: Further studies on the metabolic fate of chloral hydrate and trichoroethanol. *Bull Johns Hopkins Hosp,* 97:320–326, 1955.
76. Garrett ER, and Lambert HJ: Pharmacokinetics of trichloroethanol and metabolites and interconversions among variously referenced pharmacokinetic parameters. *J Pharm Sci, 62:*550–572, 1973.
77. Bernstine JB, Meyer AE, and Bernstine RL: Maternal blood and cerebral fluid estimation following the administration of chloral hydrate during the puerperium. *Am J Obstet Gynecol,* 73:801–804, 1957.
78. Baziri ND, et al: Hemodialysis in the treatment of acute chloral hydrate poisoning. *South Med J,* 70:377–378, 1977.
79. Merry J: Withdrawal fits. *Lancet,* 1:96, 1968.
80. Beier LS, Pitts WH, and Gonick HC: Metabolic acidosis occurring during paraldehyde intoxication. *Ann Intern Med,* 58:155–158, 1963.
81. Sinai SH, and Crowe JE: Cyanosis, cough and hypotension following intravenous administration of paraldehyde. *Pediatrics,* 57:158–159, 1976.
82. Burstein CL: The hazards of paraldehyde administration. *JAMA, 121:*187–189, 1943.
83. Kaye Sand Haag HB: Study of death due to combined action of alcohol and paraldehyde in man. *Toxicol Appl Pharmacol,* 6:316–320, 1964.
84. Hitchcock P, and Nelson EE: The metabolism of paraldehyde. *J Pharmacol Exp Ther,* 79:286–294, 1943.
85. Lang DW, and Borgstedt HH: Rate of pulmo-

nary excretion of paraldehyde in man. *Toxicol Appl Pharmacol,* 15:269–274, 1969.
86. Gardner HL, Levine H, and Budansky M: Concentration of paraldehyde in the blood following its administration during labor. *Am J Obstet Gynecol,* 40:435–439, 1940.
87. Maxwell MH: The indications for and the limitations of peritoneal dialysis. *Bull New Jersey Acad Med,* 6:341, 1960.
88. Gutman RA, Burnell JM, and Solak F: Paraldehyde acidosis. *Am J Med,* 42:435–440, 1967.
89. Mendelson J, et al: A study of addiction to nonethyl alcohols and other poisonous compounds. *Q J Stud Alcohol,* 18:562–580, 1957.
90. Knott DH, and Beard JD: A new approach to the treatment of acute withdrawal from alcohol. *Psychosomatics,* 9:311–313, 1968.
91. Beard JD, and Knott DH: Fluid and electrolyte balance during acute withdrawal in chronic alcoholic patients. *JAMA, 201:*135–139, 1968.
92. Hanes FM, and Yates A: An analysis of four hundred instances of chronic bromide intoxication. *Arch Intern Med,* 85:783–794, 1950.
93. Hodges HH, and Gilmour MT: The continuing hazard of bromide intoxication. *Am J Med,* 10:459–462, 1951.
94. McDonal CE, Owens D, and Bolman WM: Bromide abuse: A continuing problem. *Am J Psychiatry, 131:*913–915, 1974.
95. Soremark R: The biological half-life of bromide ions in human blood. *Acta Physiol Scand,* 50:119–123, 1960.
96. Opitz JM, Grose FR, and Haneberg B: Congenital effects of bromism? *Lancet,* 1:91–92, 1972.
97. Craven EB: The clinical picture of bromide poisoning. *Am J Med Sci, 186:*525–532, 1933.
98. Carney WMP: Five cases of bromism. *Lancet,* 2:523–524, 1971.
99. Raskind MA, Kitchell M, and Alvarez C: Bromide intoxication in the elderly. *J Am Geriatr Soc,* 26:222–224, 1978.
100. Nuki G, et al.: Four cases of bromism. *Br Med J,* 2:390–391, 1966.
101. Baer RL, and Harris H: Types of cutaneous reactions to drugs. *JAMA, 202:*710–713, 1967.
102. Wieth JO, and Funder J: Treatment of bromide poisoning. *Lancet,* 2:327–329, 1963.
103. Millins JL, and Rogers RS: Furosemide as an adjunct in the therapy of bromism and bromoderma. *Dermatologica, 156:*111–119, 1978.
104. Adamson JS Jr, Flanigan WJ, and Ackerman GL: Treatment of bromide intoxication with ethacrynic acid and mannitol diuresis. *Ann Intern Med,* 65:749–752, 1966.
105. Blume RS, MacLowry JD, and Wolfe SM: Limitations of chloride determination in the diagnosis of bromism. *N Engl J Med,* 279:593–595, 1968.
106. Schmitt GW, Maher JF, and Schreiner GE: Ethacrynic acid enhanced bromuresis: A comparison with peritoneal dialysis and hemodialysis. *J Lab Clin Med,* 68:913–922, 1966.
107. Merrill JP, and Weller JM: Testament of bromism with the artificial kidney. *Ann Intern Med,* 37:186–190, 1952.

108. Bailey DN and Jatlow PI: Methyprylon overdose: Interpretation of serum drug concentrations. *Clin Toxicol,* 6:563–569, 1973.

109. Burstein N, and Stauss HK: Attempted suicide with methyprylon. *JAMA,* 194:1139–1140, 1965.

110. Haider I, and Oswald I: Late brain recovery processes after drug overdose. *Br Med J,* 2:318–322, 1970.

111. Pellegrino ED, and Henderson RR: Clinical toxicity of methyprylone (Noludar). Case report and review of twenty-three cases. *J Med Soc NJ,* 54:515–518, 1957.

112. Pancorbo AS, et al: Hemodialysis in methyprylon overdose: Some pharmacokinetic considerations. *JAMA,* 237:470–471, 1977.

113. Xanthaky G, et al: Hemodialysis in methyprylon poisoning. *JAMA,* 198:1212–1213, 1966.

114. Mandelbaum JM, and Simon NM: Severe methyprylon intoxication treated by hemodialysis. *JAMA,* 216:139–140, 1971.

115. Chang TMS, et al: Methaqualone, methyprylon, and glutethimide clearance by the ACAC microcapsule artificial kidney: In vitro and in patients with acute intoxication. *Trans Am Soc Artif Intern Organs,* 19:87–91, 1973.

116. Jensen GR: Addiction to Noludar: A report of two cases. *N Z Med J,* 59:431–432, 1960.

117. Berger H: Addiction to methyprylon: Report of case of 24-year-old nurse with possible synergism with phenothiazine. *JAMA,* 117:63–65, 1961.

118. Jorgensen EO, and Jensen VB: Acute glutethimide poisoning. *Dan Med Bull,* 22:263–268, 1975.

119. McBay AJ, and Katsas GG: Glutethimide poisoning: A report of four fatal cases. *N Engl J Med,* 257:97–100, 1957.

120. Decker WJ, Thompson HL, and Arnerson LA: Glutethimide rebound. *Lancet,* 1:778–779, 1970.

121. Hansen AR, et al: Glutethimide poisoning: A metabolite contributes to morbidity and mortality. *N Engl J Med,* 292:250–252, 1975.

122. Charytan C: The enterohepatic circulation in glutethimide intoxication. *Clin Pharmacol Ther,* 11:816–820, 1970.

123. Holland J, et al: Drugs ingested in suicide attempts and fatal outcomes. *NY State J Med,* 75:2343–2349, 1975.

124. Maher JF, Schreiner GE, and Westervelt, FB: Acute glutethimide intoxication I. Clinical experience (22 patients) compared to acute barbiturate intoxication (62 patients). *Am J Med,* 33:70–82, 1962.

125. Brown DG, and Hammill JF: Glutethimide poisoning: Unilateral pupillary abnormalities. *N Engl J Med,* 285:807, 1971.

126. Curry SH, et al: Disposition of glutethimide in man. *Clin Pharmacol Ther,* 12:849–857, 1971.

127. Kadar D, et al: Comparative drug elimination capacity in man—glutethimide, amobarbital, antipyrine and sulfinpyrazone. *Clin Pharmacol Ther,* 14:552–560, 1974.

128. Chazan JA, and Garella SL: Glutethimide intoxication: A prospective study of 70 patients treated conservatively without hemodialysis. *Arch Intern Med,* 128:215–219, 1971.

129. Wright N, and Roscoe P: Acute glutethimide poisoning: Conservative management of 31 patients. *JAMA,* 214:1704–1706, 1970.

130. Chazan JA, and Cohen JJ: Clinical spectrum of glutethimide intoxication: Hemodialysis reevaluated. *JAMA,* 208:837–839, 1969.

131. Myers RR, and Stockard JJ: Neurologic and electroencephalographic correlates in glutethimide intoxication. *Clin Pharmacol Ther,* 17:212–220, 1975.

132. McDonald DG, et al: Experience in acute glutethimide (Doriden) intoxication: Superiority of extracorporeal dialysis over peritoneal dialysis. *Invest Urol,* 1:127–133, 1963.

133. King LH Jr, et al: A clinically efficient and economical lipid dialyzer: Use in treatment of glutethimide intoxication. *JAMA,* 211:652–653, 1970.

134. Rosenbaum JL, et al: Resin hemoperfusion: A new treatment for acute drug intoxication. *N Engl J Med,* 284:874–877, 1971.

135. Lloyd EA, and Clark LD: Convulsions and delirium incident to glutethimide (Doriden) withdrawal. *Dis Nerv Syst,* 20:524–526, 1959.

136. Lucy ED, and Domino EF: Additional evidence of the addiction liability of glutethimide in man. *JAMA,* 181:46–48, 1962.

137. Sadwin A, and Glen RS: Addiction to glutethimide (Doriden). *Am J Psychiatry,* 115:469–470, 1958.

138. Johnson FA, and Van Buren HC: Abstinence syndrome following glutethimide intoxication. *JAMA,* 180:1024–1027, 1962.

139. Abboud RT, et al: Methaqualone poisoning with muscular hyperactivity necessitating the use of curare. *Chest,* 65:204–205, 1974.

140. Ibe K: Acute methaqualone intoxication II. *Arch Toxicol,* 21:289–309, 1969.

141. Lawson AAH, and Brown SS: Poisoning with Mandrax. *Scott Med J,* 12:63–68, 1966.

142. Matthew H, et al: Mandax poisoning: Conservative management of 116 patients. *Br Med J,* 2:101–102, 1968.

143. MacDonald HRF, and Laksman AD: Poisoning with Mandrax. *Br Med J,* 1:500, 1967.

144. Proudfoot AT, et al: Peritoneal dialysis and hemodialysis in methaqualone (Mandrax) poisoning. *Scott Med J,* 13:232–236, 1968.

145. Sanderson JH, Cowdell RH, and Higgins G: Fatal poisoning with methaqualone and diphenhydramine. *Lancet,* 2:803–804, 1966.

146. Wallace MR, and Allen E: Recovery after massive overdose of diphenhydramine and methaqualone. *Lancet,* 2:1247, 1968.

147. Caridis DT, McAndrew GM, and Matheson NA: Hemodialysis in poisoning with methaqualone and diphenhydramine. *Lancet,* 1:51–52, 1967.

148. Huff BB: Methaqualone (Sopor). *Physicians' Desk Reference.* 34th Ed. Oradell, NJ, Medical Economics Co., 1980, p. 764.

149. Brown SS, and Goenechea S: Methaqualone: Metabolic, kinetic, and clinical pharmacologic

observations. *Clin Pharmacol Ther, 14*:314–324, 1973.

150. Bailey DN, and Jatlow PI: Methaqualone overdose: Analytical methodology, and the significance of serum drug concentrations. *Clin Chem, 19*:615–620, 1973.

151. Gerald MC, and Schwirian PM: Nonmedical use of methaqualone. *Arch Gen Psychiatry, 28*:627–631, 1973.

152. Madden JS: Dependence on methaqualone hydrochloride (Melsedin). *Br Med J, 1*:676, 1966.

153. Ewart RBL, and Priest RB: Methaqualone addiction and delirium tremens. *Br Med J, 3*:92–93, 1967.

154. Benady DR: Mandrax. *Br Med J, 1*:577–578, 1969.

155. Swartzburg M, Lieb J, and Schwartz AH. Methaqualone withdrawal. *Arch Gen Psychiatry, 29*:46–47, 1973.

Chapter 6

Narcotic Analgesics

Vasilios A. Skoutakis

Historically, the narcotic analgesics have provided the medical practitioner with one of the most valuable tools available in his clinical practice, the ability to alleviate pain. However, these same drugs have contributed to an astonishingly complex problem of widespread medical, social, and economic importance. For example, such problems as drug abuse, addiction, acute overdosages, and injuries and deaths due to narcotic analgesics have become a daily common occurrence, not only in the larger cities and city ghettos, but in college campuses and small towns as well.

Data from the Drug Abuse Warning Network (DAWN) indicate that during the spring quarter of 1976, 2496 drug-related deaths and 46,321 drug-related injuries were reported in 24 of the largest metropolitan areas in the United States. During that quarter, narcotic analgesic drugs were responsible for 30.3% of the deaths and 10.1% of the injuries.[1] Additional published reports also attest to the problem of abuse, addiction, acute overdosages, and deaths with the narcotic analgesic drugs.[2-12]

Due to widespread use, abuse, and overdosages of these drugs, and the increased morbidity and mortality rates among adults as well as pediatric patients, the clinician should be readily familiar with the recognition and management of the narcotic-intoxicated patient.

CASE REPORT

A 21-year-old male was rushed by his roommate to the Neighborhood Health Care Clinic, after being found at home lethargic, confused, and disoriented. A discussion with the roommate revealed that the patient had been moody and depressed for the previous 2 weeks and that he had a history of past parenteral drug abuse. At this time, however, the roommate stated that he was not able to detect any evidence (empty medicine bottles, pills, or syringes) of drug overdosage or parenteral drug abuse.

At the clinic, the patient was noted to be lethargic, cyanotic, and in moderate respiratory distress. His pupils were pinpoint and nonreactive to light. Vital signs were pulse rate, 80 beats/min; respirations, 8/min; blood pressure, 118/78 mm Hg; and temperature, 37°C. No alcoholic odor was present on the breath. Naloxone hydrochloride (Narcan), 0.4 mg, was administered intravenously. Within 2 minutes, the pupils returned to normal size, the level of consciousness improved, and breathing recovered immediately. An oral dose of magnesium citrate was given, and the patient was transported to the University of Tennessee Medical Center.

Upon arrival, the ambulance team reported that en route to the Medical Center, the patient complained of nausea and vomited once. On admission, the patient was comatose and unresponsive to painful stimuli. Vital signs at this time were blood pressure, 120/60 mm Hg; pulse rate, 105 beats/min and irregular; respirations, 7/min and shallow; and temperature, 36°C. The lungs were clear to auscultation and percussion. The abdominal examination revealed diminished bowel sounds but no tenderness. The electrocardiogram indicated nonspecific ST-segment and T-wave abnormalities. Examination of the extremities and skin failed to show any pathologic findings. Chest x-ray examination, electrolytes, urinalysis, and complete blood count results were within normal limits.

CLINICAL ASSESSMENT AND MANAGEMENT OF THE PATIENT

In this case, we were presented with a patient who had a history of parenteral drug abuse, and who had been moody and depressed for a period of 2 weeks. Physical examinations upon admission at both the Neighborhood Health Care Clinic and The University of Tennessee Medical Center revealed signs and symptoms of (1) respiratory depression, (2) impaired level of consciousness, (3) pinpoint pupils, (4) hypotension, (5) hypothermia, and (6) decreased bowel sounds. These symptoms in addition to the patient's responsiveness to the administration of naloxone, strongly suggested an overdosage with narcotic analgesic drugs. However, the differential diagnosis as to the specific agents(s) involved or the possibility of mixed drug overdosage (i.e., other CNS depressants) could not be made clinically at this time.

The appropriate management of this patient or other patients intoxicated with a narcotic analgesic drug demands consideration of the following: (1) drugs classified as narcotic analgesics, (2) manifestations and mechanisms of action of narcotic analgesic drugs in intoxicated patients, (3) pharmacokinetic properties of the narcotic analgesic drugs, (4) role of the toxicology laboratory, (5) indicated therapeutic measures, (6) manifestations and treatment of infant withdrawal, and (7) general prognosis.

DRUGS CLASSIFIED AS NARCOTIC ANALGESICS

The narcotic analgesics or opioids include the naturally occurring alkaloids and many related semisynthetic and synthetic drugs that effectively relieve pain without producing loss of consciousness, and that have the potential to produce tolerance and physical and psychological dependence.[13-17] These drugs are subject to control under Title II of the Comprehensive Drug Abuse Prevention and Control Act of 1970 (Public Law 91–513), commonly known as the Controlled Substance Act.[18]

The commonly used and abused narcotic analgesics may be classified as derivatives of (1) the natural opium alkaloids, (2) the semisynthetic opiates, and (3) the synthetic narcotic analgesic drugs.

Natural Opium Alkaloids

These drugs have long been in use and are alkaloids obtained from opium, which is the dried exudate of the unripe seed capsule of the poppy plant Papaver somniferum, indigenous to Asia Minor. At least 25 different alkaloids are found in opium. They constitute about 25% by weight of opium and fall into two distinct chemical classes, namely the *phenanthrenes* and *benzylisoquinolines*. The pharmacologic properties of the phenanthrenes and benzylisoquinolines, however, are different. The phenanthrene group contains the only two important narcotic analgesics found in opium, morphine and codeine, which are used as analgesics and cough suppressants. The main opium alkaloids found in the benzylisoquinoline group are papaverine (an intestinal relaxant), and noscapine (a cough suppressant); they lack morphine-like effects and are not subject to control under the Federal Controlled Substance Act of 1970.[18] The main al-

kaloids that occur naturally in opium, their approximate percentages, and therapeutic indications are listed in Table 6–1.

The basic phenanthrene structure found in opium is shown in Figure 6–1 (see Table 6–2). Morphine, the prototype narcotic analgesic, has hydroxyl groups (OH) at positions C-3 and C-6 of the basic phenanthrene structure. Codeine, which also is a normal constituent of opium, having analgesic and cough-suppressant properties, has a hydroxyl group at C-6, but a methoxy (OCH_3) group at C-3. Morphine also can be synthesized in the laboratory, but with difficulty. However, derivatives of morphine can be made by relatively simple modification of the morphine molecule, resulting in the production of the so-called semisynthetic opiate derivatives.

Semisynthetic Opiate Derivatives

Substitution at C-3 and C-6 of the morphine molecule by different chemical radical groups yields drugs of varying interest and importance. All of these drugs, however, possess narcotic analgesic activity. The best known and most abused semisynthetic opiate drug is diacetylmorphine or heroin. Heroin is prepared by the acetylation of morphine, resulting in esterification ($OCO-CH_3$) of both hydroxyl groups at C-3 and C-6 in the morphine molecule. Other semisynthetic opium alkaloids that have been prepared by chemical treatment of the basic morphine molecule and their structural relationships to the morphine molecule are also shown in Table 6–2.

Although substitution at C-3 and C-6 in

Table 6–1. Alkaloids of Opium.

CHEMICAL CLASS	NATURAL ALKALOID	PERCENTAGE IN OPIUM	THERAPEUTIC INDICATIONS
Phenanthrene	Morphine	10.0	Narcotic analgesic
	Codeine	0.5	Narcotic analgesic/ cough suppressant
	Thebaine	0.2	
Benzylisoquinolines	Papaverine	1.0	Smooth muscle relaxant
	Noscapine	6.0	Antitussive

Table 6–2.   The Naturally Occurring Opium Alkaloids and Opioid Antagonists as Chemically Related to Morphine.

GENERIC NAME	TRADE NAME	CHEMICAL GROUPS AND POSITIONS ON MORPHINE MOLECULE (see Fig. 6–1)			
		C-3	C-6	C-17	OTHER CHANGES*
Morphine		—OH	—OH	—CH₃	—
Heroin (Diacetylmorphine)		—OCOCH₃	—OCOCH₃	—CH₃	—
Hydromorphone (Dihydromorphinone)	Dilaudid	—OH	=O	—CH₃	1
Oxymorphone (Dihydrohydroxy-morphinone)	Numorphan	—OH	=O	—CH₃	1, 2
Levorphanol	Levo-dromoran	—OH	—H	—CH₃	1, 3
Codeine		—OCH₃	—OH	—CH₃	—
Hydrocodone (Dihydrocodeinone)	Hycodan†	—OCH₃	=O	—CH₃	1
Oxycodone (Dihydrohydroxy-codeinone)	Percodan†	—OCH₃	=O	—CH₃	1, 2
Nalorphine	Nalline	—OH	—OH	—CH₂CH₂=CH₂	—
Naloxone	Narcan	—OH	=O	—CH₂CH₂=CH₂	1, 2
Naltrexone	—	—OH	=O	—CH₂–◁	1, 2
Butorphanol	Stadol	—OH	—H	—CH₂–◇	2, 3
Nalbuphine	Nubaine	—OH	—OH	—CH₂–◇	1, 2

* Other changes in the morphine molecule are as follows:
    1—Single instead of double bond between C-7 and C-8.
    2—OH added to C-14.
    3—No oxygen between C-4 and C-5.
† These opioids are marketed in the United States only in combination with additional ingredients.

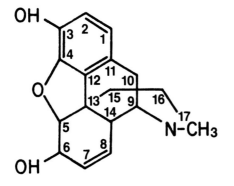

MORPHINE

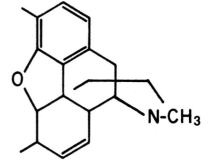

PHENANTHRENE NUCLEUS

Fig. 6–1.   Morphine and phenanthrene nucleus (see Table 6–2).

the morphine molecule yields semisynthetic opium alkaloids with narcotic analgesic activity, the substitution of an allyl group ($CH_2CH_2 = CH_2$) for the N-methyl group at C-17 of the morphine molecule produces nalorphine (Nalline), which possesses analgesic as well as narcotic antagonistic actions. Similarly, other narcotic analgesics, such as levallorphan (Lorfan) and naloxone (Narcan), have been prepared by substitutions at C-3, C-6, or C-17 of the morphine molecule. The structural relationships of morphine to its narcotic antagonists are also shown in Table 6–2.

Synthetic Narcotic Analgesics

In addition to morphine, codeine, and the semisynthetic derivatives of the natural opium alkaloids, a number of synthetic narcotic analgesic drugs have a range of pharmacodynamic actions similar to morphine (e.g., selective analgesia, respiratory depression, GI spasm, and morphine-like physical and psychological dependence). A stereochemical configuration resembling the structure of morphine molecule in three-dimensional space. and thus the ability to fit the same receptor site, is thought to be

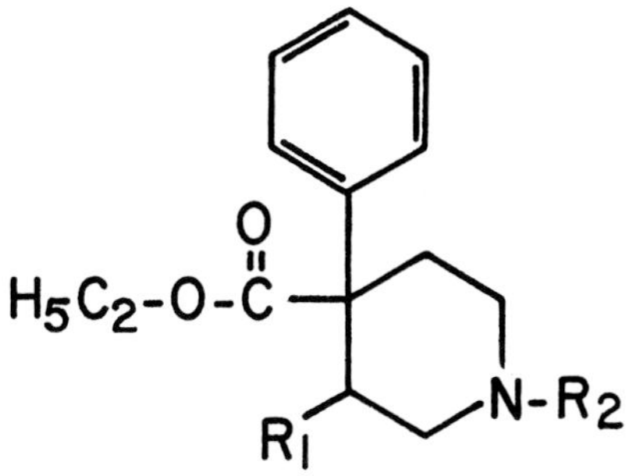

	R_1	R_2
Meperidine (Demerol)	-H	$-CH_3$
Alphaprodine (Nisentil)	$-CH_3$	$-CH_3$
Anileridine (Leritine)	-H	$-CH_2-CH_2-$⟨⟩ 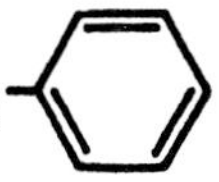
Piminodine (Alvodine)	-H	$-CH_2-CH_2-CH_2-NH-$⟨⟩ 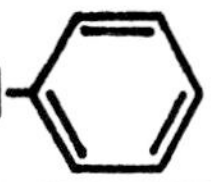
Diphenoxylate (in Lomotil)	-H	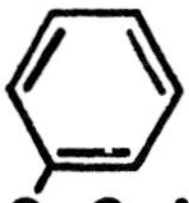 $-CH_2-CH_2-C-C≡N$ 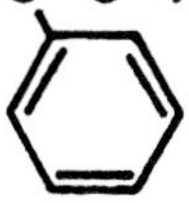

Fig. 6–2. Meperidine and related synthetic analgesics of the phenylpiperidine type.

responsible for the similarity of pharmacologic, therapeutic, and toxicologic actions between morphine and the semisynthetic and synthetic narcotic analgesic drugs.[19,20] The pharmacologic actions of these synthetic drugs also can be reversed by the use of narcotic antagonists.[21-24]

Chemically, the synthetic narcotic analgesics can be classified as (a) phenylpiperidine derivatives and (b) diphenylheptane derivatives.

Phenylpiperidine derivatives. Meperidine (Demerol) is the prototype of the phenylpiperidine-derived narcotic analgesics. Replacement of the N-methyl group of meperidine at position R_1 with different chemical radical groups produces a number of drugs with different analgesic activities and therapeutic indications. Figure 6–2 summarizes the structural relationship between meperidine and its surrogates.

Diphenylheptane derivatives. Methadone (Dolophine) is the only commercially available narcotic analgesic that is a diphenylheptane derivative. Propoxyphene (Darvon) is not considered a narcotic analgesic, but its structural, pharmacologic, and toxicologic properties are closely related to those of methadone (Fig. 6–3). Furthermore, propoxyphene is not under the control of the Federal Controlled Substances Act of 1970.[18]

The narcotic analgesic drugs vary in structural, quantitative, and even some qualitative effects. Although the degree of severity of the intoxication might be different, the symptoms, toxicologic manifestations, and therapeutic management of patients intoxicated with narcotic analgesics are similar.

MANIFESTATIONS AND MECHANISMS OF NARCOTIC ANALGESIC INTOXICATION

As in the case presented, the toxicologic manifestations of the narcotic-intoxicated patient include CNS depression ranging from stupor to a profound coma, respiratory depression possibly progressing to Cheyne-Stokes respiration and/or cyanosis, cold clammy skin and/or hypothermia, miosis, bradycardia, hypotension, flaccid skeletal muscles, decreased urinary output, and decreased GI motility. In patients with severe overdosage, apnea, circulatory collapse, cardiac arrest, and death can occur.[1,2,4,5-12] The narcotic analgesic drugs, therefore, produce their toxicologic manifestations by acting on the CNS, cardiovascular, and GI organ systems.

Central Nervous System

The effects of narcotic analgesic drugs on the CNS are complex and comprise both depressant and stimulant actions depending

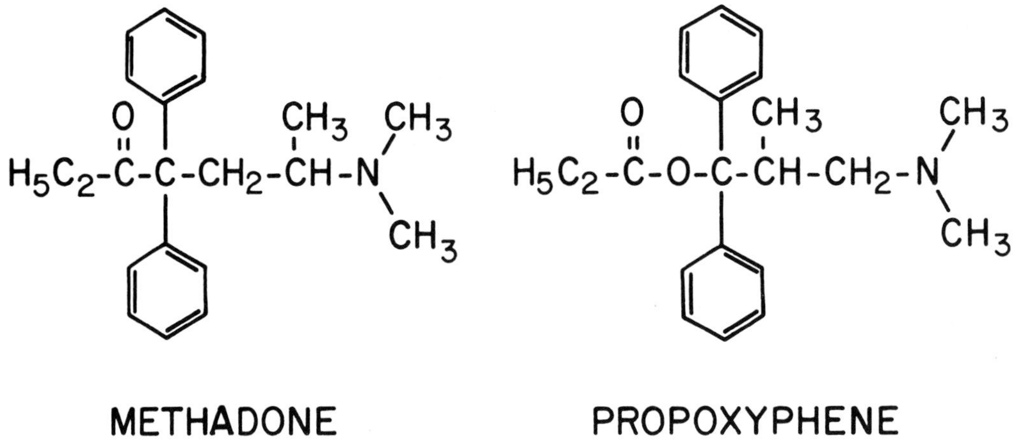

METHADONE   **PROPOXYPHENE**

Fig. 6–3. Diphenylheptane derivatives: Similarities of methadone and propoxyphene.

on the dose, the site of action, and biochemical variations among individuals. The predominant effects, however, are those of CNS depression and are manifested by analgesic and/or euphoric, sedative-hypnotic, respiratory-depressant, and endocrinologic actions. The stimulant effects are manifested by nausea and emesis, miosis, bradycardia, intestinal spasticity (see discussion of GI system), and general excitatory effects.[16,17,25-30]

Analgesic and/or euphoric effects. The strict structural requirements of narcotic analgesic drugs, their potency, stereochemistry, and the existence of agonists and antagonists all favor the proposal that the narcotic drugs exert their analgesic action by binding to specific opiate receptors in the brain and other body tissues. These binding sites are widely but unevenly distributed throughout the CNS. They are present in highest concentrations in the limbic system (frontal and temporal cortex, amygdala, and hippocampus), thalamus, striatum, hypothalamus, midbrain, and spinal cord.[31,32] The affinity of the narcotic analgesic drugs for these binding sites correlates closely with their potency as analgesics. It is postulated, therefore, that by binding to specific opiate receptors, the narcotic analgesic drugs, or endogenously produced, morphine-like peptides (endorphins), alter the central release of neurotransmitters from afferent nerves sensitive to noxious stimuli, and consequently produce their analgesic effects.[26,29,30-33]

The mechanisms by which the narcotic analgesic drugs produce euphoria, tranquility, and other alterations of mood are not clearly defined. However, the *locus ceruleus* contains both nonadrenaletic neurons and highly sensitive opioid receptors and is postulated to play a critical role in feelings of alarm, panic, fear, and anxiety. Activity in the locus ceruleus is inhibited by alpha-adrenergic agonists and by exogenously administered narcotic drugs or endogenously produced, morphine-like peptides.[17,34-36]

Sedative-hypnotic effects. The narcotic analgesic drugs in therapeutic doses produce drowsiness, lethargy, apathy, or mental confusion in both patients and normal volunteers. In the presence of pain, sedation and hypnosis may result from relief of pain and from its accompanying mental and physical exhaustion. As the dose is increased, or in cases of acute overdosages, the sedative-hypnotic effects become more pronounced and are manifested by increased drowsiness that can lead to sleep and/or profound coma. The site of the sedative-hypnotic action of narcotic analgesic drugs appears to lie in the sensory area of the cerebral cortex.[16,17,25,26,29,30]

Respiratory effects. The brain stem respiratory centers are highly sensitive to narcotic analgesic drugs and are depressed by even small doses.[16,17,25,29,30,37] The narcotic analgesic drugs depress all components of respiratory activity (e.g., rate, minute volume, tidal exchange) and may induce irregular and periodic breathing. In humans, death from narcotic analgesic overdosage is nearly always due to respiratory arrest. The mechanism by which the narcotic analgesic drugs cause respiratory depression involves a reduction in the responsiveness of the brain stem respiratory centers to increases in carbon dioxide tension (P_{CO_2}).[17,29,37,38] The mechanism of irregular and periodic breathing is believed to be related to the depression of the pontine and medullary centers, which are responsible for regulating respiratory rhythmicity.[38,39]

Endocrinologic effects. Cold, clammy skin and/or hypothermia and decreased urinary output are usually present in narcotic-intoxicated patients. The mechanism responsible for hypothermia involves the alteration or suppression of the equilibrium point of the hypothalamic heat-regulatory mechanisms.[17,25,26,28,40,41] The mechanism responsible for the decreased urinary output can be related to the release of antidiuretic hormone (ADH). This action is mediated through the hypothalamus.[17,25,40] However, the oliguria that follows during an acute overdose with narcotic analgesic drugs may also represent a direct renal effect or a hemodynamic effect.[42]

Nausea and emetic effects. Nausea and vomiting commonly occur during the initial phase of intoxication with narcotic analgesic drugs. These effects are the results of direct stimulation of the chemoreceptor trigger zone (CTZ) for emesis, in the area postrema of the medulla.[17,25,29,30] Nausea is less likely to occur, however, in the recumbent intoxicated patient. This suggests that the sensitivity of the vestibular system is also increased by the narcotic analgesic drugs.[17,25,43]

Pupil reaction. The narcotic analgesic drugs also have an effect on the pupil, causing miosis. Therefore, when a patient has had an acute overdosage, and if constriction of the pupil (miosis) is present, it is a pathognomonic sign of narcotic intoxication, since tolerance to the miotic action of the narcotic analgesic drugs does not occur. If asphyxia intervenes, however, mydriasis is commonly present, and miosis cannot be used as a pathognomonic sign of narcotic intoxication. The exact mechanism of the miotic action of the narcotic analgesic drugs is not clearly established, but it is believed to be mediated through stimulation of the third cranial nerve nucleus.[17,25,29,30,44]

Bradycardic effects. Slowing in heart rate is commonly observed in narcotic-intoxicated patients. This is the result of stimulation of vagal centers or possibly of a selective depression of the supramedullary centers, which can lead to suppression of autonomic reflexes.[16,17,25,27,30,38] Sinoauricular and atrioventricular nodal bradycardia was noted in patients anesthetized with cyclopropane who were premedicated with meperidine and morphine. The intravenous administration of atropine was followed within 30 seconds by the appearance of sinus tachycardia. Patients not receiving narcotics before cyclopropane, however, did not develop slower heart rates. This observation suggests that narcotics may increase vagal

tone and, as a consequence, a slowing in heart rate.[38,45,46]

General excitatory effects. The narcotic analgesic drugs, when ingested in large doses, can produce convulsions. The cortex seems to be directly affected, since the administration of morphine either topically or systemically produces a prolongation of induced after-discharge in the isolated cortex. Seizure-like activity also can be seen unilaterally in the electrocorticograms of dogs given large systemic doses of morphine and methadone.[18,25,26,29,30,47,48]

Cardiovascular System

In therapeutic doses, the narcotic analgesic drugs exert little or no major effects on cardiovascular function (e.g., blood pressure, cardiac rate, or rhythm).[17,38] In cases of acute intoxications, however, hypotension and cardiac arrhythmias have been described,[38,49-52] and are usually the results of hypoxia rather than the direct effects of these drugs on the cardiovascular system. Thus, administration of oxygen usually causes the blood pressure to rise despite the persistence of medullary depression.[38]

In patients severely intoxicated with narcotic analgesic drugs, however, circulatory collapse, cardiac arrest, and deaths have been reported,[11,12,38,53-55] and are usually the results of (1) peripheral arteriolar and venous dilatation (liberation of histamine, which leads to dilation of peripheral blood vessels and pooling of blood), (2) direct depression of the vasomotor center (central suppression of adrenergic tone, which blunts the reflex vasoconstriction caused by increased P_{CO_2}), and (3) direct myocardial depression (depression in myocardial contractility and an increase in the susceptibility of the heart to potassium ions).[38,56]

Gastrointestinal System

The narcotic analgesic drugs cause a decrease in gastric motility, and an increase in the tone of the antral portion of the stomach, which delays the passage of gastric contents through the duodenum and often results in constipation.[16,17,25,27] These drugs increase the resting tone of the smooth muscle of the small and large intestine almost to a point of spasm and decrease propulsive peristaltic movements. The tone of the ileocecal valve and the anal sphincter also is greatly increased. These actions also contribute to the constipating effects of these drugs.[17,25,27] The tone of the bronchial smooth muscle and of the smooth muscle of the biliary tract is also greatly augmented and, as a result, bronchial and biliary secretions are decreased or inhibited.[17,25]

PHARMACOKINETIC PROPERTIES OF THE NARCOTIC ANALGESIC DRUGS

The narcotic analgesic drugs are readily absorbed from the GI tract, as well as from the nasal mucosa (e.g., heroin sniffing), the lungs (e.g., opium smoking) and after subcutaneous or intramuscular administration. The effect of a given dose, however, is lower after oral ingestion, nasal sniffing, or smoking as compared to parenteral administration because of the significant "first pass effect," which results in vastly different amounts of the narcotic analgesic drugs being metabolized by the liver immediately after absorption.[25,57,58]

The distribution of narcotic analgesic drugs is similar to that of organic bases in general. Thus, drugs pass through membranes in undissociated form. The acidic compounds, which are mostly ionized at blood pH, tend to be distributed extracellularly and to be excreted rapidly in the urine. In contrast, basic compounds exist in sufficient quantities in the undissociated form at pH 7.4 to favor penetration into cells and as a result are less available for excretory mechanisms.

Indeed, shortly after absorption, the narcotic analgesic drugs become concentrated in tissues, especially kidney, liver, skeletal muscle, lung, and spleen, and the concentrations therein quickly exceed those in blood.[59] The fact that opiate-dependent babies are born to addicted mothers serves also as dramatic proof of the passage of opiates through the placenta.[60,61] Furthermore, the levels of these drugs in the CNS have been reported to correlate well with the onsets, intensities, and durations of their analgesic effects,[62,63] although a barrier to the passage of these drugs from the blood into the CNS exists such that the concentrations found in the brain are low.[64,65]

Narcotic analgesics are metabolized primarily in the liver, the major site being the microsomes in the endoplasmic reticulum. These drugs are also metabolized in the CNS, kidneys, lungs and placenta. The narcotic analgesic drugs undergo conjugation with glucuronic acid, hydrolysis, oxidation, and/or N-dealkylation. They are excreted primarily in the urine in the unchanged form and as metabolites. Small amounts are also excreted in the feces.[16,17,25,58,66-69]

ROLE OF THE TOXICOLOGY LABORATORY

Although with certain drug overdosages, the services of the toxicology laboratory can assist the clinician, in the case of a narcotic-intoxicated patient the services of the toxicology laboratory are of limited value or unnecessary for the following reasons. (1) In narcotic overdose cases, even if the agent ingested is not known or the history is questionable or unavailable, the administration of naloxone will quickly provide the information necessary to confirm the suspected diagnosis. (2) Determination of a lethal dose and/or therapeutic or lethal levels is useless, not only because of the concept of tolerance and the great variability in active drug concentrations found in street preparations, but because the quantitative identification of these drugs is done with great difficulty, and time is a major factor.

(3) The therapeutic approaches in the treatment of these patients will be the same regardless of the narcotic agent involved and the dosage ingested or administered. (4) Frequent monitoring of serum drug levels to assess the patient's progress while hospitalized is unnecessary because the intermittent or continuous administration of naloxone according to the patient's clinical manifestations will negate the actions of the narcotic agent. Emergency toxicologic measurements can be costly to the patient, and generally they are not justified in many narcotic overdose situations.

The services of the toxicology laboratory are necessary or advisable, however, when the patient has had a multiple drug overdose, when a multiple or mixed overdose has been suspected, or when the patient is not responding to the administration of naloxone. Additionally, toxicology laboratory analysis may be advisable in cases of heroin overdosages, for identification of possible adulterants (e.g. strychnine, phencyclidine, quinine), which may require specific therapeutic interventions.

In the case presented, results of a qualitative analysis of the urine were positive for morphine. Upon further questioning, the patient admitted that he had injected a "fix" (one dose) of heroin 2 hours prior to admission. Furthermore, the overdose was attributed to misinformation regarding the concentration of the heroin purchased from the street.

Early studies of narcotic metabolism indicated that heroin is rapidly deacetylated to morphine in many tissues and is then excreted primarily in the urine as free morphine and its glucuronide conjugate (with recovery of up to 60% of an intravenous dose).[58,66,68,69] Heroin infusion studies in man have indicated that morphine excretion occurs up to 40.5 hours following termination of drug administration, allowing derivation of a theoretical maximum heroin disposition of 6.0 mg/93 kg/hr.[70] Therefore, during acute overdose situations, frequent monitoring of these patients for up to 48 or 72 hours for the detection, prevention, and/or correction of possible complications, in addition to intermittent naloxone administration, is essential.

INDICATED THERAPEUTIC MEASURES

The approach to the management of the narcotic-intoxicated patient can be divided into five phases: (1) emergency measures, (2) nonspecific therapy, (3) specific therapy, (4) symptomatic care and prevention and treatment of possible complications, and (5) detoxification.

Emergency Measures

The key principle in the treatment of the narcotic-intoxicated patient is to concentrate on support of the vital functions before any other treatment measures are attempted. The patient, therefore, should be assessed promptly upon arrival in the emergency room and the need for immediate intervention determined. If the patient is apneic, for example, he should be intubated with a cuffed endotracheal tube and attached to a respirator. If the patient is hypotensive, an intravenous line should be inserted, and fluid therapy replacement should be initiated. Hypotension usually responds to correction of hypoxia and moderate fluid replacement. Fluids should not be administered too vigorously, however, or problems with pulmonary congestion may ensue, since these patients are not fundamentally volume depleted. On rare occasions, plasma expanders or pressor amines may be required for the control of blood pressure. The use of CNS stimulants should be avoided.

Once the vital functions are adequate or supported, available historical data should be gathered, and a physical examination should be performed. Subsequently, 10 ml of arterial blood should be collected for blood gas determination and 20 ml of venous blood for biochemical, hematologic and toxicologic analysis. An EKG and chest x-ray examination should be performed. If comatose, the patient should be catheterized and 350 ml of urine collected and sent to appropriate laboratories for urinalysis and drug screen for opiates and sedative-hypnotics. The information obtained from the physical examination and the laboratory will constitute the data base for future decisions and the formulation of a treatment plan.

In the present case, once the patient's vital signs (e.g., respiration, blood pressure, pulse rate, and body temperature), level of consciousness, deep tendon reflexes, and pupil size and reactivity were assessed and recorded, the oropharynx was suctioned, a sample of arterial blood for blood gas determination was promptly drawn, and a cuffed endotracheal tube was inserted and connected to 90% oxygen. (A word of caution regarding the administration of oxygen: One of the mechanisms of narcotic-induced depression of respiration is decreased sensitivity of brain stem receptors to rising P_{CO_2}. Therefore, some patients will be utilizing the hypoxic respiratory drive as a stimulus to breathe. If oxygen is given injudiciously or withdrawn abruptly, the hypoxic stimulus may be absent or may disappear, and the patient may become apneic. In severe overdosages with narcotic analgesic drugs, the use of a mechanical respirator is advisable.)

Subsequently, access to the circulation was established via an intravenous line, blood was obtained for hematologic (Hemo-10 with differentials), biochemical (SMA-12), and basic toxicologic screening (opiates and sedative-hypnotics), and dextrose (5% in ½-normal saline solution at a rate of 175 ml/hr) was administered. In addition, an EKG and an x-ray examination were performed, the patient was catheterized, and 350 ml of urine was collected and sent to the laboratory for urinalysis and drug screening for opiates and sedative-hypnotics.

Nonspecific Therapy

The overall objective of nonspecific therapy is the prevention of further absorption of the ingested drug. Therefore, if drug ingestion has occurred within the previous 4 to 6 hours, emesis should be initiated unless the patient is comatose, convulsing, or without the gag reflex. The narcotic analgesic drugs reduce gastric emptying time and peristalsis, and a large quantity of the ingested dose may remain in the stomach. In addition, revival of the patient may reinstitute peristalsis and cause further absorption of the ingested drug. Therefore, initiation of emesis following revival of the intoxicated patient is recommended.

Syrup of ipecac should be used to induce emesis. The pediatric dose is 15 ml and the adult dose is 30 ml; these should be given with two or more glasses of water. Emesis will usually occur within 30 minutes. If emesis does not occur, the dose of syrup of ipecac can be repeated, but not more than twice.

If contraindications to emesis exist, endotracheal intubation should precede gastric lavage and should be followed by the administration of activated charcoal (30 to 50 g) in a water slurry, given orally or through the lavage tube. A cathartic such as sodium sulfate or magnesium sulfate (250 mg/kg) also should be administered, orally or through the lavage tube, to promote the evacuation of the ingested drug. The initial gastric contents (approximately 300 ml) should be collected and sent to the toxicology laboratory for analysis in cases of unknown intoxications or multiple ingestions.

Specific Therapy

Presently, three narcotic antagonists are available, which the clinician may use to confirm the diagnosis or reverse the coma, respiratory depression, miosis, and convulsions produced by the narcotic analgesic agents. These are (1) nalorphine, (2) levallorphan, and (3) naloxone.[16,17,21–24,71] However, although all three drugs are narcotic antagonists, the pharmacologic actions of nalorphine and levallorphan are quite different from those of naloxone. These differences become important when the clinician has to decide which agent to use, particularly when dealing with unknown intoxicants.

Nalorphine and levallorphan have almost identical pharmacologic actions. Both agents can reverse the respiratory-depressant effects produced by the narcotic analgesic drugs, with the exception of pentazocine. However, when given in the absence of narcotic analgesics, both nalorphine and levallorphan produce effects like those of narcotic analgesics (e.g., analgesia, respiratory depression, pupillary constriction, and physical dependence following chronic administration). In addition, both of these drugs will produce withdrawal symptoms in the narcotic-dependent individual.[17,21–24,38,71–73] Therefore, they are classified as partial rather than pure antagonists of narcotic analgesic drugs, and their use is not recommended for the treatment of narcotic analgesic poisonings.

Naloxone was the first pure antagonist to be discovered, and is the recommended drug of choice for the treatment of narcotic intoxications, including narcotic depression of the newborn and narcotic analgesia.[17,21–24,71,72] Furthermore, although naloxone is similar to morphine, it does not possess morphine-like activity and is not controlled under the Federal Controlled Substances Act of 1970.[18] Naloxone is a specific antagonist for all narcotic analgesics, including pentazocine, and is capable of reversing the respiratory depression and psychotomimetic disturbances induced by nalorphine and levallorphan.[17,21–24,71,72] In addition, naloxone is capable of reversing the coma, respiratory depression, pupillary constriction, and convulsions produced by propoxyphene.[74,75]

The recommended initial dose of naloxone in adults is 0.4 mg IV. In neonates and children, the recommended dose of naloxone is 0.01 mg/kg of body weight, and it may be administered subcutaneously or intramuscularly.[21,23,24,71,72] Naloxone is rapidly absorbed when administered subcutaneously or intramuscularly and readily crosses the blood-brain barrier. Its duration of action is short, and the serum half-life is just over 1 hour.[76,77] The intravenous administration, however, assures the most rapid, reliable onset of action, and is the recommended route to be used.[17,21–24,71,72,76,77]

In the patient reported here, subsequent to the implementation of the immediate supportive measures at the University of Tennessee Medical Center, and because a history of drug ingestion was not available, 0.4 mg of naloxone (Narcan) were administered intravenously, with no response from the patient. This dose was followed by the administration of three additional doses of naloxone, 0.4 mg each at 6- to 8-minute intervals. Within 2 minutes of the last dose, the pupils returned to normal size, the level of consciousness improved, and breathing recovered immediately. Respiratory depression induced by sedative-hypnotic drugs or other CNS depressants would not have been reversed following the administration of naloxone.

Thereafter, a solution of 4 mg of naloxone in 1 L of D_5W (5% dextrose in water) was prepared and administered IV at 100 ml/min. The rationale for the continuous intravenous administration of naloxone in this patient was based on the following considerations. (1) Because the antagonist effects of naloxone are relatively short-lived, and because the unknown intoxicant possibly was a long-acting narcotic such as methadone, we found it necessary to administer naloxone by continuous intravenous infusion to maintain an adequate therapeutic effect. (2) The continuous infusion of naloxone decreases the incidence of respiratory arrest, which is the major cause of death in these patients, by providing steady-state CNS levels of naloxone. (3) There are no contraindications to the use of naloxone. Doses of up to 24 mg have been administered to narcotic-intoxicated patients during the entire course of hospitalization, without any side effects.[23,78,79]

In the administration of naloxone by any route (intramuscular, subcutaneous, or intravenous), however, it is extremely important that the vital signs and overall clinical condition be monitored closely and frequently. Patients who have been under the effects of large doses of narcotics for several hours, who have past medical histories of narcotic drug abuse, will have acute and chronic physical drug dependencies, and excessive doses of naloxone can precipitate withdrawal signs and symptoms.[21–24,71,72] These symptoms, or the abstinence syndrome, can be manifested as nausea, vomiting, hyperactive bowel sounds, tachycardia, mydriasis, elevated blood pressure, tachypnea, rhinorrhea, yawning, piloerection (gooseflesh), myalgias and cramps, tremors, excitement, and discomfort (see the following section on the abstinence syndrome and its treatment). These symptoms begin to subside, however, about 30 to 60 minutes after cessation of naloxone administration.

In the present case, shortly after the continuous intravenous administration of naloxone was established, the endotracheal intubation was removed from the patient, and no abstinence or withdrawal symptoms were observed during the treatment. The total intravenous dose of naloxone administered to this patient during his entire hospitalization (72 hours) was 9.5 mg.

Symptomatic Care and Prevention and Treatment of Possible Complications

Patients intoxicated with heroin or other narcotic analgesic drugs should be observed closely until they are stable. For example, any patient who requires naloxone for the reversal of respiratory depression and coma should be hospitalized for at least 24 hours. Pulmonary edema, if present, indicates hospitalization for 24 to 48 hours. In addition, hospitalization will allow the opportunity for the clinician to further evaluate the patient with regard to general medical assessment and to prevent, detect, and correct possible disorders or complications. The disorders most frequently seen during the recovery phase of heroin or other narcotic analgesic overdosages are pulmonary, cardiac, GI, and renal complications.

PULMONARY DISORDERS

In addition to decreased respiratory rate or respiratory arrest, discussed in the preceding section of this chapter, three major complications commonly occur in overdosages with heroin and other narcotic analgesic drugs: pulmonary edema, aspiration pneumonia, and embolization.[11,12,80–86]

Pulmonary edema. Since its first description by Olser,[85] narcotic-induced pulmonary edema has been cited with increasing frequency as a clinical entity and an autopsy finding.[11,12,80–86] Pulmonary edema was the most common (57%) of the complications noted in a series of 28 cases.[84] In all cases, it was clinically suspected on the basis of rales or rhonchi upon auscultation of the chest, and in all cases in which x-ray examinations were performed, this impression was confirmed. The x-ray examination most often will reveal bilateral, fluffy, ill-defined perihilar densities with a normal heart configuration. Drug-induced pulmonary edema is not peculiar to heroin. It has been reported also with morphine,[85] propoxyphene,[87] codeine,[88] and methadone.[89]

The cause of heroin-induced pulmonary edema has not been firmly established, but recent evidence implicates anoxia in connection with altered pulmonary capillary permeability. Patients with narcotic induced pulmonary edema usually respond satisfactorily to a narcotic antagonist, intubation, mechanical ventilation, and oxygen therapy. Although presently a proper clinical study is lacking, a review of the literature indicates that diuretics, digitalis, and other therapeutic regimens for the treatment of pulmonary edema are not recommended in this situation.

Aspiration pneumonia. The narcotic-intoxicated patient frequently develops aspiration pneumonia as a result of vomiting or a popular street remedy, in which an obtunded patient is forced to take milk or cocoa.[90] In these cases, the aspirated substances usually end up in the lower lobe of the right lung. The cornerstone of treatment of aspiration pneumonia consists of standard supportive measures. Some clinicians will administer steroids for 1 or 2 days to decrease the inflammatory response, but this method of treatment has not been widely accepted. The prophylactic use of antibiotics should be avoided, however, in all cases.

Embolization. This complication usually occurs as a result of distant septic foci (e.g., thrombophebitis), or because of insoluble adulterants present in heroin. Embolization, therefore, initiates bacterial pneumonitis, foreign body granuloma, and pulmonary fibrosis.[11,12,80-82] Lipoid pneumonia also may occur as a result of another folklore remedy, which consists of intravenous milk injection ("milk run"). Treatment should consist of the administration of penicillin, 20,000,000 units/day IV or, in case of staphylococci, oxacillin, 12 g/day IV. In addition, anticoagulation and,

possibly, surgical intervention should be performed if there is an abscess formation close to the vein, or if emoblization continues despite therapy.

CARDIAC DISORDERS

Arrhythmias and endocarditis are the two major cardiac complications of heroin and other abused narcotic drugs.[11,12,38,49-52, 80-86]

Arrhythmias. A variety of cardiac abnormalities have been described in narcotic analgesic overdosages, especially in heroin overdose patients, including arrhythmias, gallop rhythm, cardiac enlargement, elevated central venous pressure, low cardiac output, and left ventricular failure.[38,49-52] In the majority of overdose cases, however, arrhythmia is the most common abnormality, and it is the result of hypoxia. Arrhythmias usually can be corrected by the administration of oxygen, and specific antiarrhythmic drugs are rarely needed.

Endocarditis. Bacterial or fungal endocarditis is a well known infectious complication in intravenous drug users. The occurrence of bacterial and fungal endocarditis among drug users has been reviewed by Louria and associates,[80] and by Shapira.[82] In summary, two clinical patterns of endocarditis seem to occur in narcotic drug users and can be distinguished according to whether the lesion involves the right or left side of the heart.

Right-sided endocarditis always affects a previously normal tricuspid valve, and the pulmonary valve is not involved. Right-sided endocarditis is usually caused by Staphylococcus aureus and almost never by a fungus, an unusual organism for these patients. Streptococcus viridans is the most common organism responsible for the development of right-sided endocarditis in nonaddicts. Right-sided endocarditis is accompanied by septic pulmonary emboli in almost all cases. Embolization of a systemic organ, usually the brain, spleen, or kidney, has been described with right-sided endocarditis. The presence of septic pulmonary infarcts is a valuable clue to the diagnosis of right-sided endocarditis, since in many cases there are no physical findings to implicate the tricuspid valve.[91,92,93]

The second distinct pattern is that of left-sided endocarditis, in which physical signs of valvular disease are invariably apparent. Either the aortic or the mitral valve may be affected, but when both valves are involved simultaneously, the aortic lesion is usually the more severe. The infecting bacterial organism is usually some form of streptococcus, but other pathogens, including fungi, are common. If the endocarditis is caused by a fungus, prior valve damage is possible.

The general treatment of an addicted patient suspected of having endocarditis (fever, elevation of white blood cell count, and toxicity), is directed mainly towards the staphylococci. Any of the anti-staphylococcal penicillins (oxacillin or naf-cillin, 12 g/day, or methicillin, 24 g/day) is an adequate initial therapy. If the patient is hypersensitive to penicillin, a cephalo-sporin (e.g., cephalothin, 12 g/day) can be used. When the strain proves penicillin sensitive, then 20,000,000 units/day of aqueous penicillin are recommended.[94-96]

Several clinicians also recommend the administration of an aminoglycoside (e.g., gentamicin, kanamycin) in the initial regimen to cover gram-negative organisms and enterococci. This mode of therapy, however, is usually not needed, since gram-negative microorganisms are not frequently present in these patients. Vancomycin, 2.4 to 3.6 g/day, has been reported also to be effective, but the invariable phlebitis causes problems in addicted patients, because of the few available veins that they may have. In addition, large doses of lincomycin, 6 to 8 g/day, or clindamycin, 3 to 4 g/day, have been used successfully in patients with susceptible staphylococcal isolates.[94-96] The duration of treatment for infectious endocarditis

due to Staphylococcus aureus or some form of streptococcus is usually 4 to 6 weeks.

In patients with Candida endocarditis, amphotericin B and 5-fluorocytosine should be used.[96-98] A dose of 2 to 4 g of amphotericin B will effectively treat most mycotic infections. Amphotericin B is initially given intravenously, in a dose of 1 to 5 mg infused over a period of 4 to 6 hours daily. If the patient tolerates this dose, the total dose is increased to 10 mg daily. The daily dose is increased in 5- to 10-mg increments as tolerated by the patient, until a dose of approximately 1 mg/kg is reached. Side effects and toxicities include nausea and vomiting, fever, chills, thrombophlebitis, anemia, hypokalemia, renal tubular acidosis, liver damage, hypomagnesemia, and decreased renal function. At total dosages above 5 g, permanent residual renal damage is most likely to occur.[99,100]

5-Fluorocytosine is given in a dose of 100 to 150 mg/kg orally in four divided doses daily. Adverse reactions include nausea and vomiting, transient rises in liver enzymes, thrombocytopenia, and agranulocytosis.[96,101] Fluorocytosine should never be given alone, but only as an adjunct to amphotericin therapy. Long-term treatment of fungal infection of cardiac valves has not been always successful, and in some cases, prosthetic valve replacement is essential for the patient's survival.

GASTROINTESTINAL DISORDERS

Hepatitis, duodenal ulcers, and intestinal hemorrhage are the most commonly noted GI complications in patients abusing or addicted to narcotic analgesic drugs.[11,12,53,54,80-82,102-105]

Hepatitis. This disorder is a frequent and occasionally a recurrent, severely chronic, or lethal complication of illicit narcotic use. Steigman and associates appear to have been the first to recognize serum hepatitis as a complication of heroin abuse.[106] Since their report on 23 patients in 1950, numerous studies have documented this association.[12,80–82,102–105] Acute hepatitis is transmitted by contaminated needles, and it is the foremost cause of admissions of addicts to the medical services at municipal hospitals.

In one study, for example, Louria and associates reported that 42 of the 100 complications noted were related to hepatitis.[80] In 8 of the patients, the serum glutamic-oxaloacetic transaminase (SGOT) or -pyruvic (SGPT) transaminase levels were over 1000 units at some time during their illness, and in 7 other patients, the transaminase levels exceeded 2000 units. Serum bilirubin concentrations were also often elevated, exceeding 10 mg/100 ml in 13 patients and 20 mg/100 ml in 4 other patients. Of the 42 patients, 36 recovered completely, 1 died of acute hepatic necrosis, and 5 had hyperglobulinemia or hepatic decompensation and biopsy evidence of permanent liver disease characterized by various degrees of fibrosis upon histologic study. Death or chronic disease appeared to correlate with elevated transaminase levels, whereas there was no apparent correlation between chronicity or death and serum bilirubin concentration.

The treatment of these patients is nonspecific (e.g., bed rest for acutely ill patients, and adequate intake of food and fluids). Presently, there is no evidence that prolonged rest during convalescence is useful. Furthermore, strict isolation procedure appears unnecessary, but all caution should be used in the handling of the patient's blood. Results of the use of steroids have been unimpressive in the treatment of fulminant cases, and the role of immunosuppressive therapy for the treatment of such cases remains to be elucidated.[12,80,82,102–104]

Duodenal ulcers and intestinal hemorrhage. Duodenal ulcers are commonly seen in these patients, whose history of symptoms usually dates back to when they were active drug users. Chronic duodenal ulcers can lead to perforation or massive GI hemorrhage, and deaths have been reported to occur.[11,12,54,80,82] The duodenal ulcers usually can be managed with diet, frequent feeding, and antacids. The use of sedative-hypnotics or hypnotic-anticholinergic mixtures should be avoided, because of the possibility that these patients will start abusing these agents also.

RENAL DISORDERS

Acute tubular necrosis and renal failure, the nephrotic syndrome, acute nephritis, and urinary tract infections have been reported in patients with histories of chronic abuse of narcotic analgesic drugs, as well as in overdose situations.[11,12,80,82,107–112]

Acute tubular necrosis and renal failure. Overdosages with narcotic analgesic drugs sometimes result in acute tubular necrosis and renal failure, usually caused by hypotension, shock, or the development of rhabdomyolysis and myoglobinuria.[107–110] Hypotension or shock promotes alterations in renal hemodynamics and, because of the decreased renal blood flow and hypoxia, places these patients in a higher risk category for the development of acute tubular necrosis. In addition, the prolonged coma or tangled posture commonly observed in these patients creates an anoxic muscle crush injury, which leads to myoglobinuria and renal injury.[107] Myoglobinuria, rhabdomyolysis, and resultant renal failure without coma or crush injury also have been reported.[109,110] Supportive and symptomatic care constitutes the cornerstone of therapy for these patients. Careful attention to fluid and electrolyte balance is mandatory, and in some cases, peritoneal dialysis or hemodialysis may be required.

Nephrotic syndrome. Renal biopsy reveals most of these cases to be of the membranoproliferative, chronic glomerular, or focal sclerosis type.[111–114] The exact mechanisms by which the narcotic analgesic drugs produce these morphologic manifestations have not been elucidated. Presently, two proposed etiologic hypotheses have been reported. According to the first hypothesis, immune complexes of HB Ag (hepatitis-B antigen) are responsible, whereas in the second hypothesis, the syndrome is due to the binding of narcotic analgesic drugs by serum globulins and subsequent deposition into the glomerular basement membrane.[115,116] In any case, the hallmark of the nephrotic syndrome is increased protein in the urine, in amounts of greater than 3.5 g/24 hours. Unlike cases of "lipoid" nephrosis, these lesions are not responsive to corticosteroid therapy. Cyclophosphamide (Cytoxan) treatment, however, appears to reduce proteinuria, but its effect on glomerular function remains to be determined.

Acute nephritis. Acute glomerulonephritis is usually the result of (1) β-hemolytic streptococcal septicemia, secondary to a cellulitis from an infected injection site, or from a septic thrombophlebitis, or (2) staphylococcal or streptococcal endocarditis.[12,80–82,86] Renal failure is usually mild in degree and of brief duration, since these patients respond favorably to antimicrobial therapy. During the active treatment period, however, frequent and careful monitoring of fluid intake and output and of biochemical and hematologic indices is essential.

Urinary tract infections. Venereal disease, pelvic inflammatory disease, and urinary tract infections are common in addicted patients.[12,80–82,86] Female addicts have a high rate of venereal disease because many earn most of their money for drugs from prostitution. It is not unusual for these patients also to transmit hepatitis virus or for it to be transmitted to them through sexual intercourse. When male patients complain of urethral pain or discharge, or when females complain of pain of the lower urinary tract and/or discharge, appropriate urinary and blood samples should be collected and cultured for gonococci and/or bacterial infections. The treatment of gonococcal infection consists of 4,800,000 units of procaine penicillin administered intramuscularly, and 1 g of probenecid administered orally. For penicillin-hypersensitive patients, 2 g of spectinomycin should be administered intramuscularly. When oral therapy is required, several days of therapy with ampicillin or tetracycline can be used.[117]

In patients with urinary tract infections, once the necessary cultures have been performed, 10 to 14 days of therapy can be initiated, with either sulfisoxazole (Azo Gantrisin), 4 g/day; ampicillin, 2 g/day; or tetracycline, 1 g/day.[118]

MISCELLANEOUS DISORDERS

Complications that have been reported to occur less frequently in patients abusing heroin or other narcotic analgesic drugs, and that may also be present during acute overdose situations, include neurologic disorders (e.g., tetanus, transverse myelitis),[119,120] musculoskeletal and cutaneous disorders (e.g., osteomyelitis, septic arthritic, cellulitis, and abscesses),[121,122] and hematologic and vascular disorders (e.g., malaria, septicemia, vasculitis).[121,123] The hospitalized patient, therefore, should be followed closely for the detection and prevention of these disorders. When one is detected, appropriate therapeutic interventions should be implemented (e.g., immobilization, administration of appropriate antibiotics, and prophylactic and/or active treatment of tetanus).

Detoxification

The withdrawal symptoms or abstinence syndrome following abrupt cessation of a narcotic analgesic drug have been demonstrated in dependent or tolerant individuals, including infants, and in acutely intoxicated patients in the recovery phase of the intoxication.[11–17, 21–25, 60,61,80,82] Factors that influence the character and severity of the narcotic abstinence syndrome include the drug used, amount of daily intake, the interval between doses, the duration of abuse, and the health and personality of the individual.

The diagnosis of narcotic addiction can be made on the basis of patient's history, physical examination during admission (e.g., needle marks, pigmented streaks along superficial veins, scars), and close observation for characteristic withdrawal symptoms during the recovery phase. The symptoms that appear in the narcotic analgesic addict ·during this period include anxiety, irritability, restlessness, yawning, and a strong desire for narcotic analgesic drugs. These symptoms are intensified and are later accompanied by lacrimation, rhinorrhea, and diaphoresis. Occasionally, a restless "yen" ("craving") sleep occurs, from which the patient emerges, with all the previously described symptoms, 12 to 24 hours after the last dose. Thereafter, anorexia, cramps, myalgias, tremors, insomnia, nausea, vomiting, diarrhea, craving for sweets, and increases in pupillary size, blood pressure, heart rate, respiratory rate, and body temperature usually follow.

The piloerection, which results in skin resembling that of a plucked turkey, gives rise to the term "cold turkey" for narcotic withdrawal. Muscle spasms and involuntary leg movements give rise to the term "kicking the habit." In males, penile erections and premature ejaculations are common, and females may have occasional orgasms. The anorexia, vomiting, sweating, and diarrhea may result in weight loss and dehydration, ketosis, and disturbances in the acid-base balance. Occasionally, cardiovascular collapse may occur. Without treatment, most of the grossly observable symptoms disappear in 10 to 14 days.

The treatment of the narcotic withdrawal can be accomplished by the reintroduction of the original addicting agent if available, or by substitution of methadone. Presently, the substitution of methadone is the most commonly accepted method of treatment and consists of two major modalities: methadone detoxification and methadone maintenance.

Methadone detoxification. Isbell and Vogel were the first to study the effectiveness of methadone in narcotic detoxification.[124] Their clinical experience encouraged the United States Public Health Service Hospitals at Lexington, Kentucky and Fort Worth, Texas to adopt methadone as the most satisfactory method of allaying narcotic withdrawal hunger in the process of weaning addicts from opiates. The initial regimen called for the subcutaneous injection of methadone twice daily, and the amount of the drug was decreased in graded amounts over a 7- to 10-day period. Thereafter, a physiologically detoxified state (lack of physical dependence) was achieved by the addicted patient.

Since the early 1950s, however, other techniques employing methadone in the detoxification of addicted patients have emerged. Chambers has grouped these techniques into two major categories: inpatient withdrawal and ambulatory (outpatient) detoxification.[125] The philosophy of both programs is similar. The first goal is to stabilize the patient on a low to moderate dosage of methadone (20 to 40 mg/day) and then to gradually reduce the dose until the addicted patient no longer requires a narcotic to allay withdrawal discomfort. Usually 1 mg of methadone can substitute for 4 mg of morphine, 2 mg of heroin, or 20 mg of meperidine.[126] Reduction of the dose can be started immediately; a 20% daily reduction is well tolerated and causes little discomfort. The majority of patients can be withdrawn completely from narcotic analgesic drugs in 10 to 14 days.

During treatment with either technique, a great deal of stress is placed upon helping the addict to learn new productive behavior patterns or to re-establish old ones. The ambulatory methadone detoxification modality requires the patient to assume the largest share of responsibility for treatment and rehabilitative success, and the clinician's role is more passive. He can only administer medication and provide supportive services if the addicted patient decides to come to the clinic. Alternatively, the inpatient detoxification program can help the addicted patient to reach a drug-free state in a supportive and closely supervised environment, and for a limited time, protects him from the pressures of the street. During this process, it is hoped that the inpatient detoxification program will be able to provide adequate ancillary services (e.g., counseling, job placement), and once free of the drug, the patient will be more likely to become a productive member of society.

Methadone maintenance. The methadone maintenance program attempts to shift emphasis to social and vocational rehabilitation. Rather than provide the individual with heroin or other narcotics for intravenous use, a current concept is to offer him large oral doses of methadone. It has been proposed that methadone blocks the euphoric effects of other narcotic analgesic drugs, without itself producing euphoria. The oral dose of methadone necessary to block the euphoric effects of other narcotic analgesic drugs has been reported to be from 80 to 150 mg. This dose produces a high degree of cross-tolerance to other narcotic analgesic drugs, and thus it is extremely difficult for the addicted patient to achieve euphoric effects with the intravenous use of these other narcotic drugs.[127]

While in the methadone maintenance program, the addicted patient is stabilized on a dose that will be sufficient to suppress withdrawal symptoms associated with heroin or other abused narcotic drugs for 12 to 24 hours, but that will not produce the euphoric effects or the "nodding high" seen with the narcotic analgesic drugs. The methadone dose usually will not exceed 50 mg.[125,128]

Methadone is administered in single daily oral doses, so that there is daily contact between the health care team and the patients. It is hoped that, with the aid of daily counseling and rehabilitation, addicted patients not only will be eventually independent of methadone, but that this treatment will enable them to escape from the illicit drug scene, thereby affording them the time to review their present lifestyle, reorient their goals, rehabilitate themselves, and become drug-free individuals and productive members of society.

Although early results regarding the success of methadone maintenance programs were somewhat varied, they were generally favorable and have constituted one of the most exciting developments in the treatment of narcotic-addiction in the past decade. However, the early enthusiasm for methadone maintenance has been tarnished by the recent abuse of methadone. Presently, the role of methadone has been questioned because addicted patients have been able to obtain euphoric effects from doses of 60 to 100 mg of oral methadone administration. Furthermore, at lower maintenance doses at which methadone does not produce euphoria, addicted patients have been able to reach euphoric states through the intravenous administration of other narcotic analgesic drugs. Indeed, in some addicted patients, methadone has become not only a secondary drug of abuse, but the common cause of overdosages and death.[5,129-132]

As an alternative to methadone maintenance treatment, new investigative approaches to the treatment of narcotic addictions with agents such as long-acting methadone (LAAM),[129,133] cyclazocine,[134] naltrexone,[135] oxilorphan,[136] and endorphins[137] are presently being developed by many investigators. At this time, however, there are no conclusive data or evidence available regarding the effectiveness and safety of these agents in the prevention and/or treatment of narcotic addiction or their relative usefulness as compared to methadone maintenance treatment.

As research continues in the development of better modalities for the treatment of chronically narcotic-addicted patients, methadone maintenance will remain the mainstay of therapy. Methadone maintenance, however, is not feasible in the office practice of private physicians because they cannot provide all of the services for the various therapeutic needs of the patient (e.g., adequate facilities for the supervised collection of urine, and for frequent and accurate urine testing for the presence of morphine and other drugs, adequate staff and psychiatric services, and rigid controls of the methods of dispensing methadone, to prevent diversion to illicit sale or to possible intravenous use).

Practicing physicians, however, should cooperate with methadone maintenance programs in their communities and should offer whatever services they may be able to provide. In addition, the methadone maintenance program is subject to special regulations by guidelines of the Food and Drug Administration, the Drug Enforcement Agency, the Department of Justice, and in many instances it is subject to state regulations as well.[18] Methadone may be shipped only to programs approved by the above agencies for use in maintenance or withdrawal, or to hospital pharmacies for use as an analgesic or for inpatient withdrawal. Private practitioners are required also to file with the agencies described above for approval if they wish to develop methadone detoxification and maintenance programs.

MANIFESTATIONS AND TREATMENT OF INFANT WITHDRAWAL

Another area closely related to adult detoxification is infant withdrawal. Infants born to mothers physically dependent on narcotic drugs or who are undergoing treatment in a methadone maintenance program may also be narcotic dependent and usually exhibit withdrawal symptoms from 1 to 4 days after birth. These symptoms include generalized tremors and hypertonicity with any form of tactile stimuli, hyperalertness, sleeplessness, excessive crying, sneezing, vomiting, diarrhea, yawning, low birth weight, and occasionally fever.[61,62,138–143] Those infants with mild degrees of physical dependence may be given 0.06 to 0.5 ml of paregoric every 4 to 6 hours.[144,145] Infants with severe physical dependence may require, in addition to paregoric, methadone 100 μg to 1.2 mg daily.[144,146,147] Other agents, such as phenobarbital in a dose of 8.0 mg/kg/24 hrs divided in three to four doses daily,[139,144,148,149] and chlorpromazine in a dose of 1 to 3.5 mg/kg/24 hrs divided in three to four doses daily,[144,149,150] have also been used successfully for the treatment of withdrawal symptoms in infants. Once these are relieved, the dosage of the administered drugs should be decreased gradually and withdrawn completely over a 2- to 4-week period.

The widespread practice of giving chlorpromazine in full dosage for 10 to 14 days, and then in decreasing amounts for 1 or 2 more weeks, however, appears to be unadvisable. Other sedative-hypnotic drugs (e.g., chloral hydrate, diazepam)[144,151] have also been used successfully in the management of withdrawal symptoms in infants, but presently there is no evidence that they are more efficacious than phenobarbital.

GENERAL PROGNOSIS

Narcotic overdosage is a common cause of death among addicts as well as pediatric and adult patients. The exact cause of death due to overdose is not known, but it is associated with respiratory depression, coma, pulmonary edema, and in some occasions convulsions, which are most commonly seen with meperidine and propoxyphene. All of these toxic, life-threatening effects can be reversed by the use of narcotic antagonists, and by close monitoring of the patient for the prevention, detection and/or treatment of possible complications. Therefore, the prognosis for patients acutely intoxicated with narcotic analgesic drugs is good when appropriate therapeutic measures are applied. In patients who have been addicted to these drugs, however, the road to recovery is long and painful, although successful treatment is attainable.

REFERENCES

1. Anon: Drug related deaths and injuries. U.S. Government Printing Office, 720–12611. Drug Enforcement Administration, Washington, D.C., U.S. Department of Justice, 1977.
2. Huber DH, Stivers RR, and Howard LB: Heroin-overdose deaths in Atlanta. *JAMA*, 228:319–322, 1974.
3. Green RC, Carroll GJ, and Buxton WD: Drug addiction among physicians: The Virginia experience. *JAMA, 236*:1372–1375, 1976.
4. Hudson P, Barringer M, and McBay AJ: Fatal poisoning with propoxyphene: Report from 100 consecutive cases. *South Med J, 70*:938–942, 1977.
5. Smialek JE, et al: Methadone deaths in children. *JAMA, 238*:2516–2517, 1977.
6. Connaughton JF, et al: Perinatal addiction: Outcome and management. *Am J Obstet Gynecol, 129*:679–686, 1977.
7. Welti CV, Davis JH, and Blackbourne BD: Narcotic addiction in Dade County Florida: An analysis of 100 consecutive autopsies. *Arch Path, 93*:330–343, 1972.
8. Kersh, ES, and Schwartz LK: Narcotic poisoning: An epidemic disease. *Am Fam Physician, 8*:90–97, 1973.
9. Rumack BH, and Temple AR: Lomotil® poisoning. *Pediatrics, 53*:495–500, 1974.
10. Cushman P: Propoxyphene revisited. *Am J Drug Alcohol Abuse, 6*:245–249, 1979.
11. Cherubin C, et al: The epidemiology of death in narcotic addicts. *Am J Epidemiol, 96*:11–22, 1972.
12. Cherubin CE: The medical sequelae of narcotic addiction. *Ann Intern Med, 67*:23–33, 1967.
13. Eddy BN, et al: Drug dependence: Its significance and characteristics. *Bull WHO, 32*:721–733, 1965.
14. Seevers MH: Psychopharmacological elements of drug dependence. *JAMA, 206*:1263–1266, 1968.
15. Council on Mental Health: Narcotics and medical practice: Medical use of morphine and morphine-like drugs and management of persons dependent on them. *JAMA, 218*:578–583, 1971.
16. Murphee HB: Clinical pharmacology of potent analgesics. *Clin Pharmacol Ther, 3*:473–504, 1962.
17. Jaffe JH, and Martin WR: Opioid analgesics and antagonists. In *Pharmacological Basis of Therapeutics.* 6th Ed. Edited by AG Gilman, LS Goodman, and A Gilman. New York, Macmillan, 1980, pp. 494–534.
18. Code of Federal Regulations: *Title 21: Food and Drugs.* U.S. Government Printing Office. Drug Enforcement Administration, Washington, D.C., U.S. Department of Justice, 1979.
19. Braenden OJ, Eddy NB, and Halbach H: Synthetic substances with morphine-like effect: Relationship between chemical structure and analgesic action. *Bull WHO, 13*:937–998, 1955.
20. Barnett G, Trsic M, and Willette RE (eds): *QuaSAR: Quantitative Structure Activity Relationships of Analgesics, Narcotic Antagonists, and Hallucinogens.* National Institute on Drug Abuse, Research Monograph No. 22. U.S. Government Printing Office, Washington, D.C. 1978.
21. Martin WR: Opioid antagonists. *Pharmacol Rev, 19*:463–521, 1967.
22. Lewis JW, Bentley, KW, and Cowan A: Narcotic analgesics and antagonists. *Annu Rev Pharmacol Toxicol, 11*:241–270, 1971.
23. Evans LEJ, et al: Treatment of drug overdosage with naloxone, a specific narcotic antagonist. *Lancet, 1*:452–455, 1973.
24. Martin WR: Naloxone. *Ann Intern Med, 85*:765–768, 1976.
25. Reynolds AK, and Randal LD: *Morphine and Allied Drugs.* Toronto: University of Toronto Press, 1957.
26. Martin WR, and Sloan JW: Neuropharmacology and neurochemistry of subjective effects, analgesia, tolerance, and dependence produced by narcotic analgesics. In *Handbook of Experimental Pharmacology. Vol. 45/I, Drug Addiction I: Morphine, Sedative Hypnotic and Alcohol Dependence.* Edited by WR Martin. Berlin, Springer-Verlag, 1977, pp. 43–158.
27. Burks TF: Gastrointestinal pharmacology, *Annu Rev Pharmacol Toxicol, 16*:15–31, 1976.
28. Fishman J: The opiates and the endocrine system. In *The Bases of Addiction.* Edited by J Fishman. Dahlen Konferenzen. Berlin, Abakon Verlasgesellshaft, 1978, pp. 257–279.
29. Domino EF: Effects of narcotic analgesics on sensory input, activating system and motor output. *Res Publ Assoc Res Nerv Ment Dis, 46*:117–149, 1968.
30. Adler MW, Manara L, and Samanin R (eds): *Factors Affecting the Action of Narcotics.* New York, Raven Press, 1978.
31. Snyder SH, Pert CB, and Pasternak GW: The opiate receptor. *Ann Intern Med, 81*:534–540, 1974.

32. Simon EJ, and Hiller JM: The opiate receptor. *Annu Rev Pharmacol Toxicol, 18*:371–394, 1978.

33. Kerr FWL, and Wilson PR: Pain. *Annu Rev Neurosci, 1*:83–102, 1978.

34. Young WS, Bird SJ, and Kuhar MJ: Iontophoresis of methionine-enkaphalin in the locus coeruleus area. *Brain Res, 129*:366–370, 1977.

35. Korf J, Bunney BS, and Agajanian GK: Noradrenergic neurons: morphine inhibition of spontaneous activity. *Eur J Pharmacol, 25*:165–169, 1974.

36. Suensson TH, Bunney BS, and Agajanian GK: Inhibition of both noradrenergic and serotonergic neurons in brain by alpha-adrenergic agonist clonidine. *Brain Res, 92*:291–306, 1975.

37. Weil JV, et al: Diminished ventilatory response to hypoxia and hypercapnia after morphine in normal man. *N Engl J Med, 292*:1103–1106, 1975.

38. Eckenhoff JE, and Dech SR: The effects of narcotics and antagonists upon respiration and circulation in man: A review. *Clin Pharmacol Ther, 1*:483–524, 1960.

39. Pentiah P, Reilly F, and Borison HL: Interaction of morphine sulfate and sodium salicylate on respiration in cats. *J Pharmacol Exp Ther, 154*:110–118, 1966.

40. George R: Hypothalamus: Anterior pituitary gland. In *Narcotic Drugs: Biochemical Pharmacology*. Edited by DH Clovet. New York, Plenum Press, 1971, p. 283.

41. Winter CA, and Flataker L: The relation between skin temperature and the effect of morphine upon the response to thermal stimuli in the albino rat and the dog. *J Pharmacol Exp Ther, 109*:183–188, 1953.

42. Glauser FL, et al: Renal hemodynamics in drug-overdosed patients. *Am J Med Sci, 272*:147–152, 1976.

43. Gutner LB, Gould WJ, and Batterman RC: The effects of potent analgesics upon vestibular function. *J Clin Invest, 31*:259–266, 1952.

44. Lee HK, and Wang SC: Mechanism of morphine induced miosis in the dog. *J Pharmacol Exp Ther, 192*:415–431, 1975.

45. Johnstone M: Pethidine and general anesthesia. *Br Med J, 2*:943–946, 1951.

46. Pickering RW, et al: Some effects of meperidine (Demerol) on gastro-enteric, extrahepatic biliary and cardiovascular activity. *J Am Pharm Assoc, 38*:188–192, 1949.

47. Gilbert PE, and Martin WR: Antagonism of the convulsant effects of heroin, d-propoxyphene, meperidine, normeperidine and thebaine by naloxone in mice. *J Pharmacol Exp Ther, 192*:538–541, 1975.

48. Frenk H, McCarty BC, and Liebeskind JC: Different brain areas mediate the analgesic and epileptic properties of enkephalin. *Science, 200*:335–337, 1978.

49. Labi M: Paroxysmal atrial fibrillation in heroin intoxication. *Ann Intern Med, 71*:951–959, 1969.

50. Paranthanan SK, and Khan F: Acute cardiomyopathy with recurrent pulmonary edema and hypotension following heroin overdosage. *Chest, 69*:117–119, 1976.

51. Lipski J, Stimmel B, and Donoso E: The effect of heroin and multiple drug abuse on the electrocardiogram. *Am Heart J, 86*:663–668, 1974.

52. Abramson DH: Bigeminy and heroin intoxication. *NY State J Med, 72*:2888–2890, 1972.

53. Siegel H, Helpern M, and Ehrenreich T: The diagnosis of death from intravenous narcotics. *J Forensic Sci, 11*:1–16, 1966.

54. Helpern M, and Rho YM: Deaths from narcotism in New York City. *NY State J Med, 66*:2391–2408, 1966.

55. Froede RC, and Stahl GJ: Fatal narcotism in military personnel. *J Forensic Sci, 16*:199–218, 1972.

56. Zelis R, Flaim SF, and Eisele JH: Effects of morphine on reflex arteriolar constriction induced in man by hypercapnia. *Clin Pharmacol Ther, 22*:172–178, 1977.

57. Brunk SF, and Dell M: Effect of route of administration on morphine metabolism in man. *Clin Res, 20*:721, 1972.

58. Way EL, and Adler TK: The biological disposition of morphine and its surrogates (monograph). Geneva, World Health Organization, 1962, pp. 3–117.

59. Spector S: Quantitative determination of morphine in serum by radioimmunoassay. *J Pharmacol Exp Ther, 178*:253–258, 1971.

60. Zelson C, Rubio E, and Wasserman E: Neonatal addiction: 10 year observation. *Pediatrics, 48*:178–189, 1971.

61. Zelson C: Infant of the addicted mother. *N Engl J Med, 288*:1393–1395, 1973.

62. Miller JW, and Elliot HW: Rat tissue levels of carbon-14 labeled analgetics as related to pharmacological activity. *J Pharmacol Exp Ther, 113*:283–291, 1955.

63. Mirsa AL, et al: Differential pharmacokinetic and metabolic profiles of the stereoisomers of 3-hydroxy-N-methyl morphine. *Res Commun Chem Pathol Pharmacol, 7*:1–16, 1974.

64. Adler TK, Elliott HW, and George R: Some factors affecting the biological disposition of small doses of morphine in rats. *J Pharmacol Exp Ther, 120*:485–489, 1957.

65. Oldendorf WH, et al: Blood brain barrier penetration of morphine, codeine, heroin, and methadone after carotid injection. *Science, 178*:984–986, 1972.

66. Way EL: Distribution and metabolism of morphine and its surrogates. *Res Publ Assoc Res Nerv Ment Dis, 46*:13–31, 1968.

67. Brunk SF, and Delle M: Morphine metabolism in man. *Clin Pharmacol Ther, 16*:51–57, 1974.

68. Oberst FW: Studies on the fate of heroin. *J Pharmacol Exp Ther, 79*:266–270, 1943.

69. Mirsa AL: Metabolism of opiates. In *Factors Affecting the Actions of Narcotics*. Edited by MW Adler, L Manara, and R Samanin. New York, Raven Press, 1978, pp. 297–343.

70. Elliott HW, et al: Actions and metabolism of heroin adminstered by continuous intravenous

infusion to man. *Clin Pharmacol Ther*, 12:806–814, 1971.

71. Braude MC, et al (eds): *Narcotic Antagonists.* New York, Raven Press, 1974.

72. Kosterlitz HW, Collier HOJ, and Villarreal JE (eds): *Agonistic and Antagonistic Actions of Narcotic Analgesic Drugs.* Baltimore, University Park Press, 1973.

73. Calesnick B: Use of narcotic (opiate) antagonists. *Am Fam Physician*, 13:158–159, 1976.

74. Lovejoy FH, Mitchell AA, and Goldman P: The management of propoxyphene poisoning. *J Pediatr*, 85:98–100, 1974.

75. Kersh ES: Treatment of propoxyphene overdosage with naloxone. *Chest*, 63:112–114, 1973.

76. Ngar SH, et al: Pharmacokinetics of naloxone in rats and in man: Basis for its potency and short duration of action. *Anesthesiology*, 44:398–401, 1976.

77. Longnecker DE, Grazis PA, and Eggers GWN Jr: Naloxone for antagonism of morphine-induced respiratory depression. *Anesth Analg (Cleve)*, 52:447–453, 1973.

78. Rumack BH (ed): Management of opiates. *Poisondex.* Denver, Micromedex, Inc., August, 1980.

79. Holsbruuck JD: The antagonism of morphine anesthesia by naloxone. *Anesth Analg (Cleve)*, 50:954–959, 1971.

80. Louria DB, Hensle T, and Rose J: The major medical complications of heroin addiction. *Ann Intern Med*, 67:1–22, 1967.

81. White AG: Medical disorders in drug addicts: 200 consecutive admissions. *JAMA*, 223:1469–1471, 1973.

82. Shapira JD: The narcotic addict as a medical patient. *Am J Med*, 45:555–588, 1968.

83. Jaffe RB, and Koschmann EB: Intravenous drug abuse: Pulmonary, cardiac and vascular complications. *Am J Roentgenol*, 109:107–120, 1970.

84. Kaufman DM, and Hegyi T: Heroin intoxication in adolescents. *Pediatrics*, 50:746–753, 1972.

85. Olser W: Oedema of left lung—morphia poisoning. *Montreal Gen Hosp Rep*, 1:291–292, 1980.

86. Kurtzman RS: Complications of narcotic addiction. *Radiology*, 96:23–30, 1970.

87. Bogartz LJ, and Miller WC: Pulmonary edema associated with propoxyphene intoxication. *JAMA*, 215:259–262, 1971.

88. Sklar J, and Timms RM: Codeine-induced pulmonary edema. *Chest*, 72:230–231, 1977.

89. Frand VI, Shim CS, and Williams HM: Methadone-induced pulmonary edema. *Ann Intern Med*, 76:975–979, 1972.

90. Kaufman RE, and Levy SB: Overdose treatment: Addict folklore and medical reality. *JAMA*, 227:411–413, 1974.

91. Olsson RA, and Romansky MJ: Staphylococcal triscuspid endocarditis in heroin addicts. *Ann Intern Med*, 57:755–762, 1962.

92. Goldburgh HL, Baer S, and Lieber MM: Acute bacterial endocarditis of triscuspid value. *Am J Med Sci*, 204:319–324, 1942.

93. Bain RC, et al: Right-sided bacterial endocarditis and endarteritis. *Am J Med*, 24:98–110, 1958.

94. Cherubin CE, et al: Infective endocarditis in narcotic addicts. *Ann Intern Med*, 69:1091–1098, 1968.

95. Sapira J, and Cherubin CE (eds): *Drug Addiction: A Guide for the Clinician.* New York, Excerpta Medica Press, New York, 1975.

96. Kaye D: Changes in the spectrum, diagnosis and management of bacterial and fungal endocarditis. *Med Clin North Am*, 57:941–957, 1973.

97. Butler WT: Pharmacology, toxicity and therapeutic usefulness of amphotericin B. *JAMA*, 195:127–131, 1966.

98. Drutz DJ, et al: Treatment of disseminated mycotic injections: A new approach to amphotericin B therapy. *Am J Med*, 45:405–418, 1968.

99. Butler WT, et al: Nephrotoxicity of amphotericin B: Early and late effects in 81 patients. *Ann Intern Med*, 61:175–187, 1964.

100. Takacs FJ, Tomkiewicz ZM, and Merrill JP: Amphotericin B nephrotoxicity with irreversible renal failure. *Ann Intern Med*, 59:716–724, 1963.

101. Vandevelde AG, Mauceri AA, and Johnson JE III: 5–Fluorocytosine in the treatment of mycotic infections. *Ann Intern Med*, 77:43–51, 1972.

102. Gorodetzky CW, et al: Liver disease in narcotic addicts. I. The role of the drug. *Clin Pharmacol Ther*, 9:720–724, 1968.

103. Sapira JD, Jasinski DR, and Gorodetzky CW: Liver disease in narcotic addicts. II. The role of the needle. *Clin Pharmacol Ther*, 9:725–739, 1968.

104. Seeff LB, et al: Hepatic disease in asymptomatic parenteral narcotic drug abusers: A Veterans Administration collaborative study. *Am J Med Sci*, 270:41–47, 1975.

105. Rho YM: Infections as fatal complications of narcotism. *NY State J Med*, 72:823–830, 1972.

106. Steigman F, Hyman S, and Goldbloom R: Infectious hepatitis (homologous serum type) in drug addicts. *Gastroenterology*, 14:642–646, 1950.

107. Schreiber SN, et al: Limb compression and renal impairment (Crush Syndrome) complicating narcotic overdose. *N Engl J Med*, 284:368–369, 1971.

108. Sreepada Rao TK, Nicastri AD, and Friedman EA: Renal consequences of narcotic abuse. *Adv Nephrol*, 7:261–290, 1978.

109. Ritcher RW, et al: Acute myoglobinuria associated with heroin addiction. *JAMA*, 216:1172–1176, 1971.

110. Schwartzfarb L, Gurmukh MB, and Marcus D: Heroin-associated rhabdomyolysis with cardiac involvement. *Arch Intern Med*, 137:1255–1257, 1977.

111. Kilcoyne MM, et al: Nephrotic syndrome in heroin addicts. *Lancet*, 1:17–20, 1972.

112. Eknogan G, et al: Nephropathy in patients with

drug addiction. *Virchows Arch (Pathol Anat)*, 365:1–13, 1975.

113. Treser G, et al: Renal lesions in narcotic addicts. *Am J Med*, 57:687–694, 1974.

114. Grishman E, Churg J, and Porush JG: Glomerular morphology in nephrotic heroin addicts. *Lab Invest*, 35:415–424, 1976.

115. Welti CV, Noto TA, and Fernandez-Carol A: Immunologic abnormalities in heroin addiction. *South Med J*, 67:193–197, 1974.

116. Ryan JJ, Parker CW, and Williams RC Jr: Gamma-globulin binding of morphine in heroin addicts. *J Lab Clin Med*, 80:155–164, 1972.

117. Olansky S: Antimicrobial therapy of venereal diseases. In *Antimicrobial Therapy*. 2nd Ed. Edited by BM Kagan. Philadelphia, W.B. Saunders, 1974, pp. 253–255.

118. Carvajal HF, Daeschner CW Jr, and Warren MM: Urinary tract infections. In *Antimicrobial Therapy*. 2nd Ed. Edited by BM Kagan. Philadelphia, W.B. Saunders, 1974, pp. 355–365.

119. Cherubin CE: The epidemiology of tetanus in narcotic addicts. *NY State J Med*, 70:267–271, 1970.

120. Richter R, and Baden M: Transverse myelitis associated with heroin addiction. *JAMA*, 206:1255–1257, 1968.

121. Thompson BD: Medical complications following intravenous heroin. *Ariz Med*, 32:798–801, 1975.

122. Richter R, and Baden M: Neurological complications of heroin addiction. *Trans Am Neurol Assoc*, 94:330–332, 1969.

123. Rosenblatt JF, and Marsh H: Induced malaria in narcotic addicts. *Lancet*, 2:189–190, 1971.

124. Isbell H, and Vogel VH: The addiction liability of methadone (Amidone, Dolophine, 10820), and its use in the treatment of the morphine abstinence syndrome. *Am J Psychiatry*, 105:909–914, 1949.

125. Chambers CD: A description of inpatient and ambulatory techniques. In *Methadone: Experiences and Issues.* Edited by CD Chambers, and L Brill. New York, Behavioral Publications, 1973, pp. 185–194.

126. Jaffe JH: Drug addiction and drug abuse. In *The Pharmacological Basis of Therapeutics*. 6th Ed. Edited by AG Gilman, LS Goodman, and A Gilman. New York, Macmillan, 1980, pp. 535–584.

127. Dole VP, Nyswanter ME, and Kreek MJ: Narcotic blockade. *Arch Intern Med*, 118:304–309, 1966.

128. Goldstein A: The pharmacologic basis of methadone treatment. In *Fourth National Conference on Methadone Treatment. Proceedings.* Edited by A Goldstein. New York, National Association for Prevention of Addiction to Narcotics, 1972, pp. 27–32.

129. Resnick RB: Problems of methadone diversion and implications for control. *Int J Addict*, 12:803–806, 1977.

130. Aronow R, Paul SD, and Woolley PV Jr: Childhood poisoning: An unfortunate consequence

of methadone availability. *JAMA*, 219:321–324, 1972.

131. Zinberg NE: The crisis in methadone maintenance. *N Engl J Med*, 296:1000–1002, 1977.

132. Aronow R, Brenner SL, and Woolley PV: An apparent epidemic: Methadone poisoning in children. *Clin Toxicol*, 6:175–182, 1973.

133. Schecter A, and Schecter MJ: The role of long-acting methadone (LAAM) in the treatment of opiate dependence. In *Treatment Aspects of Drug Dependence*. Edited by A Schecter. West Palm Beach, Florida, CRC Press, 1978, pp. 33–40.

134. Brahen LS, Copone T, and Wiechert U: Chemotherapy: Cyclazocine. In *Treatment Aspects of Drug Dependence*. Edited by A. Schecter. West Palm Beach, Florida, CRC Press, 1978, pp. 51–57.

135. Schecter A, and Schecter MJ: Naltrexone in the rehabilitation of opiate addicts. *Treatment Aspects of Drug Dependence*. Edited by A Schecter. West Palm Beach, Florida, CRC Press, 1978, pp. 59–70.

136. Resnick RB, Schwartz LK, and Kestenbaum RS: Oxilorphan. In *Treatment Aspects of Drug Dependence*. Edited by A Schecter. West Palm Beach, Florida, CRC Press, 1978, pp. 71–77.

137. Clovet DH, and Verebey K: Possible use of endorphins in the treatment of opiate addiction. In *Treatment Aspects of Drug Dependence*. Edited by A Schecter. West Palm Beach, Florida, CRC Press, 1978, pp. 79–82.

138. Schneck H: Narcotic withdrawal symptoms in the newborn infants resulting from maternal addiction. *J Pediatr*, 52:584–587, 1958.

139. Goodfriend MJ, Shey IA, and Klein MD: The effects of maternal narcotic addiction on the newborn. *Am J Obstet Gynecol*, 71:29–36, 1956.

140. Strauss ME, et al: Pregnancy, birth and neonate characteristics. *Am J Obstet Gynecol*, 120:895–900, 1974.

141. Finnegan LP, et al: A scoring system for evaluation and treatment of the neonatal abstinence syndrome: A clinical and research tool. In *Basic and Therapeutic Aspects of Perinatal Pharmacology*. Edited by PL Morselli, S Garattini, and F Sereni. New York, Raven Press, 1975, p. 139.

142. Glass L, et al: Effect of heroin withdrawal on the respiratory rate and acid-base status of the newborn. *N Eng J Med*, 286:746–748, 1972.

143. Newman RG, Bashton S, and Calko D: Results of 313 consecutive live births delivered to patients in the New York City Methadone Maintenance Program. *Am J Obstet Gynecol*, 121:233–237, 1975.

144. Hill R, and Desmond MM: Management of the narcotic withdrawal syndrome in the neonate. *Pediatr Clin North Am*, 5:67–86, 1963.

145. Cobrinik RW, Hood RT, and Chusid E: The effect of maternal narcotic addiction on the newborn infant. Review of the literature and report of 22 cases. *Pediatrics*, 24:288–304, 1959.

146. Krause SO, et al: Heroin addiction among pregnant women and their newborn babies. *Am J Obstet Gynecol*, 75:754–758, 1958.

147. Cary W: Cold turkey in the new born. *Med J Aust, 18*:361–363, 1972.
148. Kunstadler R II, et al: Narcotic withdrawal symptoms in newborn infants. *JAMA, 168*:1008–1010, 1958.
149. Kahn EJ, Newman LL, and Polk GA: The course of heroin withdrawal syndrome in newborn infants treated with phenobarbital or chlorpromazine. *J Pediatr, 75*:495–500, 1969.
150. Aivazian GH: Chlorpromazine in the withdrawal of habit forming drugs in addicts. *Dis Nerv Syst, 16*:57–60, 1955.
151. Nathenson G, Golden GS, and Litt IF: Diazepam in the management of the neonatal narcotic withdrawal syndrome. *Pediatrics, 48*:523–527, 1971.

Chapter 7

Tricyclic Antidepressants

Vasilios A. Skoutakis

Since their introduction into clinical medicine in the late 1950s, the tricyclic antidepressant compounds (Fig. 7–1) have become the most widely used drugs in the treatment of depression and in the management of enuresis in children.[1,2] However, their widespread use has been associated with an increasing number of accidental ingestions in children and suicidal attempts in adults throughout the world.[1,3–5] In our area of clinical toxicology, intoxication with tricyclic antidepressants is now one of the most commonly seen types of drug overdosages, surpassing even those of barbiturates and tranquilizers.

An understanding of the clinical diagnostic considerations, the causes of the toxicologic manifestations, the appropriate required laboratory tests, and the available therapeutic measures is a requisite for the optimal management of the patient who is intoxicated by tricyclic antidepressants.

CASE REPORT

A 20-year-old white man was found semicomatose in his apartment. The ambulance team reported that the patient had three generalized seizures en route to the hospital. He was comatose upon arrival at the emergency room.

Physical examination on admission revealed a deeply comatose patient who was unresponsive to painful stimuli. All extremities were hyperactive (tonic-clonic seizures). Vital signs were blood pressure, 145/95 mm Hg;

127

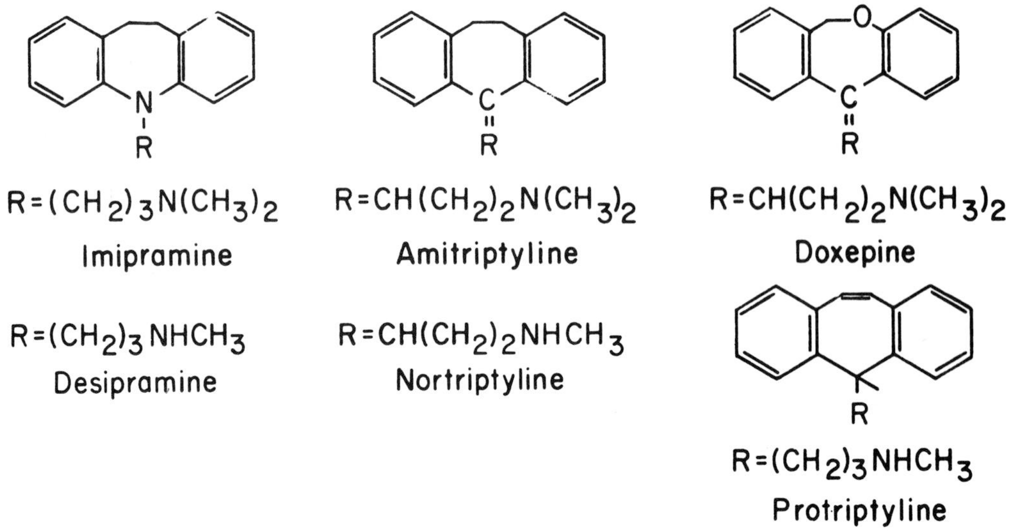

R=(CH$_2$)$_3$N(CH$_3$)$_2$
Imipramine

R=(CH$_2$)$_3$NHCH$_3$
Desipramine

R=CH(CH$_2$)$_2$N(CH$_3$)$_2$
Amitriptyline

R=CH(CH$_2$)$_2$NHCH$_3$
Nortriptyline

R=CH(CH$_2$)$_2$N(CH$_3$)$_2$
Doxepine

R=(CH$_2$)$_3$NHCH$_3$
Protriptyline

Fig. 7–1. Chemical structures of tricyclic antidepressants.

pulse, 180 beats/min and regular; respirations, 13/min; and rectal temperature, 38.5°C. There were no signs of trauma. The pupils were dilated and fixed, with minimal response to light.

The mucous membranes of the mouth were dry, and no abnormal odors could be detected. The lungs were clear to auscultation and percussion. The abdominal examination revealed diminished bowel sounds but no tenderness. His skin was warm, dry and normal in appearance. There was no evidence of past parenteral drug abuse. The electrocardiogram revealed a prolongation of the Q-T interval, widening of the QRS complexes, and ST segment and T-wave abnormalities consistent with subendocardial injury. Chest x-ray examination results, urinalysis, and complete blood count were within normal limits.

CLINICAL ASSESSMENT AND MANAGEMENT OF THE PATIENT

In the assessment of this patient, the following should be considered: (1) clinical diagnostic considerations, (2) sub-stances capable of producing the anticholinergic syndrome, (3) confirmation of the diagnosis through use of physostigmine salicylate, and the therapeutic indications and contraindications for its use, (4) causes of the toxicologic manifestations, (5) indicated laboratory tests, (6) indicated therapeutic measures, (7) end-points of therapy, and (8) general prognosis.

CLINICAL DIAGNOSTIC CONSIDERATIONS

We are presented with a patient in a coma. He does not have a history of possible drug overdose, and there is no information pertaining to that possibility. The physical examination revealed signs of (1) CNS toxicities (hyperactivity, seizures, respiratory depression, coma), (2) cardiovascular toxicities (impaired cardiac conduction, tachycardia, hypertension), and (3) peripheral manifestations of intoxication (mydriasis, hyperpyrexia, decreased bowel sounds, and dry skin and mucous membranes).

Therefore, these clinical symptoms suggest cholinergic blockade or an anticholin-

Table 7–1. Central and Peripheral Signs and Symptoms of the Anticholinergic Syndrome

BODY SYSTEMS	MANIFESTATIONS
Central nervous system	Anxiety Agitation and/or restlessness Twitching and/or jerky movements Hyperreflexia Hallucinations Seizures Coma Respiratory failure Circulatory collapse
Peripheral nervous system	Mydriasis Tachycardia Vasodilatation Urinary retention Hyperpyrexia Decreased gastrointestinal motility Decreased salivary and sweat gland secretions Decreased bronchial and nasal secretions Increased blood pressure

ergic syndrome. Table 7–1 summarizes the toxicologic signs and symptoms seen with anticholinergic agents.

SUBSTANCES CAPABLE OF PRODUCING THE ANTICHOLINERGIC SYNDROME

Acute intoxications with anticholinergic agents can occur in a number of clinical settings. For example, large numbers of alkaloids, antidepressants, tranquilizers, antihistamines, antispasmodics, antiparkinsonian agents, ophthalmic preparations, nonprescription sleeping aids, and plants have been reported to possess significant anticholinergic activity.[6-8] Table 7–2 summarizes those drugs and plants capable of producing the anticholinergic syndrome.

CONFIRMATION OF DIAGNOSIS: PHYSOSTIGMINE SALICYLATE

Physostigmine salicylate (Antilirium), a reversible anticholinesterase agent, is the drug of choice for confirmation of the diagnosis or for reversal of the anticholinergic syndrome. Unlike similar drugs, such as neostigmine, pyridostigmine, and edrophonium (Fig. 7–2), which have a quaternary amine moiety, physostigmine is a tertiary amine. For this reason, it is nonionized and lipophilic, and can cross the blood-brain barrier to exert central as well as peripheral cholinomimetic actions.[9]

Specific indications for the use of physostigmine salicylate include the presence of one or more of the following symptoms: convulsions, deep coma of unknown origin, severe agitation and hallucinations, hypertension, and cardiac arrhythmias.[8,10-13] The recommended trial dose of physostigmine salicylate in an adult is 2 mg given by slow IV injection (1 mg/min). If there is no response, another 2 mg may be given again in 20 minutes. In responsive patients, repeated doses of 1 to 4 mg may be required every 30 to 60 minutes, since physostigmine salicylate is rapidly metabolized.[12] The initial pediatric dose should be 0.5 mg given by slow IV injection. If toxic effects persist and no cholinergic effects are produced, the drug should be readministered at 5-minute intervals.[12] The relative contraindications of the use of physostigmine salicylate include (1) asthma, (2) cardiovascular disease, and (3) mechanical obstruction of the GI tract or genitourinary tract.[8,9,12]

In the present case, several minutes after the administration of physostigmine salicylate, the patient became alert and oriented. His EKG dramatically reverted to normal sinus rhythm. Upon questioning, the patient stated that he had ingested 50 25-mg tablets of amitriptyline (Elavil) in an attempt to commit suicide. Subsequently, the patient was treated with standard supportive procedures as outlined and discussed in the section on treatment.

However, over the next 6 hours the

Table 7–2. Common Drugs and Plants that May Produce the Anticholinergic Syndrome

CHEMICAL CLASSIFICATION	REPRESENTATIVE EXAMPLES
Tricyclic antidepressants	Amitriptyline HCl (Elavil) Amitriptyline HCl and perphenazine (Triavil, Etrafon) Amitriptyline HCl and chlordiazepoxide (Limbitrol) Desipramine HCl (Norpramin, Pertofrane) Doxepine HCl (Sinequan, Adapin) Imipramine HCl (Tofranil) Imipramine pamoate (Tofranil-PM) Nortriptyline HCl (Aventyl) Protriptyline HCl (Vivactil)
Antipsychotic drugs	Phenothiazines (especially thioridazine) Butyrophenones (haloperidol)
Antihistamines	Chlorpheniramine maleate (Ornade, Teldrin) Diphenhydramine HCl (Benadryl) Orphenadrine HCl (Disipal) Promethazine HCl (Phenergan)
Ophthalmic preparations	Atropine, 1% ophthalmic solution Cyclopentolate (Cyclogel) Tropicamide (Mydriacyl)
Antispasmodics	Methantheline Br (Banthine) Propantheline Br (Pro-Banthine)
Antiparkinson agents	Benztropine mesylate (Congentin) Biperiden HCl (Akineton) Ethopropazine HCl (Parsidol) Procyclidine HCl (Kemedrin) Trihexyphenidyl HCl (Artane, Pipanol, Tremin)
Proprietary (hypnotics, analgesics, antiasthmatics)	Asthmador (belladonna or stramonium alkaloids) Compoz (scopolamine, methapyrilene, pyrilamine) Excedrin-PM (salicylamide, acetaminophen, methapyrilene) Sleep-Eze (scopolamine, methapyrilene) Sominex (scopolamine, methapyrilene, salicylamide)
Belladonna alkaloids	Atropine sulfate Scopolamine HBr Tincture of belladonna Belladonna extract
Plants	Bittersweet (Solanum dulcamara) Black henbane (Hyoscyamus niger) Deadly nightshade (Atropa belladonna) Jimson weed (Datura stramonium) Jerusalem cherry (Solanum pseudocapsicum) Potato leaves, sprouts, tubers (Solanum tuberosum)

patient became less oriented and more agitated, and the EKG showed ventricular tachycardia. The slow IV administration of another 2 mg of physostigmine salicylate produced an immediate response. Normal sinus rhythm was achieved, and the pulse rate decreased from 180 to 100 beats/min.

However, the repeated blind administration of physostigmine salicylate is risky, as it may result in precipitation of cholinergic crisis, which can be manifested as bradycardia, bronchospasm, hypersalivation, increased pulmonary secretions, and possibly convulsions. If toxic

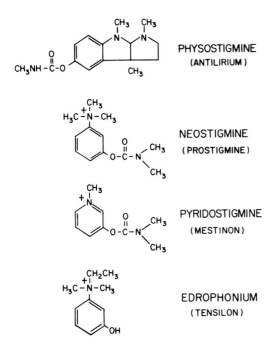

PHYSOSTIGMINE
(ANTILIRIUM)

NEOSTIGMINE
(PROSTIGMINE)

PYRIDOSTIGMINE
(MESTINON)

EDROPHONIUM
(TENSILON)

Fig. 7–2. Structures of reversible anticholinesterase agents.

cholinergic effects do result, atropine sulfate (0.5 mg for each 1 mg of physostigmine salicylate that has been administered to the patient up to that point) can be given by slow IV administration during EKG monitoring, to counteract the effects of physostigmine salicylate.[8,12]

CAUSES OF THE TOXICOLOGIC MANIFESTATIONS

The causes of the CNS, cardiovascular, and peripheral toxicities present in this patient can be related to the sedative, anticholinergic, alpha-adrenergic neuronal blocking, and quinidine-like actions of the tricyclic antidepressant agents.

Central Nervous System Toxicities

The mechanism of action by which tricyclic antidepressants cause CNS toxicities (Table 7–1) is most likely a peripheral and central blockade of acetylcholine.[9,14] Chorea, for example, may result from a

decrease in the balance of acetylcholine relative to dopamine in the basal ganglia.[10] Myoclonus, unlike chorea, might result from the decrease of serotonin uptake and subsequent increase of serotonin at the synaptic areas.[11] Respiratory depression and disturbances of body temperature, however, may result from direct effects of the tricyclics on the respiratory center in the medulla of the brain and thermoregulatory centers in the hypothalamus, respectively.[15,16]

Cardiovascular Toxicities

As in the present case, the most common cardiotoxic effects seen after acute ingestion of tricyclic antidepressants are tachyarrhythmias, impairment of cardiac conduction, and hyper- or hypotension.

Tachyarrhythmias. Although the mechanism by which the tricyclic antidepressants cause tachyarrhythmias cannot be explained fully, the vagal-blocking anticholinergic effects of these drugs are probably responsible.[16,17] Cardiac arrhythmias also may be due to blockade of norepinephrine reuptake into the sympathetic nerve endings,[14,18] or they may be secondary to respiratory or metabolic acidoses.[19]

Impairment of cardiac conduction. The mechanism by which tricyclic agents alter cardiac conduction is probably a direct depression of conduction and excitability on the cardiac tissue (quinidine-like effects).[20,21] The Q-T interval in the case presented was prolonged, probably in part owing to increased duration of electrical systole, but also in part to diminished intraventricular conduction velocity, reflected also in an increased duration of the QRS complex.

Hypertension or hypotension. Since the tricyclic antidepressants block reuptake of norepinephrine into the sympathetic nerve endings,[20] their actions can be manifested by alpha and beta receptor stimulation. The alpha effects will increase total peripheral resistance of blood vessels, and the beta effects will increase cardiac rate and decrease total peripheral resistance. Therefore, at the time of initial blockade, norepinephrine would be capable of causing an increased heart rate and mean arterial pressure, as manifested in the present case. Thereafter, since norepinephrine is blocked from being taken up into the axon, it undergoes a rapid enzymatic degradation by monoamine oxidase (MAO) and catechol-o-methyl transferase (COMT). Thus, as norepinephrine is metabolized, its vasopressor effect is lost, and hypotension occurs.[20,21]

Additional Peripheral Anticholinergic Effects

The peripheral signs of atropinism, such as dilated pupils, dry mucous membranes, warm dry skin, diminished bowel sounds, and hyperpyrexia seen in the present patient are probably due to the peripheral acetylcholine blockade caused by the tricyclic antidepressants.[14–16]

LABORATORY TESTS

As with all comatose patients in whom a drug-related cause is suspected, a route for the administration of intravenous fluids should be established, and toxicologic screening and blood analysis should be performed for glucose, electrolytes, blood urea nitrogen, complete blood count, and liver function determinations. Arterial blood gas determination is necessary to rule out any subclinical acid-base imbalance or hypoxia that might require urgent attention. In addition, a 12-lead EKG should be obtained to check for tachyarrhythmias and conduction system disturbances, as well as for continuous cardiac monitoring.

Since tricyclics are firmly bound to tissues and proteins,[23] only a few laboratories are capable of detecting the relatively low plasma and urinary levels of these drugs. The severity of the intoxication can be determined by measurement of the plasma tricyclic antidepressant level

with gas chromatography-mass fragmentography.[24] Significant toxicity and coma are usually observed when the total serum tricyclic levels are in excess of 1000 ng/ml.[24]

If the laboratory facilities are not available to measure tricyclic antidepressant levels, the most reliable sign for evaluation of the seriousness of the intoxication is the prolongation of the QRS complex in the electrocardiogram. Usually, patients with plasma drug levels greater than 1000 ng/ml will also have QRS complexes of at least 100 msec in the first 24 hours after drug ingestion.[24] The duration of the QRS complex also reflects the plasma drug level of tricyclic antidepressants in subsequent days. As the drug levels decrease, the duration of the QRS complex approaches normal values.[24]

INDICATED THERAPEUTIC MEASURES

The basic treatment procedures for the patient intoxicated with tricyclic antidepressants are (1) correction of life-threatening symptoms, (2) removal of unabsorbed drug, (3) prevention of further absorption, (4) removal of the absorbed drug, and (5) symptomatic and supportive therapy as required or indicated.

Correction of Life-Threatening Symptoms

It is essential that we treat the patient first rather than the intoxicant. Therefore, the establishment of vital organ function is necessary. If respiration is inadequate, an artificial airway should be established. The determination of inadequacy should be based on the presence of cyanosis, rate and depth of respiration, and arterial blood gas values. To correct life-threatening complications, such as CNS and cardiovascular toxicities, the use of physostigmine salicylate should be considered, as in the present case. However, because of biochemical individuality, some arrhythmias may be refractory to physostigmine salicylate therapy.

Arrhythmias refractory to physostigmine salicylate may respond to the intravenous administration of sodium bicarbonate and potassium chloride,[25] phenytoin (Dilantin),[26] or propranolol (Inderal).[27] An understanding of the rationale for use of these agents is essential. The administration of sodium bicarbonate in a dose of 2 mEq/kg is based on the evidence that the risk of arrhythmias is reduced if the serum pH is greater than 7.4.[19,25] Potassium chloride (1.5 mEq/kg/24 hrs) is given to counteract the decrease of the serum potassium level that occurs with the alkalinization.[25]

Phenytoin reverses the quinidine-like toxicity of tricyclics by accelerating atrial-ventricular conduction.[26] The phenytoin dose in adults is 100 mg IV over 3 minutes, repeated every 5 to 10 minutes until the arrhythmias respond or until a maximum of 1000 mg is given. The pediatric dose of phenytoin is 1 mg/kg by slow IV administration.[26] Propranolol also has been used with some success but should be used with caution, because it may potentiate the negative inotropic and chronotropic actions of the tricyclic compounds. Its antiarrhythmic effect may be the result of both a beta-blocking action and a direct anesthetic effect on cell membranes that effects the cardiac muscle action potential. The dosage of propranolol in adults is 1 mg IV every 2 minutes until a response occurs or until a maximum dose of 10 mg is administered. The pediatric dose is 0.1 mg IV.[27] In asthmatic patients, propranolol can increase bronchial resistance and should be used cautiously if at all.[27]

Hypotension should be treated initially with fluids. If a pressor agent is required, the indirect-acting sympathomimetic amines, such as metaraminol (Aramine) and mephentermine (Wyamine) should not be used, since the tricyclic antidepressants block their uptake into the adrenergic neuron. Norepinephrine (Levophed) in a dose of 0.1 to 0.2 μg/kg/min, or dopamine (Intropin), 3 to 5 μg/kg/min, is the recommended drug of choice, because of its direct action.

However, these agents should be used with caution, because they can induce arrhythmias as well.[20] If cardiac arrhythmias are present, and the administration of a pressor drug appears to be imperative, phenylephrine (Neo-Synephrine) in a dose of 10 mg (1 ml of 1% solution of phenylephrine added to 500 ml of dextrose) should be administered intravenously at an initial rate of 100 to 150 drops/min. When the blood pressure is stabilized, a maintenance rate of 40 to 60 drops/min usually suffices.[28]

CNS and peripheral anticholinergic toxicities (Table 7–1) usually respond to physostigmine salicylate therapy. However, if the CNS toxic manifestations are refractory to physostigmine salicylate therapy, then diazepam (0.1 to 0.3 mg/kg in a child and 10 mg in an adult) or phenytoin (1 to 3 mg/kg of body weight) may be used.[29]

Removal of Unabsorbed Drug

The techniques involved in the removal of tricyclic antidepressants still remaining in the GI tract are emesis or lavage. The decision whether to produce emesis or to initiate lavage depends on the accuracy of the initial history and the length of time between when the patient is seen and when the drug was initially ingested. Usually, if a significant amount of drug was ingested 1 hour or more prior to admission, the patient should be intubated and lavage initiated. If the patient is seen early, that is, within 30 to 45 minutes of the time of ingestion, and if he has an intact gag reflex, a trial dose of 30 ml of syrup of ipecac in adults, and 15 ml in children, followed by 8 to 10 oz of water, should be administered. If emesis is not produced within 20 to 30 minutes, lavage should be initiated.

In the present case, the patient was intubated with the assistance of an anesthesiologist, and a large-bore nasogastric tube was inserted into the stomach. Lavage was performed with isotonic saline solution used as the lavage fluid. During lavage, the patient was placed in a modified Trendelenburg position on his left side. The reason for this position is to avoid aspiration while the gastric contents are successfully emptied. Lavage was continued until the aspirate was clear; in this case, it required 2 L.

Prevention of Further Absorption

The tricyclic antidepressant compounds are primarily eliminated by metabolism in the liver. Amitriptyline, imipramine, and doxepin are demethylated to nortriptyline, desipramine, and dimethyldoxepin, respectively.[23] In addition, these parent compounds and demethylated active metabolites undergo enterohepatic cycling and are further metabolized to inactive compounds, which are excreted as glucuronides in the feces and urine.[23] Because these compounds undergo enterohepatic cycling and also prolong GI transit time, the administration of activated charcoal and a saline cathartic is recommended to promote their intestinal elimination.[30]

In the present case, activated charcoal was administered after lavage, as a 25% w/v (25 g of charcoal powder in a total volume of 100 ml) tap water suspension. This dose was repeated every 6 hours for the first 48 hours after ingestion. The rationale for this technique is related to the fact that tricyclics are basic drugs and are ion-trapped in the acid secretions of the stomach. Continued gastric suction and/or adsorption to activated charcoal would remove the drug present in the stomach. If not removed from the stomach, the drug will pass into the duodenum, become nonionized in the alkaline environment, and be reabsorbed.

Sodium sulfate, 250 mg/kg of body weight, also was administered as a cathartic, to facilitate removal of the charcoal

drug complex from the GI tract. Magnesium sulfate or magnesium citrate also can be used (250 mg/kg of body weight) for this purpose. However, in cases of impending or manifest renal failure, the magnesium-containing cathartics should be avoided because hypermagnesemia may develop and contribute to CNS depression, cardiac arrhythmias, and death.

Removal of Absorbed Drug

Elimination of the tricyclic antidepressant compounds occurs via metabolism by hepatic microsomal enzymes, and only a small percentage (3% to 5%) of unaltered drug appears in the urine.[23] Furthermore, these compounds have high lipid solubility and are rapidly distributed to body tissue sites, especially in the liver, kidney, lung, brain and heart.[23] As a result, because of the low serum concentrations and high tissue levels of these drugs, peritoneal dialysis, hemodialysis, forced diuresis, and exchange transfusions are not effective methods of facilitating their removal from the blood.[31] Theoretically, acidification of the urine would increase the percentage of drug excreted by the urine, but the possibility of systemic acidosis also enhances the cardiotoxic effects of these drugs. Therefore, removal of absorbed drug by these modes of therapy is not advisable. None of these methods was used in the present case.

Symptomatic and Supportive Care

After the initial intensive therapeutic interventions (correction of life-threatening complications and the removal and prevention of further absorption of the drug), symptomatic and supportive care constitutes the cornerstone of therapy for the patient intoxicated with tricyclic antidepressants. Deaths due to arrhythmias, however, have been reported several days after an acute ingestion.[31,32] The specific arrhythmias that have been reported are atrial tachycardia, atrial fibrillation, atrial flutter, atrioventricular block, ventricular tachycardia, ventricular flutter, multifocal extrasystoles, complete heart blocks, bundle branch blocks, and cardiac arrest.[10-12, 17,19-22,27,31,32] The reasons for these delayed cardiac arrhythmias are not clearly understood. Perhaps the delayed absorption due to anticholinergic action, coupled with enterohepatic cycline and the large volume of redistribution of the tricyclic compounds, are the causative factors. Regardless of the cause, the tricyclic-intoxicated patient requires close monitoring of fluid, electrolytes, and vital signs during the first 72 hours of hospitalization.

In the present case, except for the initial symptomatic and supportive care, the patient's hospital course was uneventful, and he was discharged 72 hours postadmission.

ENDPOINTS OF THERAPY

The crucial period of treatment is the first 24 hours. The basic therapeutic interventions are those already described: (1) administration of physostigmine salicylate to treat life-threatening anticholinergic complications, (2) removal and prevention of further absorption from the stomach by emesis or gastric lavage, (3) administration of activated charcoal for at least 48 hours, (4) general supportive measures, and (5) monitoring of the cardiovascular and respiratory systems for the first 72 hours.

GENERAL PROGNOSIS

Prognosis in tricyclic antidepressant overdosages is determined chiefly by the age of the patient, the dose, and the interval between ingestion and discovery. Sudden relapse and death have occurred after apparent recovery. However, if the patient can be sustained for the first 48 to 72 hours, survival is likely, since these drugs are largely metabolized within 72 hours.

REFERENCES

1. Ballin JC: Toxicity of tricyclic antidepressants. *JAMA, 231*:1369, 1975.
2. Poussant AF, and Ditman KS: A controlled study of imipramine (Tofranil) in the treatment of enuresis. *J Pediatr, 67*:283–290, 1965.
3. Newton RW: Physostigmine salicylate in the treatment of tricyclic antidepressant overdosage. *JAMA, 231*:941–943, 1975.
4. Brewer C: Suicide with tricyclic antidepressants. *Br Med J, 2*:110, 1976.
5. Pettit JM, and Biggs JT: Tricyclic antidepressant overdose in adolescent patients. *Pediatrics, 59(2)*:283–287, 1977.
6. Shader RI, and Greenblatt DJ: Belladonna alkaloids and synthetic anticholinergics: Uses and toxicity. In *Psychiatric Complications of Medical Drugs.* Edited by RI Shader. New York, Raven Press, 1972, pp. 103–147.
7. Greenblatt DJ, and Shader RI: Drug therapy: Anticholinergics. *N Engl J Med, 288*:1215–1219, 1973.
8. Granacher RP, and Baldessarine RJ: Physostigmine: Its use in acute anticholinergic syndrome with antidepressant and antiparkinson drugs. *Arch Gen Psychiatry, 32*:375–380, 1975.
9. Koelle GB: Anticholinesterase agents. In *The Pharmacological Basis of Therapeutics.* 4th Ed. Edited by LS Goodman and A Gilman. New York, Macmillan, 1970, pp. 442–465.
10. Burks JS, Walker JE, and Rumack BH: Tricyclic antidepressant poisoning: Reversal of coma, choreothetosis, and myoclonus by physostigmine. *JAMA, 230(10)*:1405–1407, 1974.
11. Slovis TL, et al: Physostigmine therapy in acute tricyclic antidepressant poisoning. *Clin Tox, 4(3)*:451–459, 1971.
12. Rumack BH: Anticholinergic poisoning: Treatment with physostigmine. *Pediatrics, 52(3)*:449–451, 1973.
13. Manoguerra AS, and Ruiz E: Physostigmine treatment of anticholinergic poisoning. *JACEP, 5*:125–127, 1976.
14. Hollister LE: Tricyclic antidepressants (first of two parts). *N Engl J Med, 299*:1106–1109, 1978.
15. Thompson EA: Amitriptyline overdose. *Drug Intell Clin Pharm, 7*:451–458, 1973.
16. Noble J, and Matthew H: Acute poisoning by tricyclic antidepressants: Clinical features and management of 100 patients. *Clin Tox, 2*:403–421, 1969.
17. Vohra JK: Cardiovascular abnormalities following tricyclic antidepressant drug overdosage. *Drugs, 7*:323–325, 1975.
18. Inverson LL: Inhibition of noradrenaline uptake by drugs. *J Pharm Pharmacol, 17*:62–64, 1965.
19. Brown TCK: Treatment of tricyclic overdosage arrhythmias. *Pediatrics, 54*:386–387, 1974.

20. Jefferson JW: A review of the cardiovascular effects and toxicity of tricyclic antidepressants. *Psychosom Med*, 37(2):160–179, 1975.

21. Serafimouski N, et al: Tricyclic antidepressive poisoning with special reference to cardiac complications. *Acta Anaesthesiol Scand* (Suppl), 57:55–63, 1975.

22. Sigg EB, Osborne M, and Korol B: Cardiovascular effects of imipramine. *J Pharmacol Exp Ther*, 141:237–243, 1963.

23. Gard HD, et al: Studies on the disposition of amitriptyline and other tricyclic antidepressant drugs in man as it relates to the management of the overdosed patient. *Adv Biochem Psychopharmacol*, 7:95–105, 1973.

24. Spiker DG, et al: Tricyclic antidepressant overdose: Clinical presentation and plasma levels. *Clin Pharmacol Ther*, 18(5):539–546, 1975.

25. Brown TCK: Sodium bicarbonate treatment for tricyclic antidepressant arrhythmias in children. *Med J Aust*, 2:380–382, 1976.

26. Davis JM: Overdose of psychotropic drugs-tricyclic antidepressants. *Psychiatr Ann*, 3:6–11, 1973.

27. Freeman JW, and Coughhead MG: Beta blockade in the treatment of tricyclic antidepressant overdosage. *Med J Aust*, 1:1233–1235, 1973.

28. Innes IR, and Nickerson M: Sympathomimetic drugs. In *The Pharmacological Basis of Therapeutics*. 4th Ed. Edited by LS Goodman and A Gilman. New York, Macmillan, 1970, pp. 478–523.

29. Rumack BH: Poisindex. Denver, Colorado, Micromedex, Inc., 1978.

30. Crome P, Dawling S, and Braithwaite RA: Effect of activated charcoal on absorption of nortriptyline. *Lancet*, 2:1203–1205, 1977.

31. Rasmussen J: Amitriptyline and imipramine poisoning. *Lancet*, 2:850–851, 1965.

32. Sedal L, et al: Overdosage of tricyclic antidepressants: A report of two deaths and a prospective study of 24 patients. *Med J Aust*, 2:74–79, 1972.

Chapter 8

Neuroleptics

Judy Bell
George E. Bass, Jr.
Javier I. Escobar
Vasilios A. Skoutakis

"Neuroleptics" is the preferred term for a group of drugs that are potent modifiers of behavior. These drugs have also been categorized as anti-schizophrenic, antipsychotic, major tranquilizers, and ataractics. Characteristically, they have demonstrated (1) effects on the psychoses at dosages below sedative-hypnotic levels, (2) profound effects on the autonomic nervous system, and (3) specific effects on the extrapyramidal motor system. Neuroleptics are widely used today for the treatment of psychiatric disorders. This has followed the universal recognition of drug therapy as the single most effective treatment modality for schizophrenia.[1]

The availability of neuroleptics and the emergence of community mental health programs have made possible the outpatient treatment of most psychiatric patients and have contributed to the significant decline in the number of hospitalized psychiatric patients (from 600,000 in 1955 to fewer than 200,000 in 1970).[2,3] As a result, there is a more optimistic outlook for the mentally ill today than in the 1950s.[4]

It was to be expected that increased use and availability of these drugs would result in an increased incidence of intoxications, either accidental or intentional. Neuroleptics rank highly among the drugs most commonly associated with poisonings. Patients for whom neuroleptics are prescribed tend to show low compliance, unpredictable behavior, and a relatively high suicide rate, and are thus at high risk levels for intentional self-intoxication.[5,6] The fact that many of these drugs are marketed as enteric-coated tablets and have a "candy-like" appearance that may prove tempting to youngsters, adds to the likelihood of accidental poisoning.

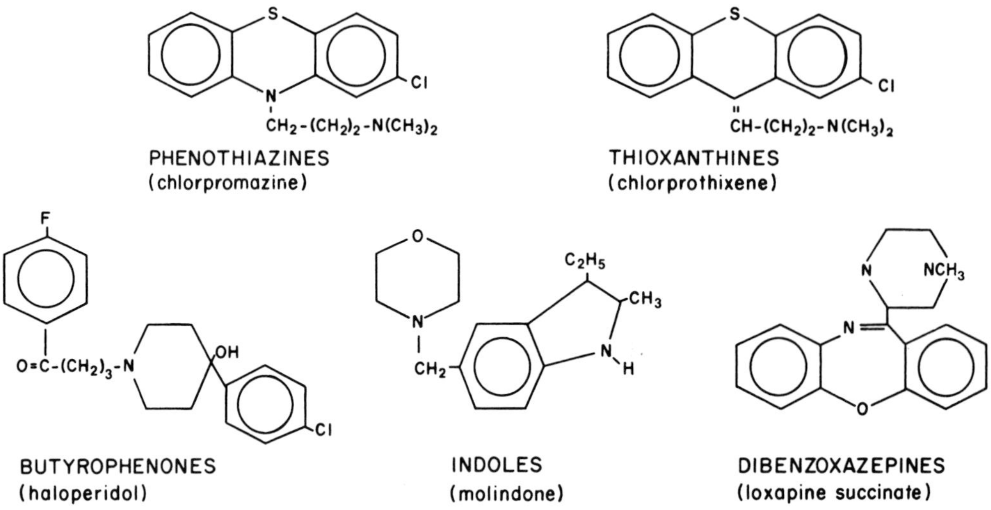

Fig. 8–1.   Major chemical classes of neuroleptic drugs.

Polypharmacy is a complicating factor in neuroleptic intoxications. Multiple drug ingestion by psychiatric patients is a common phenomenon, both during therapy and in overdose cases. This possibility may significantly confound diagnosis and treatment of such intoxications. Since neuroleptic agents have a synergistic effect with other CNS depressants, potentially fatal complications such as coma and respiratory depression may follow multiple drug overdoses. On the other hand, concomitant ingestion of neuroleptics and drugs having strong anticholinergic actions (e.g., the tricyclic antidepressants) may produce florid psychosis (CNS action) and may result in severe anticholinergic symptoms or cardiovascular difficulties (peripheral effects).

Neuroleptics used clinically fall into five major chemical classes: (1) the phenothiazines, (2) the thioxanthenes, (3) the butyrophenones, (4) the indoles, and (5) the dibenzoxazepines. These groups share many similar actions and side effects, and their overdoses are treated in the same manner. Their general chemical structures are presented in Figure 8–1. Specific

members of these groups and their daily dosages are listed in Table 8–1.

The frequency and seriousness of neuroleptic intoxications represent a public health hazard. Health care professionals should be readily familiar with the clinical diagnostic considerations, the mechanisms of the toxicologic manifestations, the appropriate tests required, and the therapeutic modalities available for the optimal management of patients intoxicated by neuroleptic drugs.

CASE REPORT

A 16-year-old male was brought to the emergency room by his older sister 8 hours after he ingested a "handful" of tablets. Prior to the overdose, the boy had become "infuriated" after he had an argument with his father. He had also shown other behavioral changes the preceding days, which had led to expulsion from school. The family reported that the boy obtained the pills from friends who called them "downers." Description of the color and shape of these pills led to a

Table 8–1.   Commonly Used Neuroleptic Drugs

ANTIPSYCHOTIC AGENT	DAILY DOSAGE RANGE* (MG)	DOSE RATIO EQUIVALENT TO 300 MG CHLORPROMAZINE
Phenothiazine		
Aliphatics		
Chlorpromazine	100–1000	300
(Thorazine)		
Triflupromazine	20–150	100
(Vesprin)		
Piperidines		
Thioridazine	30–800	300
(Mellaril)		
Mesoridazine	50–400	150
(Serentil)		
Piperacetazine	20–160	30
(Quide)		
Piperazines		
Trifluoperazine	2–30	25
(Stelazine)		
Perphenazine	2–64	28
(Trilafon)		
Carphenazine	25–400	75
(Proketazine)		
Acetophenazine	40–80	50
(Tindal)		
Butaperazine	30–50	30
(Repoise)		
Prochlorperazine	15–125	60
(Compazine)		
Thiopropazate	6–30	30
(Dartal)		
Fluphenazine	0.5–20	6
(Prolixin)		
Thioxanthene		
Chlorprothixene	10–600	300
(Taractan)		
Thiothixene	6–60	25
(Navane)		
Butyrophenones		
Haloperidol	1–100	15
(Haldol)		
Indoles		
Molindone	15–225	60
(Moban)		
Dibenzoxazepines		
Loxapine succinate	15–160	30
(Loxitane)		

* Dosage ranges derived from package inserts published in 1980 Physicians Desk Reference. Upper limits are "recommended."

suspicion of a chlorpromazine (Thorazine) overdosage.

On examination, the patient was semicomatose but responsive to painful stimuli; reflexes were intact. Vital signs were blood pressure, 90/66 mm Hg; pulse, 110 beats/min; respirations, 12/min; and temperature (rectal), 35.6°C. Mucous membranes were dry, and bowel sounds were decreased. There was no abdominal tenderness. Examination of the chest showed that lungs were clear and the cardiovascular system was normal except for tachycardia. The blood pressure fell to 80/0 and temperature to 34.4°C 30 minutes after admission. An EKG obtained shortly after admission showed prolongation of the Q-T interval, wideninig of the QRS complex, and flattening of the T-wave. Chest x-ray examination results were normal; results of laboratory evaluations, such as biochemical (SMA-12) and hematologic (Hemo-10 with differentials) indices, including urinalysis, were all within normal limits.

CLINICAL ASSESSMENT AND MANAGEMENT OF THE PATIENT

In this particular instance, we were fortunate to have clues to the drug's identity. In general, however, a thorough assessment and successful management of the neuroleptic-intoxicated patient will require systematic consideration of the following points: (1) manifestations and mechanisms of neuroleptic toxicity, (2) assessment of the severity of the intoxication, (3) appropriate management and treatment, (4) measures available to decrease toxicity, (5) endpoints of therapy, and (6) general prognosis.

MANIFESTATIONS AND MECHANISMS OF NEUROLEPTIC TOXICITY

The clinical picture of a neuroleptic overdose may be variable, ranging from mild drowsiness to life-threatening symptoms such as coma and respiratory depression. Initially, the intoxicated patient may exhibit agitation, hyperactivity, psychotic symptoms, or seizures which precede the onset of CNS depression. In the majority of cases, however, the most frequent immediate manifestations of acute neuroleptic overdose are somnolence and orthostatic hypotension.

In the fully developed neuroleptic intoxication, the main toxicologic effects involve the CNS, the cardiovascular system, and the peripheral (autonomic) nervous system, as evidenced in the case presented above (i.e., CNS toxicities such as Grade 1 coma and respiratory depression, cardiovascular toxicities such as hypotension and EKG abnormalities, and peripheral toxicities such as dry mucous membranes, decreased bowel sounds, mydriasis, and hypothermia).

The mechanisms of the CNS, cardiovascular, and peripheral toxicities seen with neuroleptic overdoses, as in the case presented, can be related to the anticholinergic properties, alpha-adrenergic blockade, quinidine-like action, and antidopaminergic action of the neuroleptic drugs.[5-11]

Central Nervous System

Neuroleptics affect the CNS at all levels, producing CNS depression. Their most specific effects take place at the reticular activating system (RAS), the hypothalamus, the limbic system, especially the amygdala, hippocampus and nucleus accumbens septi, and the basal ganglia.[12]

Reticular activating system. The RAS controls the overall degree of CNS activity. The RAS of the brain stem is basically responsible for wakefulness.[13] Neuroleptics cause only a slight increase in the threshold for arousal produced by direct electrical stimulation in the RAS of the brain stem. Toxic doses of neuroleptics depress this function. Therefore, the intoxicated patient may exhibit a state ranging from sedation to coma, depending on the dose ingested and other complicating factors. Coma is a rare complication of neuroleptic intoxication in adults, but is seen frequently in children.

Severe CNS depression in young children has been reported following ingestion of as little as 100 mg of chlorpromazine.[14] A 1-year-old child became comatose and apneic after swallowing 200 mg of chlorpromazine.[14] A 3-year-old child died after ingesting 800 mg of the same drug.[14] An article by Kahn and Blum reported that six infants (aged 9 to 22 weeks) admitted to a particular hospital in a 7-month period developed sleep apnea, resulting in sudden infant death syndrome (SIDS).[15] These cases were attributed to the administration of alimenazine and promethazine syrup.

Respiration is a vital function that may be affected by the neuroleptic's action on the RAS of the brain stem. The respiratory center of the medulla is not affected by clinical doses of neuroleptics, but is directly depressed by toxic amounts of these drugs.[7] Ventilatory assistance is required in some cases. A newborn of a schizophrenic mother receiving fluphenazine developed respiratory depression, owing to the fact that the drug crosses the placental barrier.[5]

An unusual case report cites a middle-aged female who developed respiratory depression during rapid tranquilization (neuroleptization) with chlorpromazine and who died suddenly without any other abnormal physical signs.[14] There have been other reports of respiratory complications, especially with children.[6] In a review by Barry and associates, tachypnea was noted in some patients, with no explanation as to its cause,[5] but has not been noted by others. However, this potentially lethal complication of neuroleptic overdose should be kept in mind.

Hypothalamus. The hypothalamic nuclei activate, control, and integrate peripheral autonomic mechanisms, endocrine activity, and many other somatic functions. The hypothalamus plays a special role in the control of the vasomotor system. Stimulation of this area results in vasoconstriction, whereas neuroleptic-induced depression of the same area produces vasodilation (inhibition of vasoconstrictor tone), resulting in clinically significant hypotension.

Since the temperature-regulating center is also located within the hypothalamus, neuroleptics ingested in toxic amounts may upset this center, leading to hypo- or hyperthermia.[5]

Limbic system. The antipsychotic efficacy of neuroleptics is assumed to result from blockade of dopaminergic receptors within the mesolimbic pathway. Areas of the limbic system are thought to be primarily responsible for mood and behavior. "Reward" and "punishment" centers are thought to be located within certain structures of the limbic system. Neuroleptic-induced decreases in affective reactivity may be a result of the neuroleptics' action on these centers. The more sedating neuroleptics (e.g., aliphatic phenothiazines) will calm the hyperactive individual, whereas the "activating" agents (e.g., thioxanthenes) tend to stimulate the catatonic individual. In toxic doses, neuroleptics may produce exaggerated responses involving sedation or hyperactivity, according to the model proposed above.

Large doses of neuroleptics may induce spontaneous motor activity within the amygdala.[7] Seizures may be observed, since these drugs have the ability to lower the seizure threshold. This is a potential problem especially for those patients with (a) a pre-existing seizure disorder, (b) abnormal EEG without a history of seizures, (c) pre-existing CNS pathology, (d) history of electroconvulsive therapy, (e) rapid increases in drug dosage, or (f) history of parenteral administration of neuroleptic drugs.[16]

Basal ganglia. Neuroleptics produce a blockade of dopamine receptors in the

Table 8–2.   Neuroleptic-Induced Extrapyramidal Symptoms

CLASSFICATION	SIGNS AND SYMPTOMS

Parkinsonian reactions	Akinesia
	   Immobility of face
	   Slow, monotonous speech
	   Rigidity, immobility, "cog-wheel" sign
	   Disturbed posture
	   Shuffling, festinating gait
	Tremor
	   Pill-rolling movements of hands and fingers
	   Regular rhythmic to-and-fro oscillations of extremities
	Increased salivation

Dystonic reactions	Dystonias
	   Oculogyric crisis, fixed upward gaze, eye-walling
	   Neck twisting and torticollis
	   Jaw spasm, inability to open and close mouth
	   Lip spasm, inability to purse to whistle
	   Tongue spasm, protrusion and curling
	   Facial distortions, bizarre grimaces
	   Throat spasm, difficulty in speech and swallowing
	   Shoulder raising
	   Opisthotonus, arching of back, hyperextension of neck and trunk
	Dyskinesias
	   Clonic involuntary contractions of muscle groups
	   Blinking, facial tics, and twitches
	   Chewing movements, lip smacking
	   "Rabbit syndrome;" aimless movements of tongue
	   Shoulder shrugging, pedaling movement of legs

Akathisia reactions	Akathisia
	   Inability to sit still
	   Continuous agitation and restless movement
	   Rocking and shifting weight while standing
	   Shifting of legs and tapping of heel while sitting

Tardive dyskinesia reactions	Hyperkinesias: lingual and facial BLM triad
	   Smacking and licking of lips, sucking and chewing movements,
	      rolling and protrusion of tongue
	   Grimaces
	   Spastic facial distortions
	Choreoathetoid movements of extremities
	   Clonic jerking of fingers, ankles, and toes
	   Tonic contractions of neck and back muscles

striatum (nigrostriatal pathway) within the basal ganglia, which commonly results in extrapyramidal symptoms (EPS).[16] These are characteristic motor disturbances and are listed and described in Table 8–2.

The dystonic reactions are commonly seen with acute neuroleptic ingestion, especially with haloperidol and the piperazine phenothiazines. As a rule, dystonias are side effects of treatment initiation and may be seen after a single dose. Young males are particularly susceptible. Medical personnel, when unaware of neuroleptic intake, may attribute signs of dystonia to epilepsy, encephalitis, or meningitis.[9,16] Proper tests must be performed to rule out these possibilities.

Akathisia and parkinsonism usually occur during the first several weeks of therapy. When these symptoms are manifest, dosage of the neuroleptic ought to be titrated. If this fails to control severe EPS, administration of an antiparkinsonian agent or substitution by a less potent neuroleptic is the required procedure. Akathisia and drug-induced parkinsonism, as well as tardive dyskinesia, occur most frequently in elderly females.[16] Although acute ingestion of neuroleptics has the potential to produce these symptoms, they are more reflective of chronic toxicity.

Cardiovascular System

The effects of neuroleptics on the cardiovascular system are complex, and mechanisms related to their pharmacologic/toxicologic actions are not fully understood. The cardiovascular effects can be divided into two major categories: peripheral (blood pressure and pulse rate) and central (EKG abnormalities and arrhythmias).

Blood pressure and pulse. Hypotension is one of the most common side effects of neuroleptic drugs and is almost universally present with high doses.[9] It is most frequently caused by the aliphatic and piperidine phenothiazines. Centrally mediated vasomotor reflex inhibition, alpha-adrenergic blockade in the periphery, and a local vasodilatory action of the arterial walls are all contributing factors.[8,10] Epinephrine, which has both alpha- and beta-adrenergic actions, reverses the pressor response because of the alpha-adrenergic blockade produced by the neuroleptics, and beta-adrenergic stimulation predominates. Therefore, administration of this catecholamine causes a further drop in blood pressure.

On the other hand, norepinephrine and dopamine, which are alpha-receptor stimulators, prolong the pressor response when given in doses large enough to overcome the alpha blockade.[10,16] A moderate fall in systolic blood pressure is commonly seen, but the decrease in the diastolic reading is almost universal. A transient rise in pulse rate is usually noted.[8] Hypotensive patients are more subject to

cardiac arrhythmias and should be closely monitored.

Interestingly, a recent article by Cummingham described instances of hypertension in small children with acute ingestions of haloperidol.[18] This increase in blood pressure was of delayed onset and tended to be severe. It is recommended that children with accidental neuroleptic overdoses be observed in the hospital for a minimum of 2 days. The mechanism of action for this paradoxical adverse effect is not known.

EKG abnormalities. Various degrees of conduction impairment produced by large doses of neuroleptics are attributable to their quinidine-like activity. Any or all of the following signs may be present in the EKG: blunting and/or notching of the T-wave, prolongation of the Q-T interval, increased convexity of the ST-segment, and U-waves of high amplitude.[8,19] Thioridazine and its analogs are the most common offenders in this respect; chlorpromazine and trifluoperazine may cause similar changes, but do so less frequently.[20] Thioridazine and mesoridazine may produce characteristic distortions of the T-wave (e.g., blunting and widening), which at times constitute the only significant EKG abnormality.[8,17]

A local anesthetic effect on the myocardium may also occur with neuroleptics, similar to that produced by lidocaine. The effects produced, which are related to dose and potency of the neuroleptic, are prolongation of the refractory period (decreased heart rate), delay in intraventricular conduction time (widened QRS), and decreased excitability of the SA node and myocardium ("dropped" or "missed" beats, cardiac arrhythmias, and varying degrees of heart block).[17]

Arrhythmias. The exact mechanism for neuroleptic-induced arrhythmias is not well understood. However, increased plasma levels of catecholamines and anticholinergic effects are thought to be responsible.[10] Thioridazine is the agent most commonly responsible for ventricular arrhythmias. Most fatalities are seen at doses that significantly exceed the usually recommended therapeutic range.[8,19] The balance between the blocking effects of chlorpromazine on adrenergic receptors and the high norepinephrine levels in the blood might be disturbed, especially since chlorpromazine does not block all receptors equally.

Neuroleptics block dopaminergic receptors both pre- and postsynaptically, and the alpha-adrenergic receptors postsynaptically. Such an imbalance potentially could trigger fatal arrhythmias.[21] It has also been suggested that arrhythmias and myocardial damage are not the direct results of phenothiazine's action, but may be related to the high levels of circulating norepinephrine (the heart binds relatively little chlorpromazine compared to other tissues).[22]

Tachycardia is common. Vagal stimulation compensates for drug-induced hypotension and decreased peripheral vascular resistance. Deaths usually have been due to ventricular fibrillation or cardiac arrest.[10,17,19,23] Individuals with preexisting cardiovascular disorders or hypokalemia are at high risk levels for serious cardiovascular complications and the possibility of death.

Autonomic Nervous System

The neuroleptics act upon the autonomic nervous system, producing anticholinergic side effects, alpha-adrenergic blockade, adrenergic potentiating effects, and antiserotonin effects. The following symptoms are commonly seen with phenothiazines during both overdoses and clinical treatment, and are attributed primarily to their anticholinergic effects: decreased bowel sounds, dryness of mouth and mucous membranes, pallor, nasal congestion, difficulty in urination, miosis and/or mydriasis, and blurred vision. Hypothermia and hyperthermia have been mentioned previously as CNS effects (actions on the hypothalamus). Sweating is common with thioridazine and is sometimes associated with acute dystonic reactions.

ASSESSMENT OF THE SEVERITY OF THE INTOXICATION

The toxicologic manifestations and severity of acute neuroleptic intoxication can be adequately assessed during the first 12 to 24 hours through monitoring of vital signs and symptoms, biochemical and hematologic indices, EKG, x-ray evaluation, and serum neuroleptic concentrations, in this case, of chlorpromazine. A reliable history regarding the amount ingested, time of ingestion, and clinical condition of the patient may also be helpful in the prognostication of the severity or outcome.

Physical Examination

Neuroleptics are well absorbed orally, and the intoxicated patient will usually develop symptoms within the first several hours after ingestion. Physical examination on admission will provide a baseline for observations of the clinical status throughout the course of treatment. Since phenothiazines undergo enterohepatic circulation (e.g., vast metabolism), a large volume of distribution, and a long sojourn within the body, adverse effects can appear hours or days after an acute or severe overdose.

Correction of Life-Threatening Symptoms

This is the single most important consideration. The medical personnel must immediately assess the respiratory function by checking the tidal volume, respiratory rate, and the degree of cyanosis present if any, and by obtaining the arterial blood gas values as soon as possible, to determine if systemic acidosis has ensued. Establishment of respiration must be made and an artificial airway created if necessary.

Other vital signs must be checked. The neuroleptic-intoxicated patient is likely to be in shock due to drug-induced vasomotor collapse, further complicated by the strong alpha-adrenergic blockade. Appropriate therapy for hypotension is to place the patient in the Trendelenburg position and, if necessary, to administer fluids, plasma protein fraction (Plasmanate), or blood to expand the circulatory volume. For more severe cases, vasopressors may be needed to allow for adequate perfusion of the tissues and to restore cardiac output. Norepinephrine (0.1 to 0.2 μg/kg/min by IV infusion, usually 5 mg in 1 L of D$_5$W or D$_5$NS),[11] or dopamine (5 to 10 μg/mg/min, which may be increased as necessary up to 20 μg),[24] is the drug of choice, but metaraminol or phenylephrine could also be considered. Dopamine has the advantage of stimulating the myocardial beta receptors, without inducing tachycardia or dilating the blood vessels supplying the kidney so that there is no further decrease in urinary output. Arrhythmias can be induced by the catecholamines, however, and caution as to their use is essential.

If arrhythmias are present, phenytoin is the agent of choice to reverse depressed AV conduction caused by the quinidine-like effect of the drug. The adult dosage is 9 to 11 mg/kg, or more conveniently, 100 mg IV over 3 minutes, repeated every 5 minutes until arrhythmias have ceased and a maximum of 1000 mg has been given. The pediatric dose is 1 mg/kg, also given by slow IV infusion.[11] This method of administration avoids the risk of a sinus slowing, profound hypotension, and/or cardiac arrest. If a high degree of AV blockage is present, a pacemaker may be utilized in the right ventricle.[11]

The state of consciousness, pupillary size and reactivity, and deep tendon reflexes should be recorded at the first examination and at frequent intervals throughout the course, in order to assess neurologic status. Convulsions may be treated with IV diazepam, 0.1 to 0.3 mg/kg in children and up to 10 mg in adults.[21] This dose may be repeated 2 hours later if needed.

If the patient is unresponsive to diazepam, phenytoin may be given (1 to 3 mg/kg or 150 to 250 mg bolus by slow IV infusion). This may be repeated 30 minutes later in a dose of 100 to 150 mg if necessary. Short-acting barbiturates have been used, but they can potentiate respiratory depression. Physostigmine, which is more commonly used with anticholinergic and tricyclic antidepressant overdoses, was shown to reverse coma in a 2½-year-old boy who ingested five 100-mg tablets of chlorpromazine. This is the first reported instance of the use of physostigmine for a phenothiazine-induced CNS depression.[14]

Dosage Considerations

A review of over 100 cases of chlorpromazine intoxication revealed that patients with nonsevere intoxications took an average dose of 1.4 g of chlorpromazine, whereas those with severe poisonings took an average of 6.2 g.[6] Fatal dosages have been reported in the wide range of 15 to 150 g/kg. Children are more susceptible to toxicity. Lethal doses for young children have been reported to be as low as 350 mg.[25] In contrast, adults have survived doses of 10 g.[6] Dosages of 5 g or more of chlorpromazine usually produce CNS depression and acute EPS (mainly dystonias). In the case of massive overdoses, the clinical picture is characterized by seizures, dystonic reactions, hypotension, hyperthermia, arrhythmias, and in extreme cases, coma and respiratory depression.

ROLE OF THE LABORATORY

Any patient for whom an overdose of neuroleptic drugs is known or suspected should have blood drawn for analysis immediately, certainly before any additional medication is given. A complete blood count, total blood chemistry, and toxicologic screening should be obtained.

Techniques for measuring neuroleptics in blood have been developed in the last few years. Presently, however, their clinical applications are limited.[26] Determination of plasma levels is helpful in the case of toxic ingestions, although the majority of laboratories are not yet equipped to provide this service. Techniques available for quantitation of plasma drug levels have been totally inadequate until recently.

The relatively undeveloped state of knowledge is due primarily to lack of sensitivity and/or specificity for accurate measurement of the low levels of drug found in the plasma. These levels rarely exceed a few hundred nanograms per milliliter, regardless of the quantity ingested. Toxic levels of chlorpromazine in blood are considered to be above 300 mg/ml.[27,28] Returns from emesis and gastric lavage will often be the best fluids for analysis.[24,29]

Urine samples are important for toxicologic purposes. The Forrest colorimetric test provides a relatively quick detection of phenothiazines in urine.[11] This test will not detect most other drugs (the notable exception being tricyclic antidepressants in the dichromate test solution). Table 8–3 contains a description of the test solutions, procedures, and resultant colors.[28,30] The colors must be interpreted carefully because they may change with time and are more a reflection of average daily doses rather than of acute overdose concentrations. This test may identify phenothiazines in urine long after a therapeutic or toxic ingestion. Some phenothiazines have been detected in the urine up to a month after discontinuation.[7] False positives have been reported with urobilinogen. Haloperidol, a butyrophenone, can not be detected by the Forrest test.[11]

Other urine screening tests available in many laboratories include thin layer chromatography (TLC) and enzyme multiplied immunological techniques (EMIT). These tests are useful and allow concurrent detection of several drugs. However, both procedures may also yield false positives, and results must be interpreted carefully. If no laboratory facilities are available, reagent strips (Phenistix) may be used for colorimetric purposes. As stated previously, gas chromatography procedures are now available in some laboratories for quantitative determination of most neuroleptics.

Since other CNS depressants potentiate phenothiazine intoxication, laboratory confirmation of the presence of barbiturates, nonbarbiturate sedative-hypnotics, minor tranquilizers, alcohol, and opiates is important. If the patient gives a reliable history, or if his account is verified and he is not in an acute condition, laboratory screening may be limited to alcohol and barbiturates.

The phenothiazines are one of the few classes of drugs that are radiopaque. Other such agents include iron-containing salts and chloral hydrate. An acronym used to remember radiopaque drugs is "CHIP" (chloral hydrate, iron, phenothiazines). An abdominal x-ray examination will often indicate whether significant amounts of the drug are still present in the GI tract.[5]

An electrocardiogram is essential to assess the patient's cardiac status. Frequent monitoring is advisable since arrhythmias may develop later. Through chronological comparison of laboratory values (e.g., arterial blood gas values, blood chemistry values, EKGs) and the clinical symptoms, a prognosis can be estimated and a judgement made as to the form of therapy to be initiated or modified. If sensitive instruments are available for detection of the drug in urine or plasma, periodic analysis will help determine the rate at which the drug is being absorbed, metabolized, and most importantly, eliminated.

Table 8–3. Forrest Tests for Simple Visual Color Readings of Psychoactive Drugs in Urine

DRUG	TEST SOLUTION	PROCEDURE	RESULTING TEST COLORS			
			+	++	+++	++++
(1) Chlorpromazine (Thorazine)	20 parts 5% ferric chloride; 80 parts 10% sulfuric acid	Mix 1 ml urine with 1 ml test solution; read within 20 seconds.	Pink	Purple	Dark Blue	Dark Gray
		Daily dosage (mg)	100–300	300–600	600–900	900 & over
(2) Promazine (Sparine) and Mepazine (Pacatal)	Same as above	Same as above	Rose	Red	Brown	Dark Gray
		Daily dosage (mg)	100–300	300–600	600–900	900 & over
(3) Thioridazine (Mellaril)	2 parts 5% ferric chloride; 98 parts 30% sulfuric acid	Mix 1 ml urine with 1 ml test solution; read within 30 seconds.	Light Pink	Pink	Dark Pink	Blue
		Daily dosage (mg)	75–150	150–450	450–800	800 & over
(4) Imipramine (Tofranil)	25 parts 0.2% potassium dichromate; 25 parts 30% sulfuric acid; 25 parts 20% perchloric acid; 25 parts 50% nitric acid	Mix 0.5 ml urine with 1 ml test solution; read within 20 seconds.	Light Green	Yellow-Green	Green	Blue-Green
		Daily dosage (mg)	25–50	50–75	75–150	150–250
(5) Most Phenothiazines Vesprin Prolixin Trilafon Compazin Dartal Stelazine Tindal Mellaril Pacatal Phenergan Sparine etc. Thorazine	"FPN" Universal Test 5 parts 5% ferric chloride; 45 parts 20% perchloric acid; 50 parts 50% nitric acid	Mix 1 ml urine with 1 ml test solution; read immediately. Disregard all colors appearing after delay of 10 seconds or more.	Peach (+)	Pink (++)	Dark Pink (+++)	
		Daily dosage (mg)	20–70	70–120	120–200	
			Rose (4+)	Purple (5+)	Dark Gray (6+)	
		Daily dosage (mg)	200–400	400–800	800–2000	

From Forrest FM, Forrest IS, and Mason AS: A review of rapid urine tests for phenothiazines and related drugs. *The American Journal of Psychiatry*, Vol. 118:10, pp. 300–307, 1961. Copyright 1961, The American Psychiatric Association. Reprinted by permission.

In the case presented, a "stat" urine drug screen revealed positive results when urine is tested for phenothiazines. Abdominal x-ray examinations revealed a few radiopaque tablet-like densities scattered throughout the small intestine, further confirming the intoxicant.

INDICATED THERAPEUTIC MEASURES

Measures Designed to Decrease Absorption

Emesis. Emesis should be initiated if the patient has not lost the gag reflex, is conscious, and is not seizing. Emesis is performed by administration of syrup of ipecac in a dose of 10 ml for small children (under 5 years old) and 15 to 30 ml for older children and adults, followed by a glass of water (necessary for ipecac to act). A second dose may be given in 30 minutes if the first administration is nonproductive. Induction of emesis has been shown to be an appropriate means of removal, notwithstanding the antiemetic action of these drugs.[5]

Lavage. Lavage should be instituted after the patient has been intubated with a nasogastric hose of the largest diameter permissible (no less than 28 French),[23] to allow passage of the neuroleptic tablets. The phenothiazines are lipid-soluble but are not rapidly absorbed from the GI tract. They also delay gastric emptying owing to their anticholinergic effects. Thus, it is possible for significant amounts of the drug to be removed hours after ingestion has taken place.[5]

Isotonic saline solution is preferred, but water may also be used in adults. About 300 ml of fluid for adults and 10 ml/kg for children should be used in each wash. The patient should be placed on his left side with his head down over the table and the foot of the bed elevated to prevent aspiration, unless a cuffed endotracheal tube is used. Lavage should continue until the return fluid is clear. All aspirate should be saved for analysis, with the first liter kept separate from the others.[24]

Charcoal. Activated charcoal may be administered while the lavage tube is still in place. Any drug remaining in the stomach will be adsorbed by the charcoal, and the complex will then be eliminated. The usual dose is 5 to 10 times the amount ingested, or 30 to 50 g in a water slurry. If emesis occurs, another dose should be given.

The phenothiazines are similar to the tricyclic antidepressants in that both undergo extensive enterohepatic circulation, prolong GI transit time, and are ion-trapped, basic drugs in the stomach's acidic environment. Therefore, the rationale of repeated administration of activated charcoal every 6 hours for the first 48 hours after ingestion of tricyclic antidepressants would hold true for the phenothiazines.[31] Any drug that has passed into the duodenum will be absorbed there because of the alkaline pH of the small intestine and the basicity of the drug (making it nonionized in this environment).

Catharsis. A saline cathartic is needed to further eliminate any drug left in the GI tract. The agent of choice is sodium or magnesium sulfate, 250 mg/kg of body weight. The magnesium salt should be used with caution, however, since hypermagnesemia may develop and contribute to CNS depression, cardiac arrhythmias, and death.[32] It is also to be avoided in the presence of renal failure, a potential danger to severely intoxicated patients.[21]

Symptomatic and Supportive Care

This is most essential for the intoxicated patient after correction of life-threatening symptoms. Acute dystonic reactions are frequently cited in the literature. Haloperidol and the piperazines are the more frequent precipitating agents. Treatment of choice for dystonia is diphenhydramine, 1 to 5 mg/kg, up to a maximum of 50 mg given IV over 2 minutes.

Antiparkinsonian agents may also be used, but anticholinergic toxicity may be potentiated. The agent in this category that may be given parenterally is benztropine, 2 mg IV or IM, or biperiden, 2 mg IV or IM. Acute dystonia is usually rapidly reversed after a single injection; this response can serve as a diagnostic tool.

If the patient is asymptomatic in all other respects after the injection, he may be sent home with a 3-day supply of oral medication. Commonly prescribed drugs are biperiden, 2 mg three times a day; proclidine, 2.5 to 5 mg three times a day; trihexyphenidyl, 2 mg two or three times a day; diphenhydramine, 25 mg three times a day; and benztropine, 1 to 2 mg two times a day. This oral medication follow-up is necessary because the reactions are likely to recur within 24 hours.[5]

In brain-damaged individuals, a single ingestion of phenothiazines may cause intractable dystonia, as occurred in a 10-year-old, mentally retarded child.[33] Treatment with diphenhydramine and benztropine produced only minimal improvement, suggesting that neuroleptic drugs tend to cause permanent damage.

Hydration should be restored with fluids, and electrolyte balance should be closely monitored and kept within normal limits. Mild hypokalemia may occur and may cause synergism sufficient to produce arrhythmia. One thioridazine overdose was fatal with a potassium level of 3.3 mEq/L.[17] Death on the sixth hospital day was caused by renal failure in one 47-year-old female after a thioridazine overdose.[5]

If hypothermia is severe, it may be relieved by blankets or appropriate covering. However, care should be taken to prevent hyperthermia, since the temperature-regulating system of the hypothalamus is disturbed, and the patient will tend to approach the ambient temperature. One intoxicated patient was reported to have a temperature as low as 31°C.[25]

After apparent recovery, the patient should be monitored for a period of 72 hours because of the drug's prolonged half-life and the possibility of the patient relapsing into a state of respiratory failure, cardiac arrhythmias, or shock.[5]

Severe hypersensitivity reactions, although rare, may be seen after phenothiazine ingestion. The two most important ones are agranulocytosis and hepatitis. Therefore, follow-up evaluation of blood profiles and tests of liver and renal function should be performed. A 59-year-old male developed active chronic hepatitis 8 months after an overdose of chlorpromazine,[14] and cholestatic jaundice has been reported in 2% to 4% of patients taking phenothiazines.[7] It is thought that this is due to a continuation of the drug's initial effects on the liver.

MEASURES TO DECREASE TOXICITY

Hemodialysis. Hemodialysis and peritoneal dialysis are of little value with the phenothiazines and other neuroleptics, due to the high degree of protein binding and wide distribution of these drugs in various body tissues.[11] In one study, ^{35}S-tagged phenothiazines were given to patients undergoing hemodialysis. Little of the drug was found to pass through the cellophane membrane.[5]

Forced diuresis. Small amounts of free drug are excreted in the urine, but greater amounts are found in the bile and feces. In one study, 24-hour urine collections in patients over a 30-week period showed the average excretion of unchanged drug to be only 1%.[9] A 24-year-old male who had taken 200 mg of trifluoperazine was treated with forced diuresis, and only 16 mg were recovered in 7.5 L of urine. The majority was recovered in the feces.[6] Obviously, forced diuresis is of little help, and no beneficial results are cited in the literature.[6,9,22]

Charcoal perfusion. The utility of charcoal perfusion for removal of neuroleptics has not been investigated, but there are reasons to think it may have some value in the treatment of intoxication.

ENDPOINTS OF THERAPY

The first 24 hours are the most important for initiation of therapy. Basic measures are aimed at treatment of life-threatening complications, removal and prevention of further absorption from the stomach by emesis or gastric lavage, administration of charcoal for at least 48 hours, general supportive treatment, and monitoring of the patient's status for the first 72 hours.

In the case presented, recovery was uneventful after removal of the drug from the GI tract and administration of fluids for hypotension. The patient was discharged after a 4-day hospital stay, with a referral for psychiatric consultation.

GENERAL PROGNOSIS

Serious complications or deaths due to neuroleptic overdoses are low in adults, but relatively common in children.[35] Prognosis is generally good, and most overdoses are nonfatal, resolving within 24 hours. Nevertheless, the severity of symptoms is variable and is determined in each individual by age, dose, and interval between ingestion and initiation of treatment. The first 72 hours postingestion are the most crucial, and frequent monitoring and treatment of the patient are required. After this period, if there are no serious complications, the outcome is usually favorable.

REFERENCES

1. Hollister LE: Antipsychotic medications and the treatment of schizophrenia. In *Psychopharmacology*. Edited by JD Barchas, PA Berger, RO Ciaranello, and GR Elliot. New York, Oxford University Press, 1977, p. 131.
2. Bassuk EL, and Gerson S: Deinstitutionalization and mental health services. *Sci Am, 238(2)*:46–58, 1978.
3. Greenblatt M: Drugs, schizophrenia and the third revolution. In *Psychopharmacology: A Generation of Progress*. Edited by MA Lipton, A DiMascio, and KF Killam. New York, Raven Press, 1978, pp. 1179–1185.
4. Berger PA: Medical treatment of mental illness. *Science, 200*:947–981, 1978.
5. Barry D, Meyskens FL, and Becker CE: Phenothiazine poisoning: A review of 48 cases. *Calif Med, 118*:1–5, 1973.
6. Davis JM: Overdosage of psychotropic drugs. *Dis Nerv Sys, 29*:157–164, 1968.
7. Jarvik ME: Drugs used in the treatment of psychiatric disorders: The phenothiazine derivatives. In *The Pharmacological Basis of Therapeutics*. 4th Ed. Edited by LS Goodman and A Gilman. New York, Macmillan, 1970, pp.155–169.
8. Ebert MH, and Shader RI: Cardiovascular effects of psychotropic drugs. *Conn Med, 33(11)*:695–702, 1969.
9. Rivera-Calimlim L: Pharmacology and therapeutic application of the phenothiazines. *Ration Drug Ther, 11(4)*:1–8, 1977.
10. Alexander CS, and Nino A: Cardiovascular complications in young patients taking psychotropic drugs. *Am Heart J, 78(6)*:757–769, 1969.
11. Rumack BH (Ed): Phenothiazines and related drugs. *Poisindex*. Denver, Colorado, Micromedex, Inc., May, 1978.
12. Barchas JD, et al: Behavioral neurochemistry: Neuroregulators and behavioral states. *Science, 200*:964–973, 1978.
13. Guyton AC: Activation of the brain—The reticular activating system. In *Textbook of Medical Physiology*. 5th Ed. Philadelphia, WB Saunders, 1976, pp. 729–731.
14. Whyman A: Phenothiazine death: An unusual case report: *J Nerv Ment Dis, 163(3)*:214–216, 1976.
15. Kahn A, and Blum D: Possible role of phenothiazines in sudden infant death. *Lancet, 2(8138)*:364–365, 1979.
16. Sovner R, and DiMascio A: Extrapyramidal syndromes and other neurological side effects of psychotropic drugs. In *Psychopharmacology: A Generation of Progress*. Edited by MA Lipton, A DiMascio, and KF Killam. New York, Raven Press, 1978, pp. 1021–1032.
17. Donlon PT, and Tupin JP: Successful suicides with thioridazine and mesoridazine: A result of probable cardiotoxicity. *Arch Gen Psychiatry, 34*:955–957, 1977.
18. Cunningham DG: Hypertension in acute haloperidol poisoning. *J Pediatr, 95(3)*:489–490, 1979.
19. Crane GE: Cardiac toxicity and psychotropic drugs. *Dis Nerv Sys, 31*:534–539, 1970.
20. Huston JR, and Bell GE: The effect of

thioridazine and chlorpromazine on the EKG. *JAMA, 198*:16–20, 1966.

21. Carlsson C, Dencker SJ, Grinby G, and Haggendal J: Noradrenaline in blood-plasma and urine during chlorpromazine treatment. *Lancet, 1*:1208, 1966.

22. Forrest IS, Bolt AG, and Serra MT: Distribution of chlorpromazine metabolites in selected organs of psychiatric patients chronically dosed up to the time of death. *Biochem Pharmacol, 17*:2061–2070, 1968.

23. Greenblatt DJ, Allen MD, Koch-Wesen J, and Shader RI: Accidental poisoning with psychotropic drugs in children. *Am J Dis Child, 130*:507–511, 1976.

24. Rumack BH: Management of acute poisoning and overdose. In *Management of the Poisoned Patient*. Edited by BH Rumack and AR Temple. Princeton, Science Press, 1977, pp. 250–280.

25. Hollister LE: Overdoses of psychotherapeutic drugs. *Clin Pharmacol Ther, 7*:142–144, 1968.

26. May PRA, and Putten TV: Plasma levels of chlorpromazine in schizophrenia. *Arch Gen Psychiatry, 35*:1081–1087, 1978.

27. Curry SH, et al: Chlorpromazine plasma levels and effects. *Arch Gen Psychiatry, 22*:289–296, 1970.

28. Rivera-Calimlim L, et al: Clinical response and plasma levels: Effect of dose, dosage schedules, and drug interaction on plasma chlorpromazine levels. *Am J Psychiatry, 133*:646–652, 1976.

29. Berry DJ, and Grove J: Emergency screening for drugs commonly taken in overdoses. *J Chromatog, 80*:205–219, 1973.

30. Forrest FM, Forrest IS, and Mason AS: A review of rapid urine tests for phenothiazines and related drugs. *Am J Psychiatry, 118*:300–307, 1961.

31. Skoutakis VA: Rational management of tricyclic antidepressant poisonings. *Clin Toxicol Consul, 1(1)*:15–23, 1979.

32. Maxwell MH, and Kleeman CR: *Clinical Disorders of Fluid and Electrolyte Metabolism*. 2nd Ed., New York, McGraw-Hill, 1972, pp. 650–651.

33. Angle CR, and McIntre MS: Persistent dystonia in a brain-damaged child after ingestion of phenothiazine. *J Pediatr, 73*:124–126, 1968.

34. Russell RI, Allan JG, and Patrick R: Active chronic hepatitis after chlorpromazine ingestion. *Br Med J, 1*:755–756, 1973.

35. Peele R, and Von Loetzen IS: Phenothiazine deaths: A critical review. *Am J Psychiatry, 130*:306–308, 1973.

Chapter 9

Lithium

Javier I. Escobar
Vasilios A. Skoutakis

Lithium's therapeutic effect on symptoms of mania was first reported by Cade in 1949,[1] and its effectiveness over placebo was demonstrated by Schou in 1954.[2] However, The United States Food and Drug Administration did not approve of the use of lithium until 1970. This delay was partially due to historical disrepute stemming from the unsuccessful use of lithium as a sedative (lithium bromide),[3] its therapeutic claims for treatment of such disorders as gout, hypertension, and epilepsy in the nineteenth and twentieth centuries,[3] and the catastrophic complications that followed the use of lithium chloride as a salt substitute in the 1940s.[4]

Marketing difficulties due to lithium's low profit potential (drug companies' hesitation to market unpatentable products) also contributed to the delay.[5] Presently, in the United States, lithium carbonate is the only salt available. It is marketed under three different trade names: Eskalith (Smith, Kline and French, capsule), Lithane (Roerig, tablet), and Lithonate (Rowell, capsule); and also under its generic name (Philips Roxane, capsule). In all cases, the unit dosage form contains 300 mg of lithium carbonate.

In the last 5 years, lithium has been resoundingly accepted by American psychiatrists as the drug of choice for treatment of manic-depressive disorders.[5,6] This increased use of lithium salts, however, has resulted in an increase of lithium toxicities, both from untoward effects of therapy and as intentional overdoses. Clinicians should become familiar with the recognition and management of patients chronically or acutely intoxicated with lithium, since this intoxication is potentially lethal.[4,7-10]

CASE REPORT

A 24-year-old female was taken to the emergency room by her mother because of a drug overdose. Upon questioning, she reported the ingestion of 150 capsules (300 mg each) of lithium carbonate 2 hours previously because "there was not sense in going on." Prior to her arrival in the ER, she vomited twice, and had one episode of diarrhea. She denied taking any other drugs or alcohol.

The patient had been hospitalized 2 years previously following an intentional overdose with chlorpromazine (Thorazine) during one of her depressive episodes. Because of those recurrent affective episodes, the patient had been placed on lithium maintenance therapy and had been seen at monthly intervals at the mental health clinic. For the last few months, her treatment had consisted of 1500 mg of lithium carbonate and 200 mg of chlorpromazine per day.

Physical examination on admission revealed a well-developed, well-nourished, anxious female, complaining of nausea, vomiting, and diarrhea. Dryness of the mouth and coarse tremor of fingers were observed. Vital signs at this time were blood pressure, 120/78 mm Hg; respirations, 20/min; temperature (oral), 37.9°C; and pulse rate, 82/min. Other results of physical and initial laboratory evaluation, including chest x-ray examination, EKG, urinalysis, and biochemical (SMA-12) and

Table 9–1. Laboratory Findings during Hospitalization Following Lithium Intoxication

STUDIES	6/10/78[a]	6/10/78[b]	6/10/78[c]	6/10/78[d]	6/11/78[e]	6/16/78[f]
BUN (mg/dl)	16	30	18	16	16	14
Creatinine (mg/dl)	1.0	1.4	1.3	1.2	1.1	1.2
Calcium (mg/dl)	9.0	—	—	9.1	9.1	9.0
Phosphorus (mg/dl)	3.1	—	—	3.1	3.1	3.1
Sodium (mEq/L)	138	134	142	142	140	138
Chloride (mEq/L)	96	98	102	102	102	100
Potassium (mEq/L)	3.5	3.6	4.0	4.5	4.5	4.0
Bicarbonate (mEq/L)	24	25.5	26	24	24	24.5
Blood glucose (mg/dl)	110	124	118	105	105	100
Hematocrit (%)	41	41	41	41.5	40.2	42
WBC (no/mm³)	10,000	13,000	14,000	18,000	14,000	9,500
Urinary pH	5.0	7.0	7.8	7.0	7.0	6.0
Specific gravity	1.018	1.020	1.021	1.018	1.020	1.021
Arterial blood gases						
pH	7.45	7.41	7.45	7.41	7.45	7.45
P_{CO_2} (mm Hg)	42	36.5	40	45	40	40
P_{O_2} (mm Hg)	90	70.8	85	85	88	94
Intake (ml/24 hours)	680	2,200	2,200	2,950	1,900	2,400
Output (ml/24 hours)	600	2,000	1,800	3,140	1,840	2,610
Serum drug levels (mEq/L)						
Lithium	1.86	4.8	1.8	3.8	1.1	1.8
Stage of coma	1	3	2	3	0	0
Blood pressure	120/78	120/70	120/80	120/70	120/80	120/84
Temperature (°C)	37.9	38.0	37.0	38.8	38.0	37.5

[a] Admission: Supportive care, forced diuresis, and alkalinization of urine started.
[b] Six hours postadmission: Hemodialysis was initiated for eight hours.
[c] Hemodialysis was stopped.
[d] Ten hours post-first hemodialysis.
[e] End of second six-hour hemodialysis.
[f] Patient's biochemical, hematologic, and clinical status prior to discharge.

hematologic (Hemo-10 with differentials) indices were all within normal limits (Table 9–1).

CLINICAL ASSESSMENT AND MANAGEMENT OF THE PATIENT

From a review of this patient's complaints and major clinical findings from initial physical and laboratory evaluations, only a few clinical manifestations of lithium toxicity were apparent (e.g., nausea, vomiting, diarrhea, dryness of the mouth, and coarse tremor of fingers).

In order to properly assess and treat a lithium-intoxicated patient, however, adequate understanding of the following points is required: (1) immediate therapeutic interventions and differential diagnosis of lithium toxicity, (2) significance of the toxicology laboratory results, (3) various manifestations and mechanisms of lithium toxicity, (4) appropriate therapeutic management, (5) general prognosis, (6) prevention of future toxicities.

IMMEDIATE THERAPEUTIC INTERVENTIONS AND DIFFERENTIAL DIAGNOSIS

No specific antidote is available for the treatment of the lithium-intoxicated patient. Therefore, standard supportive measures established for other psychotropic overdoses are the keystones to successful management.

In the present patient, after the vital signs were assessed and recorded, access to the circulation was established via an intravenous line, and blood was obtained for hematologic, biochemical, and lithium serum level determinations (Table 9–1). At this time, which was 2½ hours postingestion, 30 ml of syrup of ipecac were administered orally, followed by 240 ml of water to evacuate the lithium from the stomach. Thereafter, because this patient had described a massive drug ingestion,

Table 9–2. The Principal Side Effects of Lithium Overdosage

PRODROMES TO INTOXICATION	INTOXICATION
Lithium levels < 2.0 mEq/L	Lithium levels > 2.0 mEq/L
Sluggishness	Severe and protracted impairment of consciousness
Languidness	Increased muscle tone
Drowsiness	Hyperactive tendon reflexes
Coarse tremor or muscle twitching	Epileptic seizures
Loss of appetite	Wide-open eyes
Vomiting	Transient neurologic asymmetries
Thirst	Various EKG abnormalities
Polyuria	Electroencephalographic (EEG) changes
Diarrhea	Renal abnormalities
EKG abnormalities (T-wave abnormalities)	Respiratory depression Hyperpyrexia

and because the initial signs and symptoms were consistent with the prodromes of lithium overdosage (Table 9–2), she was admitted to the intensive care unit (ICU) for observation.

Twenty minutes after the administration of syrup of ipecac, the patient vomited twice. Examination of the vomitus revealed yellowish particles, which upon scrutiny proved to be the contents of lithium carbonate capsules. Thereafter, supportive and symptomatic care was implemented, and forced alkaline diuresis was instituted to facilitate excretion of lithium.

In cases where the clinician is confronted with a suspected acute lithium overdose or the possibility of a multiple drug overdose, and the patient is in the comatose state, immediate supportive and therapeutic measures must be instituted to support life, e.g., assurance of adequate oxygenation, maintenance of normal vital signs and urinary output with administration of intravenous fluids, correction of acid-base and fluid electrolyte imbalances, and assessment of different organ systems through blood gas determination, x-ray examination, EKG, urinalysis, and hematologic and biochemical determinations. Thereafter, information obtained from the history, physical examination, differential diagnosis, and laboratory analyses should be used in the assessment and diagnosis of the comatose patient.

History. Aside from particular details as to the time, place, quantity, and name of the drug ingested, significant history regarding trauma, hypertension, seizure disorder, diabetes, previous psychiatric treatment, previous suicide attempts, and recent traumatic experiences should be obtained from family members if possible, or from records of a previous hospital admission, if available.

Physical examination. Lithium intoxication primarily affects the central nervous system, and at times it mimics neurologic disorders such as organic brain syndrome, encephalitis, epilepsy,[4,7,10,11-14] and heat stroke.[15] Therefore, the physical examination should include assessment of the patient's state of consciousness, determination of vital signs, inspection of skull for possible trauma, examination of pupil size and reactivity, search for signs of increased intracranial pressure, or brain trauma (e.g., pupillary edema, hemotympanus).

Examination of abdomen (e.g., organ enlargement), heart (e.g., arrhythmias, gallop), lungs (e.g., adequacy of ventilation), rectum (e.g., occult blood), urinalysis, and determinations of hematologic and biochemical indices may yield important diagnostic information regarding the comatose patient. Causes of coma other than drug ingestions also must be ruled out. These include hypoglycemia, hyperglycemic ketoacidotic coma, head trauma, postictal state, spontaneous intracranial hemorrhage, and, less commonly, malignant hypertension, cerebrovascular accident, hepatic and uremic comas, meningo-

encephalitis, hyper- or hypocalcemia, hyper- or hyponatremia, myxedema, or addisonian crisis.

Differential diagnosis. In drug-related cases and in those involving comatose patients, other psychotropic drugs, particularly barbiturates, opiates, tricyclic antidepressants, and neuroleptics, must be considered in the differential diagnosis. In general, the slow progression and long duration of the intoxication,[7-10] as well as the presence of myoclonic "jerks" (contraction of large muscular groups) during lithium overdosage, aid in the differential diagnosis.

Lithium and barbiturate or opiate overdoses could be differentiated on clinical grounds based on the observation that patients with lithium overdoses may be able to react to stimuli and even give brief answers to questions at the "height" of their intoxication, whereas with severe opiate or barbiturate overdoses, this is not the case. Also, increased muscular tone, coarse tremor, and myoclonic jerks are seen more often during lithium overdoses.

Lithium and tricyclic overdoses may be clinically differentiated according to severity and quality of cardiovascular changes, since EKG abnormalities, heart arrhythmias, or heart failure are much more common during intoxication with tricyclic antidepressants than during lithium overdoses.[16] Seizures are also more common during overdoses with tricyclic antidepressants.[16] The duration of symptoms is another clue to the differential diagnosis, since intoxication with tricyclics generally resolves within 1 or 2 days, whereas severe lithium overdoses extends over longer periods of time.[7,10]

Lithium and neuroleptic overdoses may be clinically differentiated based on blood pressure, extrapyramidal toxicities, and EKG abnormalities. Hypotension is one of the most common toxicologic effects seen with neuroleptic agents.[17] Extrapyramidal toxicities, as well as EKG abnormalities, also are usually more prominent in patients intoxicated with neuroleptic agents than in those intoxicated by lithium.[17]

ROLE OF THE TOXICOLOGY LABORATORY

In cases in which the history, clinical manifestations, and initial diagnostic measures are inconclusive or doubtful, confirmation and assessment of the severity of the intoxication can be made possible by chemical analysis of serum[3,5,7,10,18-21] or urine.[22] The usual practice has been to measure serum lithium concentrations. Recently, however, lithium estimation in several other tissues has been investigated. These include urine,[22] red blood cells,[23] and saliva.[24] In spite of these other techniques, the determination of serum lithium concentrations is the standard practice in most places, and it is found to be accurate, acceptable, and convenient.[3,5-7,10,18-21]

In cases where lithium intoxication is suspected, a 5-ml venous blood sample, collected in a tube without anticoagulants, should be sent to the toxicology laboratory. Two relatively simple procedures, flame photometry and atomic spectrophotometry, are available for lithium level determinations. Lithium concentration is reported in mEq/L. Either laboratory procedure yields rapid and accurate results, aiding in the prompt diagnosis and treatment of the lithium-intoxicated patients.[10,21]

In the present case, the urine drug screen results were negative for all psychotropic drugs, except lithium. A serum lithium concentration of 1.86 mEq/L was also obtained upon admission (Table 9-1) and gave support to a clinical diagnosis of lithium overdosage. The symptoms (Table 9-2) were interpreted as early signs of lithium toxicity resulting from the absorptive "rise" of lithium and its irritating effect on the GI mucosa. These symptoms and the patient's history of a massive lithium ingestion alerted the clinicians to the likelihood of a severe lithium overdose.

SIGNIFICANCE OF THE LABORATORY RESULTS

Lithium salts have a narrow therapeutic window and a relatively small margin of safety. Toxicity usually develops when the lithium levels go beyond the upper limit of the therapeutic range, generally considered to be between 0.6 and 1.5 mEq/L.[3,5-7,10,18,21-25]

Lithium toxicity can result from (1) an acute single overdose, as in the case reported, (2) "cumulative" overdose in a patient on lithium treatment, or (3) decreased lithium excretion in a patient receiving therapeutic dosages. The latter may be due to reduced sodium or water intake, or intercurrent illness, especially in the presence of reduced renal output.[10] Regardless of the primary cause, a hallmark of lithium toxicity is the slow progression of symptoms, possibly due to lithium's slow accumulation and passage into the intracellular space.[18-21,26]

Two main types of unwanted lithium effects can be distinguished (Table 9-2). The first is represented by symptoms such as GI irritation, tremor of hands, thirst, and polyuria. These symptoms, which also were present in the case reported, usually tend to occur at "therapeutic" lithium concentrations (below 2.0 mEq/L) and generally constitute more of an annoyance than a serious threat to the individual patient. The second type of complication is lithium intoxication, generally related to the accumulation of lithium serum concentrations above 2.0 mEq/L, and chiefly characterized by CNS toxicities (Table 9-2).[3,5-10,18-21,25,27,28]

In the case presented, the first change in the patient's consciousness was observed 6 hours after admission. Although her eyes would open when stimulated, she did not respond to questions. Increased muscle tone and hyperactive deep tendon reflexes also were present at this time. The electrocardiogram revealed prolongation of the Q-T interval. Arterial blood gases at this time were P_{O_2}, 70.8 mm Hg; P_{CO_2}, 36.5 mm Hg; pH, 7.41, and HCO_3^- (bicarbonate, 25.5 mEq/L. Serum BUN and creatinine were 30 and 1.4 mg/dl respectively.

The serum lithium concentration was 4.8 mEq/L. Serum sodium and potassium concentrations at this time were 134 and 3.6 mEq/L respectively. The remaining biochemical and hematologic results are shown in Table 9–1. Because of the high lithium serum concentrations, the pa-

tient's rapidly deteriorating condition, and elevated serum BUN and creatinine, hemodialysis was promptly instituted (Fig. 9–1).

After 8 hours of hemodialysis, the serum lithium concentration decreased to 1.8 mEq/L. However, 10 hours after the hemodialysis procedure was discontinued, the serum lithium concentration increased again to 3.8 mEq/L. Therefore, the next day hemodialysis was again instituted for 6 hours. The patient started to respond to questions after the completion of the second 6 hours of hemodialysis. The serum lithium concentration at this time was 1.1 mEq/L (Fig. 9–1). Supportive and

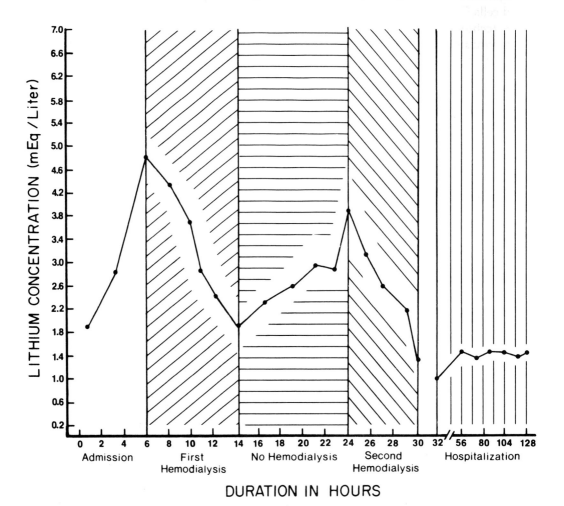

Fig. 9–1. Serum lithium levels before, during, and after hemodialysis.

symptomatic care was implemented after hemodialysis, and the patient made a gradual though slow recovery without sequelae.

MANIFESTATIONS AND MECHANISMS OF LITHIUM TOXICITY

Both therapeutic and toxic levels of lithium affect multiple organ systems and cause changes ranging from mild abnormalities to severe toxic-necrotic states, depending on the level of the lithium ions present. It affects particularly those organ systems with ion transport and polypeptide hormone action (e.g., catecholamines).[3,5,7,10,18,25,27,28] Before the manifestations and mechanisms of lithium toxicity are discussed, therefore, a brief review of neurophysiology and neurochemistry may be necessary.

During neurotransmission, as part of the process of neuronal depolarization, sodium enters the cells as potassium exits. When the neuron is at rest, a sodium pump (ATP-dependent) transports the sodium ion back across the cell membranes. In both therapeutic and toxic doses lithium, unlike sodium, is not rapidly pumped out of the cells by the active pump mechanism. It therefore tends to accumulate, perhaps making the tissue less excitable. In affective disorders (e.g., mania and depression) it has also been proposed that residual (intra-neuronal) sodium is increased, leading to potential extraneuronal "leakage" of biogenic amines.[29]

This description of the neurophysiologic and neurochemistry processes, plus the demonstration of increased lithium retention during mania, suggests that lithium's alterations of the electrolyte balance may be related to its therapeutic action.[3,5,6,10,18,19,25,27,38] Lithium also interferes with the action of hormones (e.g., catecholamines) that affect excitability.[3,5,6,18,19,25,27,28]

For example, lithium partially inhibits the positive chronotropic effect of epi-

Table 9–3. Some Hormone Responses Mediated by Adenyl Cyclase and cAMP

TISSUE	HORMONE	RESPONSE
Kidney:		
Medulla	ADH	Water reabsorption
Cortex	Parathyroid hormone (PTH)	Phosphate excretion and calcium reabsorption
Bone	PTH	Calcium reabsorption
Skin	Melanocyte-stimulating hormone (MSH)	Darkening
Adrenal	ACTH	Corticosteroid secretion
Ovary	LH	Progesterone secretion
Thyroid	TSH	T_4 secretion
Stomach	Gastrin	Hydrochloric acid secretion
Adipose	ACTH Glucagon Epinephrine	Fat release
Liver	Epinephrine	Glucose release
Muscle	Epinephrine	Glucose release and contractility
Heart	Epinephrine	Contractility and excitability
Brain	Epinephrine Norepinephrine Dopamine Acetylcholine Serotonin	Excitability and synaptic transmission

nephrine and inhibits the pressor effects of norepinephrine. Lithium may produce such effects by interfering with the stimulation of adenyl cyclase to produce cAMP, through which these hormones affect metabolism, heart rate, and peripheral resistance. These actions of lithium are thought to result in "buffering" of the aminergic system against chemical perturbations and may also contribute to lithium's prophylactic effect on affective illness.[5,6,18,19,25,27,28] Some hormone responses mediated by adenyl cyclase and cAMP are listed in Table 9–3.[28]

The different organ systems that are particularly involved in lithium intoxications and the possible mechanisms responsible for the toxicologic manifestations seen in these patients, as in the case presented, are discussed in the following sections.

Gastrointestinal System

Although both lithium and sodium cross the mucosal cell membrane into the cell, only sodium is pumped out efficiently. The inability of the cation pumps to extrude lithium as efficiently as sodium may account for the complex effects of lithium on intestinal sugar and water transfer. Substitution of lithium for sodium decreases intestinal absorption of both glucose and water. This direct interference with both solute and water absorption may produce nausea, vomiting, and diarrhea in patients treated with lithium. These symptoms and side effects may also result from lithium's irritating effect on the GI mucosa, or its interference with the effect of GI hormones such as gastrin, whose action may involve stimulation of adenyl cyclase and generation of cAMP.[5,18,19,25,27,28]

Cardiovascular System

The toxic effects of lithium on the heart are related to direct ionic substitution in transport processes, because specific cationic distributions and fluxes are im-

portant determinants of the behavior of excitable membranes, as in the cardiac conduction system.[3,5,6,18,19,25,27,28] As in other cells, lithium and sodium readily enter the cardiac cell, but lithium is not effectively removed. Instead, lithium replaces intracellular potassium, which gets diffused into the surrounding medium. These electrolyte changes probably account for the usually reversible T-wave abnormalities (T-wave depression and, less commonly, T-wave inversion),[7,10,30,31] as noted during the admission in the case presented, and for rare cases of myocardial irritability noted during chronic lithium therapy in man.[32]

Serum hypokalemia also may be associated with a prolonged Q-T interval in patients with severe lithium ingestions,[33] as manifested in the case presented, approximately 6 hours postadmission. Once the serum lithium concentrations are decreased and have entered the therapeutic range, the EKG-exhibited abnormalities are reversible, as in the case presented and as seen in other reported cases.[7,10,18,30,34]

Central Nervous System

Lithium in acute ingestion and/or chronic toxicities primarily effects the CNS. It produces a wide variety of toxic effects on the CNS, ranging from mild clouding of the sensorium to deep unresponsive coma.[5,7,10,18,19,25,27,28,34–36]

Intoxication develops gradually and is preceded by toxic manifestations such as fine tremor of hands, gastric irritability, thirst, polyuria, polydipsia, nausea, and vomiting (Table 9–2). This group of side effects coincides with peaks in the blood lithium and is most related to the rate of change in blood lithium concentration.[5,7,10,18–21,25–27]

The clinical picture of fully developed lithium intoxication is usually dominated by severe and protracted impairment of consciousness. Seizures, dysarthria, sluggishness, confusion, sommolence, increased muscle tone, hyperactive deep tendon reflexes, EKG, electroencephalo-gram (EEG) changes, and anuria are usually noted in these patients.[5,7,10,18,19,25,27,28,30,34-36] Some of these toxic effects were manifested in the case presented approximately 6 hours postadmission. The endpoint of these symptoms is stupor and coma. Therefore, when severe lithium intoxication has been suspected, the most important parameter to monitor, in addition to serum lithium concentrations, is CNS function, since the primary manifestation is CNS depression, as in barbiturate intoxication.

Lithium-induced EEG changes are largely reversible and correlate well with neurotoxicity. These changes are characterized by slow wave activity (3- to 7-hertz waves), increased amplitude, and increased delta activity.[36]

The mechanism by which lithium exerts its toxic effects upon the CNS is not clearly understood. It is believed that in both therapeutic and toxic concentrations, lithium affects nerve excitation, synaptic transmission, and neuronal metabolism by (1) acting as an imperfect substitute for other cations that normally participate in processes of ionic transfer or distribution to maintain the proper electrolyte gradients or osmotic steady states, and (2) inhibiting responses mediated by adenyl cyclase that stimulate cAMP production, resulting in an alteration of the critical physiologic environment, i.e., hormones, required for other cellular processes (Table 9-3).[3,5,6,18,19,25,27,28] In addition, perhaps during acute or chronic intoxications, lithium might decrease seizure threshold, and as a result, CNS toxic manifestations may occur.[36]

Renal System

Subtoxic and toxic doses of lithium regularly induce polyuria and polydipsia in patients.[5,7,10,18,37,38] The mechanism by which lithium induces polyuria and polydipsia is believed to be related to its inhibition of ADH-sensitive adenyl cy-clase in the renal medulla.[19,27,28,39,40] The development of polyuria, like water loading, however, does not lead to any changes in serum lithium concentrations.[18,41-44] Furthermore, the development of polyuria is not dangerous in itself, but the impairment of renal concentrating ability may involve risk of dehydration.[44,45]

Under normal circumstances, the thirst mechanism secures a water intake that is in excess of the water requirement. However, if the water intake decreases below the water requirements, as may happen during fever, psychic disease or, during lithium intoxication, dehydration develops. As a result of the dehydration, glomerular filtration and clearance of lithium decrease, and serum lithium concentration increases.[42-45] The increase of serum lithium concentration leads to further inhibition of the reabsorption of water in the kidney, which in turn aggravates the dehydration.[44,45]

Lithium also interferes with the renal handling of sodium, and during lithium intoxication, loss of body sodium usually occurs.[42-47] The lithium-induced sodium deficiency is presumably responsible for some hormonal changes, such as an increase in plasma renin concentration and the production of aldosterone,[48,49] as well as lithium's depressive effect on the glomerular filtration rate (GFR),[44,45] which is not reversed by infusion of isotonic sodium chloride.[42-45] The increased sodium requirements due to renal and extrarenal losses can result in a decrease in lithium clearance and an increase in serum lithium concentration.[42,43,45] The increased serum lithium concentration leads to a further increase in the requirements of sodium, and a vicious circle is started.[44,45]

In patients with fully developed lithium intoxications, the serum sodium concentration is a useful variable in the determination of the ratio between sodium and water in the extracellular space, but gives no information about the absolute magnitude of a sodium and water deficiency.[7,10,18,19,43-45] Serum sodium concentrations in lithium-intoxicated patients, however, are usually decreased, as manifested in the case presented (Table 9–1).

Renal histologic changes (sclerotic glomeruli and tubular damage), as well as development of acute renal failure, have been reported in cases of lithium intoxication.[7,25,35,45,50-52] Usually, the serum BUN and creatinine concentrations are increased during the beginning of the intoxication and decreased when the patients recover as in the case presented (Table 9–1). The lithium-induced renal toxicologic manifestations (sclerotic glomeruli and tubular damage) might be related to possible direct effects of the drug, whereas the transient increase in BUN and serum creatinine may be related to dehydration, leading to a lowered GFR or to the direct depressive effect of lithium on the GFR.[45-48]

Hansen and associates found that the inability of the nephron to concentrate the urine during lithium treatment was correlated to the occurrence of histologic changes (sclerotic glomeruli and tubular changes).[45] This gives rise to the yet unanswered question of whether reduced ability to concentrate the urine should be regarded as a warning sign that requires a reduction of the lithium dose or even cessation of lithium treatment.

TREATMENT OF THE LITHIUM-INTOXICATED PATIENT

Apart from the immediate therapeutic interventions and diagnostic considerations discussed in the preceding section (i.e., institution of supportive measures to ensure adequate oxygenation, correction of acid-base and electrolyte imbalance, maintenance of normal vital signs, assessment of different organ systems through biochemical and hematologic measurements, urinalysis, EKG and EEG evaluations, and determinations of serum lithium concentrations), the successful management of the lithium-intoxicated patient requires (1) prevention of further absorption of lithium, (2) facilitation of the removal of absorbed lithium, and (3) symptomatic and supportive care as indicated.

Prevention of Further Absorption

The methods involved in the prevention of absorption of lithium from the GI tract are (a) emesis or lavage, and (b) administration of a saline cathartic, but *not* activated charcoal.

Emesis and/or lavage. If the patient is alert, gastric evacuation of lithium can be performed by the oral administration of syrup of ipecac, followed by 240 ml of water in order to evacuate the lithium from the stomach. Syrup of ipecac has a lag time of 20 to 30 minutes before vomiting is initiated. The dosage of syrup of ipecac is 30 ml for adults and 15 ml for children (under 15 years).

Excellent results are usually obtained by the use of syrup of ipecac. However, if vomiting does not occur within the first 30 minutes, readministration of an additional oral dose of syrup of ipecac is recommended. Administration of apomorphine to induce emesis is not a rational alternative to syrup of ipecac and should not be used, because of its potentially serious side effects, such as CNS depression, cardiac arrhythmias, convulsions, and cardiovascular collapse.[53]

When the ingestion of lithium has produced coma, the patient should be intubated and lavage initiated. Isotonic saline solution can be used as the lavage fluid. During lavage, the patient must be placed in a modified Trendelenburg position on his left side, with the foot of the bed slightly elevated. This technique is recommended to prevent aspiration while gastric contents are being emptied. The endpoint of the lavage should be the appearance of clear gastric aspirate for 2 L.

In the case presented, the oral administration of 30 ml of syrup of ipecac followed by 240 ml of water resulted in two emeses within a 20-minute period. Examination of the vomitus revealed yellowish particles, which upon scrutiny proved to be the contents of lithium carbonate capsules.

Saline cathartics. The purpose of the administration of saline cathartics is to facilitate the intestinal transit of unabsorbed lithium, thus reducing the transit time and the amount reabsorbed. Activated charcoal does not bind lithium, so its use as a GI adsorbent is not indicated unless a multiple drug intoxication is suspected.[55] In case of a multiple drug ingestion, the dosage of charcoal should be 1 g/kg of body weight mixed with enough water to produce a fine slurry with the consistency of thick soup.

In the case presented, two doses of sodium sulfate, each 250 mg/kg of body weight were also administered during the first 6 hours postadmission to further facilitate removal of lithium from the GI tract. Magnesium sulfate and magnesium citrate should not be used as saline cathartics, because renal damage has been reported with acute lithium overdosages as well as with chronic lithium administration. In cases of impending or manifest renal failure, hypermagnesemia can potentiate the toxic effects of lithium, such as CNS depression and cardiac arrhythmias.[54]

Facilitation of the Removal of Absorbed Lithium

Prior to a discussion of the methods available to remove absorbed lithium from the body, essential facts about lithium's pharmacokinetic properties, renal handling, and the various factors that influence its clearance will be presented, in order to prevent complications in the treatment of lithium-intoxicated patients.

Lithium is administered in the form of the lithium carbonate salt. In the body, lithium exists as a small ion with a single positive electric charge. The behavior of this ion is similar to that of sodium.[5,18,19,25,27,28]

Lithium is rapidly but sometimes variably absorbed from the GI tract. Single oral doses produce peak blood concentrations after 2 to 4 hours. On the average, a dose of 300 mg of lithium raises the serum level by 0.2 to 0.4 mEq/L. The effect is linear, such that higher doses give proportionally higher serum levels.[20,21,26]

The lithium ion is not bound to plasma proteins and is distributed unevenly, with high concentrations in kidney tissue, moderate concentrations in muscle, bone, and liver, and low concentrations in brain tissue.[5,18,19,25,27,28] Following intoxication, these sites may act as reservoirs (see section on dialysis). The ratio of serum concentration to cerebrospinal fluid concentration for lithium is usually between 3/1 and 4/1 during chronic administration.[20,21,26] Lithium is transported actively across many cell membranes, reaching equilibrium after about 5 days of regular dosing.

Lithium is excreted almost exclusively by the kidneys. Insignificant amounts are excreted in sweat and feces. The lithium ion is filtered freely through the glomerular membrane, and about 80% of the filtered lithium is actively reabsorbed in the renal tubules. No specific mechanism for reabsorption or secretion of lithium is present in the kidneys.

Lithium is reabsorbed in the same way as sodium, but with varying efficiency in the different parts of the nephron. Under normal body conditions, the lithium clearance remains fairly constant (10 to 30 ml/min), but it may fall after reduction in the GFR, during inhibition of distal sodium reabsorption, and during intake of a diet with low sodium content.[5,18,19,25,27,42–44] These conditions accordingly involve extra risk in the development of lithium intoxication.

At both toxic and therapeutic concentrations, lithium is reabsorbed mainly in the proximal tubules together with sodium. In addition, a small amount may be reabsorbed in Henle's loop. When sodium excretion is low, lithium may be reabsorbed to a significant degree also in the distal parts of the nephron.[42-44]

With a single dose of lithium, 50% is excreted within 5 to 8 hours.[20,21] In patients on maintenance lithium therapy, elimination follows first-order kinetics, and the average serum half-life is 24 hours. However, the whole body or "biologic" half-life is longer than 24 hours, owing to the more stable extravascular stores of lithium, particularly in muscle and bone.[7,10,19-21,26,27] At equilibrium, the stable extravascular stores are never mobilized, and the kinetics are essentially those of a single compartment model.

However, after the intake of lithium is stopped (e.g., following an intoxication), a more complex model is necessary, because a rebound phenomenon usually occurs, with a paradoxical rise in serum lithium levels after an initially successful reduction. Redistribution of lithium from storage sites to the vascular space is probably the etiologic factor (see section on dialysis).[10,20,21,26]

The two methods currently used to facilitate the removal of absorbed lithium from the body are forced alkaline diuresis and peritoneal dialysis or hemodialysis.

Forced alkaline diuresis. Apart from maneuvers that influence the GFR, few factors influence serum lithium clearance. For example, water loading that leads to more than a 10-fold increase of urine flow, and a corresponding dilution of the urinary concentration does not affect serum lithium clearance.[41-44] Similarly, administration of potassium chloride, sodium chloride, thiazides, furosemide, ethacrynic acid, and spironolactone does not affect serum lithium clearance.[7,10,18,19,41-44]

In fact, administration of large doses of sodium chloride in severely poisoned patients may produce lung or brain edema.[42,43] The ineffectiveness of these agents in the promotion of lithium elimination further suggests that lithium, unlike sodium, is not reabsorbed in all parts of the nephron, and that there are no specific mechanisms present in the kidneys for the reabsorption or secretion of lithium.

A significant increase in renal lithium clearance has been reported, however, with the use of osmotic diuretics (e.g., mannitol, urea),[7,10,18,42-44,56] alkalinization of urine (e.g., sodium bicarbonate, sodium lactate, or acetazolamide),[42,43,57] and aminophylline.[42,43] The actions of mannitol or urea within the kidney depend upon the concentration of osmotically active particles in solution. The water retained in the proximal tubule produces an increased concentration gradient for the sodium ion and perhaps the lithium ion, and limits sodium and lithium reabsorption. Consequently, urine flow increases.

Since lithium is not reabsorbed in the distal part of the nephron, osmotic diuretics enhance its excretion.[18,19,42-44] The increase of the lithium excretion after the administration of either sodium bicarbonate, sodium lactate, or acetazolamide (a carbonic anhydrase inhibitor) might be due to an obligatory excretion of cation with unreabsorbed bicarbonate anion, since reabsorption of bicarbonate takes place mainly in the proximal tubules.[18,19,42-44] The exact mechanism of aminophylline's action is unknown, but it is believed that aminophylline might have a direct effect on the kidney tubules, or that it might increase renal blood flow and GFR and thus promote lithium excretion.[18,19,42-44]

Our experiences have been that in mild cases of lithium intoxication, with no serious renal or cardiovascular impairment, and serum lithium concentrations not greater than 3.5 mEq/L, the concomitant administration of (1) mannitol, 25 g given by slow IV four times daily, (2) aminophylline, 500 mg given by slow IV push every 6 hours, and (3) sodium bicarbonate, 50 mEq/L given by slow IV push every hour to maintain the urinary pH above 7, has resulted in a significant increase in urinary excretion of lithium and in the overall improvement of the clinical condition of patients.

Dialysis. Both peritoneal dialysis and hemodialysis have been reported to be effective in facilitating the removal of lithium from intoxicated patients.[58-60] However, the most efficient method is hemodialysis. Indications for dialysis include (1) ingestion of a potentially fatal dose of lithium, (2) kidney failure, (3) progressive increase in lithium concentrations greater than 3.5 mEq/L, and (6) prolonged coma.

Dialysis may have to be continued for at least 4 to 6 hours after serum lithium concentrations have returned to the therapeutic range, because a rebound increase in serum lithium concentration upon discontinuation of dialysis has been reported,[8,60] as in the case presented. This rebound effect is probably due to the redistribution of lithium from other body tissues.

In the case presented, hemodialysis was effective in reducing the serum lithium concentrations, and also in improving the overall clinical condition. Data obtained during the two hemodialysis procedures are shown in Figure 9-1.

Symptomatic and Supportive Care

Following correction of life-threatening symptoms and institution of measures to minimize lithium absorption and to enhance its excretion, symptomatic and supportive care constitutes the keystone of successful management.

Permanent neurologic, cardiac, hepatic, and renal abnormalities have been reported, as results of lithium intoxications.[7,10,11-14,25,60] Since lithium can affect multiple organ systems, causing changes ranging from mild abnormalities to severe toxic-necrotic states, closed

monitoring of lithium levels, electrolytes, urinalysis, EEG, EKG, and biochemical and hematologic indices is essential. Vital signs should be recorded every 4 hours. Electrolytes should be replaced as needed, and urinary output of at least 5 to 6 L per day should be maintained, in order to facilitate the actions of the different therapeutic regimens discussed in the preceding section and, thus, lithium excretion.

The gravest cases of lithium intoxications are characterized by coma, epileptic seizures, and pulmonary complications.[5,7-10,11-14,25,60] If treatment is inadequate or delayed death can result from a combination of the effects described.[7,10] Usually, however, deaths are attributed to pulmonary complications, including pneumonia and respiratory failure.[7,10] Therefore, careful evaluation of the vital signs, hematologic indices (e.g., Hemo-10 with differentials), blood culture, chest x-ray examination, urine and sputum cultures, and even lumbar puncture should be performed to rule out active infection foci. If an infection is present, it should be treated aggressively with antibiotics, and other appropriate measures should be instituted.

Agitations and hyperactivity, as well as epileptic seizures, are potential complications, and deaths have been reported. An EEG should be obtained in such cases, since EEG changes are a good index of CNS toxicity. The intravenous administration of either phenobarbital, 100 mg, diazepam, 10 mg, or phenytoin, 100 mg as needed can be used to control hypertonicity, convulsions, and seizures if present.[7,10,12-14]

In the case presented, the patient was discharged from the hospital 6 days postadmission, without any evidence of neurologic involvement, cardiac, hepatic or renal damage, or biochemical or hematologic abnormalities. The serum lithium concentration at this time was 1.5 mEq/L (Table 9-1).

GENERAL PROGNOSIS

The outcome of an acute lithium overdosage is generally determined by the amount ingested, the time interval between ingestion and treatment, the patient's age and physical condition, and the selection of appropriate therapy. In a patient with normal renal function, serum lithium levels will be expected to decrease by 50% each day. Cardiovascular disturbances or the presence of neurologic dysfunction (e.g., seizure disorder) complicate the prognosis.

Additional complications, such as infections, cardiovascular collapse, deep coma, and respiratory depression, are also important elements of the general prognosis. The availability of hemodialysis for emergency treatment significantly aids in the outcome of severe intoxications. In clinically fully developed lithium intoxication, although the patient might be out of danger within the first 24 to 48 hours, the recovery is a slow process, and the patient has to be hospitalized for an average of 4 to 6 days.

PREVENTION OF FUTURE TOXICITIES

Determinants of the safety and success of lithium therapy are based on the clinicians' thorough knowledge and understanding of lithium's pharmacologic, pharmacokinetic and toxicologic properties, as well as the various factors that might influence lithium toxicity. Toxicities due to lithium, therefore, can be prevented or minimized by patient selection, determination of lithium serum concentrations, awareness of factors related to changes in lithium concentrations, and awareness of lithium's effects in utero, on breast feeding, and on other body systems.

Patient selection. The use of lithium is contraindicated in patients with renal disease,[42-44] unreliable or suicidal patients, and those with severe cardiovascular disease. Lithium therapy should be used *cautiously* in the pregnant patient,[61] breast-feeding mothers,[61,62] elderly patients,[42-44] patients on dietary sodium restriction or diuretic therapy,[10,42-44] patients with thyroid disease,[64,65] mild kidney disease,[42-44] heart disease,[5,30-34] or organic brain syndrome.[5,10,11-14,25]

Once the physical examination and patient selection has been initiated, the following tests should be performed in all patients prior to beginning of lithium therapy: complete blood count, urinalysis, T_4 (mean free thyroxine), electrocardiogram, electrolytes, blood urea nitrogen and serum creatinine. These tests should be repeated on a monthly basis thereafter to ensure adequate therapy and to prevent or minimize toxicities and complications.

Determination of lithium serum concentrations. Regular determinations of lithium concentrations and careful adjustment of the lithium dosage are important tools in the prevention of lithium intoxication.[3,5-7,10,18-21,25] The recommended daily dosage schedule for lithium is 300 mg three times daily. Peak lithium concentrations occur 1 to 3 hours after pills are swallowed.

Therefore, in order for a lithium blood level to be valid, the blood samples should be drawn when the patient is in the postabsorptive state (e.g., 12 hours after the last dose). The therapeutic range of lithium for mania is 0.6 to 1.5 mEq/L. Severe toxicity can be expected when serum lithium concentrations are greater than 2.0 mEq/L. Concentrations above 4.0 mEq/L can be fatal.[20,21]

Factors related to changes in lithium concentrations. Possible reasons for increased lithium concentrations are (1) decreased tolerance for lithium as cells become "loaded," in remission of mania attacks, (2) sodium loss in cases of diarrhea, administration of diuretics, and restricted respiration secondary to strenuous exercise or illness with fever, (3) sodium diuresis in postpartum patients, and (4) decreased excretion of lithium in cases of kidney disease or, in elderly patients, because of a fall in the GFR.[5,7,10,18,19, 25,27,42–45]

Factors related to decreased lithium concentrations are: (1) high salt or high bicarbonate intake, because excess sodium causes increased lithium excretion, and (2) pregnancy, with decreases due to redistribution of lithium throughout body tissues and in utero.[61–64]

Lithium's effects in utero, on breast feeding, and on other body systems. Congenital malformations have been reported in infants exposed to lithium in utero.[61] Reports from the Register of Lithium Babies have indicated that 13 out of 143 babies had congenital abnormalities, most of which were cardiovascular abnormalities.[61] Because of the potential of toxicity to the fetus, lithium should be avoided during pregnancy (especially the first trimester) unless the potential benefits outweigh the hazards.

Breast feeding by lithium-treated mothers also is not advisable, because lithium appears in the breast milk in concentrations of 30% to 50% of the mother's blood level, and as a result, toxicities and/or intoxications might develop.[62,63] The clinician also should be aware that accidental or deliberate ingestion of lithium during pregnancy is not an indication for therapeutic abortion.[64]

In the course of lithium maintenance therapy, thyroid function in some patients may be altered.[28,65,66] Lithium decreases T_4 production and serum T_4 levels, and by negative feedback secondarily increases thyroid-stimulating hormone (TSH) production, release, or both. The secondarily elevated TSH levels could stimulate thyroid growth, producing the goiter observed in some patients treated with lithium.[28] Goiters usually disappear once lithium is discontinued, or when thyroxine, 100 to 200 μg daily, is administered concomitantly with lithium.[67] The mechanism by which lithium pro-

duces these effects is not clearly understood. An action on the anterior pituitary and the thyrotropin/thyrotropin-releasing-hormone axis has been proposed, possibly with a diminished sensitivity of the thyroid to thyrotropin.[66,68] The effects may also result from lithium's effect on the hormone-sensitive adenyl cyclase system.[28]

REFERENCES

1. Cade JF: Lithium salts in the treatment of psychiatric excitement. *Med J Aust,* 36:349–352, 1943.
2. Schou M, et al: The treatment of manic psychosis by the administration of lithium salts. *J Neurol Neurosurg Psychiatry,* 17:250–260, 1954.
3. Malelzhy B, and Blackly P: *The Use of Lithium in Psychiatry.* Cleveland, CRS Press, 1971.
4. Corcoran AC, Taylor RD, and Page IH: Lithium poisoning from salt substitutes. *JAMA,* 139:685–689, 1949.
5. Baldessarini R, and Lipinski J: Lithium salts: 1970–1975. *Ann Intern Med,* 83:527–533, 1975.
6. American Psychiatric Association Task Force on Lithium Therapy: The current status of lithium therapy: Report of the APA task force. *Am J Psychiatry,* 132:997–1001, 1975.
7. Hansen HE, and Amdisen A: Lithium intoxication: Report of 23 cases and review of 100 cases from the literature. *Q J Med,* 47:123–144, 1978.
8. Chapman AJ, and Lewis G: Fatal self-poisoning with lithium carbonate. *Can Med Assoc J,* 112:868–870, 1975.
9. Herrero AF: Lithium carbonate toxicity. *JAMA,* 26:1109–1110, 1973.
10. Schou M, Amdisen A, and Trap-Jensen J: Lithium poisoning. *Am J Psychiatry,* 125:112–129, 1968.
11. Agulnik PI, DiMascio A, and Moore P: Acute brain syndrome associated with lithium therapy. *Am J Psychiatry,* 129:621–623, 1972.
12. Shopsin B, Johnson G, and Gershon S: Neurotoxicity of lithium: Differential drug responsiveness. *Int Pharmacopsychiatry,* 5:170–182, 1970.
13. McCawley A, Schachnow NK, and Mandell S: Survival in lithium intoxication, status epilepticus, and prolonged coma. *NY State J Med,* 75:407–409, 1975.
14. Warick LH: Lithium poisoning: Report of a case with neurologic, cardiac and hepatic sequelae. *West J Med,* 130:259–263, 1979.
15. Granoff AL, and David JM: Heat illness syndrome and lithium intoxication. *J Clin Psychiatry,* 39:102–107, 1978.
16. Skoutakis VA: Management of acute tricyclic antidepressant poisonings. *Clin Toxicol Consult,* 1:15–23, 1979.
17. Barry D, Meyskens FL, and Becker CE: Phenothiazine poisoning: A review of 48 cases. *Calif Med,* 118:1–5, 1973.

18. Schou M: Lithium: Elimination rate, dosage control, poisoning, goiter, mode of action. *Acta Psychiatr Scand (Suppl)*, 207:49–54, 1969.

19. Schou M: Pharmacology and toxicology of lithium. *Ann Rev Pharmacol Toxicol*, 16:231–243, 1976.

20. Amdisen A: Monitoring of lithium treatment through determination of lithium concentration. *Dan Med Bull*, 22:277–291, 1975.

21. Amdisen A: Serum level monitoring and clinical pharmacokinetics of lithium. *Clin Pharmacokinet*, 2:73–92, 1977.

22. Amdisen A: The estimation of lithium in urine. In *Lithium Research and Therapy*. Edited by FN Johnson. New York, Academic Press, 1975, pp. 181–195.

23. Lyttkens L, Soderberg U, and Wetterberg L: Relation between erythrocyte and plasma concentrations as an index in psychiatric disease. *Ups J Med Sci*, 81:123–128, 1976.

24. Sims A, White AC, and Garvey K: Problems associated with the analysis and interpretation of saliva lithium. *Br J Psychiatry*, 132:152–154, 1978.

25. Schou M, et al: Pharmacology and clinical problems of lithium prophylaxis. *Br J Psychiatry*, 116:615–619, 1970.

26. Terhaag B, et al: The distribution of lithium into cerebrospinal fluid, brain tissue and bile in man. *Int J Clin Pharmacol Biopharm*, 16:333–335, 1978.

27. Schou M: Biology and pharmacology of lithium ion. *Pharmacol Rev*, 9:17–58, 1957.

28. Singer I, and Rotenberg D: Mechanisms of lithium action. *N Engl J Med*, 289:254–260, 1973.

29. Cooper A: The biochemistry of affective disorders. *Br J Psychiatry*, 113:1237–1264, 1967.

30. Dembers RG, and Heninger GR: Electrocardiographic T wave changes during lithium carbonate treatment. *JAMA*, 218:381–386, 1971.

31. Kochar MS, Wang RI, and D'Cunhi GF: Electrocardiographic changes simulating hypokalemia during treatment with lithium carbonate. *J Electrocardiol*, 4:371–373, 1971.

32. Tangedahl TN, and Gau GT: Myocardial irritability associated with lithium carbonate therapy. *N Engl J Med*, 287:867–869, 1972.

33. Jacob AI, and Hope RR: Prolongation of the Q-T interval in lithium toxicity. *J Electrocardiol*, 12:117–119, 1979.

34. Wilson JR, et al: Reversible sinus-node abnormalities due to lithium carbonate therapy. *N Engl J Med*, 294:1223–1224, 1976.

35. Laveder S, Brown JN, and Berill WT: Acute renal failure and lithium intoxication. *Postgrad Med J*, 49:277–279, 1973.

36. Small JC, and Small IF: Pharmacology: Neurophysiology of lithium. In *Lithium: Its Role in Psychiatric Research and Treatment*. Edited by S Gershon and B Shopsin. New York, Plenum Press, 1973.

37. Angrist B, et al: Lithium induced diabetes insipidus-like syndrome. *Compr Psychiatry*, 11:141–146, 1970.

38. MacNeil S, and Jenner FA: Lithium and polyuria. In *Lithium Research and Therapy*. Edited by FN Johnson. New York, Academic Press, 1975, pp 473–484.

39. Forn J: Lithium and the cyclic AMP. In *Lithium Research and Therapy*. Edited by FN Johnson. New York, Academic Press, 1975, pp. 485–497.

40. Forrest JN Jr.: Lithium inhibition of cAMP-mediated hormones: A caution. *N Engl J Med*, 292:423–424, 1975.

41. Smith DF: Renal lithium clearance during dehydration and rehydration with water or 0.9% NaCl in the rat. *Acta Physiol Scand*, 90:427–430, 1974.

42. Thomsen K, and Schou M: Renal lithium excretion in man. *Am J Physiol*, 215:823–827, 1968.

43. Thomsen K: Renal lithium elimination in man and active treatment of lithium poisoning. *Am J Psychiatry*, 207 (Suppl):83–84, 1969.

44. Thomsen K, and Olesen OV: Participating factors and renal mechanisms in lithium intoxication. *Gen Pharmacol*, 9:85–89, 1978.

45. Hansen HE, et al: Renal function and renal pathology in patients with lithium-induced impairment of the renal concentrating ability. *Proc Eur Dial Transplant Assoc*, 14:518–527, 1977.

46. Baer L, Glassman AH, and Kassir S: Negative sodium balance in lithium carbonate toxicity. *Arch Gen Psychiatry*, 29:823–827, 1970.

47. Radomski JF, et al: The toxic effects, excretion and distribution of lithium chloride. *J Pharmacol Exp Ther*, 100:429–444, 1959.

48. Kierkegaard-Hansen A: The effect of lithium on blood pressure and on plasma renin substrate and renin in rats. *Acta Pharmacol Toxicol*, 35:370–378, 1974.

49. Baer L, et al: Mechanisms of renal lithium handling and their relationship to mineralocorticoids. *J Psychiatr Res*, 8:91–105, 1971.

50. Hestbech J, et al: Chronic renal lesions following long-term treatment with lithium. *Kidney Int*, 12:205–213, 1977.

51. Evan AP, and Ollerich DA: Ultrastructure of kidneys from lithium carbonate therapy. *Am J Anat*, 134:97–106, 1972.

52. Dias N, and Hocken AG: Oliguric renal failure complicating lithium carbonate therapy. *Nephron*, 10:246–249, 1973.

52. Berry FA, and Lambdin MA: Apomorphine and levallorphan tartrate in acute poisonings. *Am J Dis Child*, 105:160–163, 1963.

54. Alfrey AC, et al: Hypermagnesemia after renal homotransplantation. *Ann Intern Med*, 73:367–371, 1970.

55. Edwards KDG, and McCredie M: Studies on the binding properties of acidic, basic and neutral drugs to anion and cation exchange resins and charcoal in vitro. *Med J Aust*, 1:534-538, 1967.

56. Hurting HI, and Dyson WL: Lithium toxicity enhanced by diuresis. *N Engl J Med*, 290:748–749, 1974.

57. Forrest JAH: Forced alkaline diuresis for lithium intoxication. *Postgrad Med J*, 51:189–191, 1975.

58. Wilson JHP, et al: Peritoneal dialysis for lithium poisoning. *Br Med J*, 2:749–750, 1971.

59. Amdisen A, and Skjoldborg H: Hemodialysis for lithium poisoning. *Lancet*, 2:213, 1969.

60. Von Hartitzsch B, et al: Permanent neurologic sequelae despite hemodialysis for lithium intoxication. *Br Med J*, 4:757–759, 1972.

61. Weinstein MR, and Goldfield M: Cardiovascular malformations with lithium use during pregnancy. *Am J Psychiatry, 132*:529–531, 1975.

62. Baldessarini R: *Chemotherapy in Psychiatry.* Cambridge, Harvard University Press, 1977.

63. Schou M, and Amdisen A: Lithium and pregnancy. III. Lithium ingestion by children breast fed by woman on lithium treatment. *Br Med J,* 2:138, 1973.

64. Schou M, et al: Lithium and pregnancy. I. Report from the register of lithium babies. *Br Med J,* 2:135–136, 1973.

65. Villeneuve A, et al: Effect of lithium on thyroid in man. *Lancet,* 2:502, 1973.

66. Segal RL, Rosenblatt S, and Eliasoph I: Endocrine exophthalmos during lithium therapy of manic-depressive disease. *N Engl J Med, 289*:136–140, 1973.

67. Schou M, Amdisen A, and Baastrup PC: The practical management of lithium treatment. *Br J Hosp Med,* 6:615–619, 1970.

68. Kirkegaard C, Lauridsen UB, and Nerup J: Lithium and the thyroid. *Lancet,* 2:1210, 1973.

Chapter 10

Anticonvulsants

Gilbert J. Burckart
Sharon R. Ternullo

The group of compounds having anticonvulsant activity represents a diversity of chemical structures and toxicologic potentials. The toxicity of these drugs was evident even with the introduction of the bromides in the nineteenth century. Few other classes of therapeutic drugs can claim the frequency of chronic intoxication, requiring acute medical care and hospitalization, of the anticonvulsants. Their widespread availability within the home makes them prime components of accidental or suicidal drug ingestions. Since therapy often involves multiple drugs, interactions are common and often complicate the acute ingestion. A thorough knowledge of drug metabolism, active metabolites, and drug elimination is essential in the management of the intoxicated patient. This chapter will therefore address the toxicity of the major anticonvulsants that are not reviewed elsewhere in this text.

CASE REPORT

A 4-month-old black female was admitted for sleepiness and diarrhea. The child had been placed on phenobarbital and phenytoin at 6 weeks of age for a generalized tonic-clonic seizure. Work-up at that time had been negative. Approximately 1 month prior to admission, the dose of phenobarbital had been increased from 5 to 6.5 mg/kg/day, and phenytoin had been increased from 5 to 10 mg/kg/day.

Five days prior to admission, the mother noted the onset of loose watery stools without fever, cough, or vomiting. A public health nurse instructed the mother to give the child clear liquids. Two days prior to admission, the child became more sleepy than usual and was unresponsive to voices or stimulation.

On admission, the child was lethargic and sleepy. There was no history of ingestion or trauma. The child's vital signs were temperature, 37.2°C; pulse rate, 104/min; respirations, 32/min; blood pressure, 94/62 mm Hg; and weight, 6.4 kg. General examination revealed an unresponsive infant with no spontaneous movement. Deep tendon reflexes were 3+ and equal bilaterally. Pupils were small, equal, and reactive to light.

The patient responded to pain, and cranial nerves were intact. The remaining physical examination results were within normal limits. Arterial blood gas analysis revealed a pH of 7.24, Pco_2 of 41, Po_2 of 74, and oxygen saturation of 92%. Chest x-ray examination results were normal. Serum electrolytes, glucose, and calcium were normal.

CLINICAL ASSESSMENT AND MANAGEMENT OF THE PATIENT

The patient's symptoms suggested several possible causes. Drowsiness and lethargy pointed to CNS involvement, the causes of which could have been an infectious process, a tumor or other space-occupying mass, trauma, or toxicologic insult. The age of this patient and a history of loose watery stools would have suggested an infectious process, yet the infant was afebrile. Physical examination and history provided no evidence of a traumatic event. Although the child did have a seizure previously, the lack of focal findings or seizures suggested that an acute exacerbation of the CNS disease was not the cause.

In this patient, the history of treatment with anticonvulsant drugs and the report of a recent dosage alteration favored a diagnosis of drug toxicity. Anticonvulsant

serum level determinations, available at most hospitals, aided in the confirmation of the diagnosis. The patient's serum concentrations were phenytoin, 63 μg/ml and phenobarbital, 40 μg/ml.

The determination of whether the intoxication is acute or chronic is of secondary importance to the following acute management considerations: (1) initial symptoms and complications that may occur with phenytoin intoxication, (2) necessary laboratory tests and significance of their results, (3) indicated therapeutic measures, (4) prognosis with phenytoin intoxication, and (5) toxicities of and therapeutic approaches to other available anticonvulsants.

INITIAL SYMPTOMS AND COMPLICATIONS OF PHENYTOIN INTOXICATION

The classical symptoms of phenytoin intoxication include nystagmus, ataxia, and mental disturbances. In adults, these symptoms are associated with serum levels of 20 μg/ml, 30 μg/ml, and 40 μg/ml, respectively. In young children and some mentally retarded patients, however, initial symptoms such as nystagmus, dizziness, dysarthria, blurred vision, and diplopia are often absent or difficult to evaluate, which makes the diagnosis more difficult. Lehtovaara found wide variations in the postrotational nystagmus observed in patients receiving phenytoin.[1] Buchthal and associates and Friedman and associates reported that only 74% to 86% of patients with phenytoin serum levels between 30 and 60 μg/ml had signs of toxicity.[2,3]

Other neurologic symptoms may be present. Pupils are often dilated. Reflexes my be brisk in the initial phase of toxicity, only to become sluggish during the depressed phase after massive doses of the drug.[4] Electroencephalography with both acute and chronic phenytoin intoxication has indicated slowing of alpha waves, whereas more severe intoxications may result in an EEG pattern dominated by high-voltage slow waves.[5,6] An agitated coma state is common in acute ingestions, and seizures may occur.

Other autonomic and endocrinologic findings have been observed after phenytoin intoxication. Urinary incontinence has been reported in association with phenytoin toxicity.[4] Hyperglycemia due to impaired insulin release has occurred in association with both chronic and acute ingestions.[7,8,9] In one reported case, a blood glucose level of 726 mg/dl in a 20-month-old male who ingested approximately 70 to 80 mg/kg of phenytoin led to an initial misdiagnosis of diabetes mellitus.[8]

A variety of movement disorders have been associated with phenytoin toxicity in both adults and children. Transient hyperkinesia has been reported after a single intravenous infusion of phenytoin.[10] Asterixis has been connected with intoxication during phenytoin therapy.[11] Two patients who were recovering from brain surgery developed a transient hemiparesis with phenytoin serum levels over 34 μg/ml.[12]

During chronic therapy, extrapyramidal signs such as dystonic posturing, tremor, involuntary tongue protrusion, lip smacking, head nod, fish-mouthing, gross flinging and flailing movements of the extremities, facial grimacing, and athetosis have been reported in children and adults.[13-18] These symptoms could be mistaken for a phenothiazine-induced reaction.

A wide variety of other phenytoin-induced effects have occurred. Right bundle-branch block has been reported in an adult after an acute ingestion of approximately 5 g of phenytoin and 2.5 g of phenobarbital.[19] A case of panmyeloid hypoplasia has been suggested as a dose-dependent toxicity.[20] High doses of phenytoin early in therapy seem to increase the incidence of a generalized skin rash in children.[21,22]

Because of the diversity of symptoms it can produce, phenytoin toxicity can be misdiagnosed as botulism,[23] hysteriform neurosis,[24] and degenerative CNS disease.[25] A thorough history is necessary to separate the toxicologic effects of phenytoin from other suspected disease entities.

A complete history may indicate whether the patient is at a high risk level for phenytoin toxicity. A recent dosage change, as in the case presented, would increase suspicion of toxicity. Liver disease has been shown to result in accumulation of the unmetabolized drug, with resultant toxicity.[26] The acute onset of neurologic symptoms in a young child from a home where phenytoin is present, or in an epileptic adolescent undergoing family adjustment problems, would put phenytoin intoxication high on the list of differential diagnostic possibilities.

Other drugs can effect the metabolism or protein-binding characteristics of phenytoin, either inducing toxicity during chronic therapy or complicating an acute ingestion. Halothane,[27] diazepam,[28] sulthiame,[29] chloramphenicol,[30,31,32] warfarin, cycloserine, disulfiram, para-amino-salicylic acid, and isoniazid[33,34] have been implicated in the induction of toxicity during chronic phenytoin therapy. Intoxication has also resulted from a change in the dosage form of phenytoin from the calcium salt to the free acid.[35] An outbreak of phenytoin intoxication has occurred secondary to a change in the capsule excipient by one manufacturer.[36]

A determination of whether an acute ingestion of phenytoin is suicidal or accidental is usually not difficult; however, there have been reported cases in which intoxication has resulted from deliberate contamination of beverages[37] or street drugs.[23]

NECESSARY LABORATORY TESTS AND THEIR SIGNIFICANCE

Because of the inhibition of insulin release by phenytoin, acutely intoxicated patients should have a urine sample checked for glucose. Significant glucosuria would dictate the need for additional monitoring of serum glucose and electrolytes.

Serum electrolytes should be monitored in the severely intoxicated patient. Both hypo- and hypernatremia have been reported. Though phenytoin is known to inhibit the secretion of antidiuretic hormone,[38,39] the relevance of this effect after acute ingestion has not been established.

An understanding of the pharmacokinetics of phenytoin should influence the interpretation of serum phenytoin levels and therapeutic decisions following an overdose. Drug absorption is slow owing to limited solubility in GI contents and occurs after 6 to 12 hours.

At lower doses of the drug, elimination from the body appears to follow a linear first-order process. The rate at which the drug is eliminated increases as the concentration of the drug in the body increases, and the elimination half-life of the drug remains constant. With higher doses, the plasma level increases disproportionately to the dose (Michaelis-Menten or enzyme saturation kinetics). Figure 10–1 shows the routes of elimination of phenytoin from the body.

The formation of HPPH by enzymatic hydroxylation is responsible for the zero-order kinetics observed during the acute ingestion of large doses of phenytoin in children,[40,41,42] and in chronic intoxication in adults.[43,44] The presence of zero-order kinetics explains the persistence of high plasma concentrations and symptoms after acute ingestions for a period longer than would be expected from the adult half-life of 22 hours.

The presence of enzyme saturation kinetics also explains why levels decrease slowly at first following a large ingestion, but more rapidly as the serum concentration decreases. A high degree of individual variability in the rate of phenytoin metabolism occurs. Children metabolize the drug more rapidly and with more variability than adults. Black males seem to metabolize phenytoin more rapidly than white males.[45]

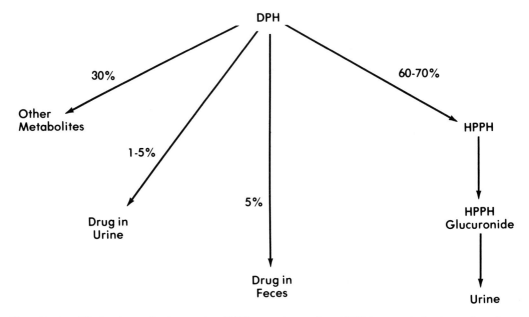

Fig. 10–1. Elimination of phenytoin. DPH = phenytoin; HPPH = 5-(p-hydroxyphenyl)-5-phenylhydantoin.

The serum phenytoin level may not represent the drug actively involved in production of cerebellar symptoms. Wilder and associates observed that the plasma/CSF ratio at equilibrium was 11/1 (the approximate ratio of total/free phenytoin in plasma).[46] Animal studies have shown much higher phenytoin levels in neural tissue than in blood. The cerebellum and brain stem have higher phenytoin concentrations than the cerebral cortex.[47]

These findings would explain the clinical appearance of nystagmus and ataxia before mental changes are observed as a result of phenytoin intoxication. Since phenytoin is highly protein bound (about 90%) in serum, the total/free phenytoin ratio will be affected by the amount of protein and other endogenous or exogenous agents, such as urea nitrogen or salicylates, that may compete for protein binding.

In a patient who exhibits toxicity despite low serum levels of phenytoin, a serum albumin or free phenytoin level determination may be helpful. The Boston Collaborative Surveillance Program found that about 11% of patients with albumin levels lower than 3.0 g/dl developed signs of phenytoin toxicity, whereas only about 4% of those patients with serum albumin equal to or greater than 3.0 g/dl were similarly affected.[48] The difference is due to an increased circulating level of free or unbound phenytoin, which may be approximated by measurement of the amount of the drug in cerebrospinal fluid or saliva.[49,50]

Assay methods vary from hospital to hospital, and an understanding of them is essential for proper use of serum level data. Some assays for phenytoin, such as radioimmunoassay and the EMIT system, are specific, whereas others are subject to interference by other chemical substances. The method of Svensmark and Kristensen, for example, is not specific for phenytoin.[51] Other drugs such as ethosuximide, primidone, mephenytoin, metharbital, bishydroxycoumarin, and phenylbutazone all interfere with the assay. Even the amount of oil of cloves and oil of sassafras absorbed from a teething lotion has been reported to interfere with this assay and to produce a falsely positive serum phenytoin level.[52] In conclusion, serum phenytoin concentrations must be interpreted in relation to the assay method, the sampling time, the dose, and the possibility of protein-binding alterations.

INDICATED THERAPEUTIC MEASURES

Correction of Life-Threatening Symptoms

Seizures and respiratory failure may occur as a result of acute phenytoin intoxication. Seizures will usually respond to diazepam, in a dose of 0.1 to 0.3 mg/kg IV (up to 10 mg in an adult), and repeated as necessary. Respiratory stimulants have been used without demonstrated efficacy and are contraindicated. Respiratory assistance, oxygen, and suctioning may be needed for coma due to phenytoin intoxication and/or secondarily due to diazepam administration. One death due to acute phenytoin intoxication has been partially attributed to cerebral edema secondary to hypoxia.[53]

Minimization of Absorption

Procedures that aid in achieving this goal are emesis or lavage, administration of activated charcoal, and a saline cathartic.

Emesis should be induced with syrup of ipecac if the patient is alert. After 12 hours postingestion, the likelihood of a significant return is not great. Gastric lavage should be reserved for those patients who are already comatose, in danger of becoming obtunded within 60 minutes, or without the gag reflex.

Saline cathartics should speed the intestinal transit of unabsorbed drug and minimize the contact time of the drug with sites of absorption. Either magnesium citrate (4.0 ml/kg) or magnesium sulfate (250 mg/kg) should be used. The dose of cathartic may have to be repeated until a charcoal-containing stool is passed.

The usual dose of activated charcoal is 5 to 10 times the estimated ingested dose of phenytoin. Since this estimation is often difficult, 30 to 50 g should be administered in a child and 50 to 100 g should be given to an adult. Since activated charcoal is used for its capacity to adsorb phenytoin and prevent GI absorption, it should be given as a slurry in water or combined with crushed ice.

Neuvonen and associates reported that 50 g of activated charcoal, taken either immediately after the ingestion of 500 mg of phenytoin or 1 hour postingestion, reduced absorption by 98% and 80% respectively.[54] It also decreased peak serum concentrations by 98% and 60%. These may be overestimates of activated charcoal's efficiency, however, owing to the concentration-dependent kinetics followed by phenytoin.

Facilitation of the Removal of Absorbed Phenytoin

Previous attempts to improve renal excretion of phenytoin by either forced diuresis or modification of urine pH have not significantly altered the course of the intoxications. Even after an acute ingestion of 300 mg/kg, when conversion of phenytoin to HPPH had been completed, only 9% of the total drug in the urine after 6 hours was the unmetabolized compound. In 24 hours, the DPH/HPPH ratio had dropped to only 2%.[42]

Peritoneal dialysis has been reported to have resulted in clinical improvement in two acute phenytoin intoxications. Tenckhoff and associates have reported a drop in phenytoin blood levels from 112 to 7.5 µg/ml after 16 hours of dialysis.[55] Analysis of the dialysate, however, revealed only "a trace" of phenytoin. The authors speculated that the hyperglycemia

due to the intoxication or dialysis may have had a palliative effect on cerebral edema.

Blair and colleagues reported a drop of serum phenytoin from 150 to 30 µg/ml during 35 hours of peritoneal dialysis, but only 775 mg of phenytoin was recovered in the dialysate.[56] Wilson and associates point out, however, that in a man weighing 70 kg, with an assumed volume of distribution of 0.61 L/kg, this amount of phenytoin would coincide with a decrease in plasma levels of about 18 µg/ml, rather than the 120 µg/ml difference reported.[57]

Hemodialysis has been reported to increase the elimination of phenytoin from the body,[58,59] and to result in clinical improvement of symptoms. The phenytoin dialysate concentrations are not reported in one case where plasma levels decreased from 116 to 79 µg/ml after 3.5 hours of dialysis.[59] Theil and associates reported a drop in plasma phenytoin from 50 to 4 µg/ml after dialysis, but attempts to measure the drug concentrations in the dialysis bath were unsuccessful.[58] Martin and colleagues reported that only 2% to 4% of an intravenous dose of phenytoin was recovered from uremic patients in the dialysate.[60] This amount would contribute little towards improving the overall elimination of the drug.

On a theoretical basis, dialysis should not be expected to be effective in increasing the clearance of phenytoin. Phenytoin is higly bound to tissue, and approximately 90% of the drug present in the blood is bound to plasma proteins. The rapid clearance rates obtained in the anecdotal reports are poorly documented and do not consider that increased elimination could be due to Michaelis-Menten pharmacokinetics. Addition of albumin to the dialysate adds considerably to the expense of the treatment, and its efficacy has not been adequately documented. In general, dialysis should be considered only in extreme intoxications and not as part of routine management.

The importance of maintaining fluid and electrolyte balance cannot be underestimated. Three reported cases of acute phenytoin ingestions of up to 300 mg/kg have been successfully managed solely by intravenous fluids and observation. Therefore, the appropriate therapy for an acute phenytoin ingestion involves good supportive care in the following areas: (1) control of seizures, (2) assurance of adequate oxygenation, (3) minimization of drug absorption, and (4) maintenance of fluid and electrolyte balance. Successful treatment of chronic intoxications frequently can be handled by withdrawal of the drug and, after an appropriate time perod, reinstitution of therapy at an adjusted dose.

PROGNOSIS WITH PHENYTOIN INTOXICATION

The prognosis for the acute and chronic forms of phenytoin intoxication is good. With conservative management, patients have recovered from doses of up to 300 mg/kg without apparent sequelae.[42]

Despite the frequency of childhood seizure disorders and the availability of phenytoin to young children, reports of fatal toxicities are few. Only three pediatric deaths have been reported due to acute ingestions. The amounts ingested were determined in two of these cases to be approximately 100 mg/kg[53] and 160 mg/kg.[61] The third fatality was a 16-year-old girl who ingested an unknown amount of phenytoin.[62] The cause of death in one patient was probably hypoxia-induced cerebral edema.[53] A second death may also have been preventable, since the cardiac tachyarrythmias developed after the patient had been treated with amphetamine sulfate, caffeine and sodium benzoate, and nikethamide.[62]

Two other deaths have been reported as allegedly due to acute phenytoin overdosage. However, both adult males had blood levels of only 4 to 5 μg/ml at the time of autopsy.[63] Although acute phenytoin toxicity usually persists for 4 to 5 days, more prolonged convalescence periods have been reported.[57,58]

In animals, chronic intoxication with phenytoin has been associated with lesions located in the cerebellum, especially in the Purkinje cells. Postmortem examinations in humans who had received large doses of phenytoin have shown changes similar to the animal studies.[64,65] Acute ingestions of phenytoin have not been reported to produce irreversible symptoms or any findings compatible with Purkinje cell degeneration or atrophy.

TOXICITIES OF AND THERAPEUTIC APPROACHES TO OTHER ANTICONVULSANTS

The hydantoins. Although there are four hydantoin analogs, phenytoin is the prototype with which each is compared with respect to efficacy and toxicity. Mephenytoin (Mesantoin) causes fewer GI symptoms, less ataxia, and less gingival hyperplasia than phenytoin. However, mephenytoin has a greater tendency to cause drowsiness and a higher incidence of dermatitis, anemia, hepatitis, and agranulocytosis during chronic administration.

Ethotoin (Peganone) is observed to induce rashes, anorexia, vomiting, nystagmus, and ataxia less often than phenytoin. Gum hyperplasia and hirsutism have not been reported with ethotoin. The significance of these differences is uncertain in acute ingestion, and reports of significant single-drug intoxication with mephenytoin or ethotoin are not available. The principles of management are the same as those discussed for phenytoin in the preceding section.

Valproic acid. Valproic acid (Depakene) is a relatively new and frequently used anticonvulsant. Although valproic acid was originally thought to be quite innocuous, several case reports to the contrary have appeared. Its two primary toxic manifestations are related to its effect on concentrations of biogenic amines in the central nervous system and to its metabolism by the liver.

The anticonvulsant activity of valproic acid may be partially mediated through an elevation of brain gamma-aminobutyric acid (GABA), which has an inhibitory synaptic action.[66] The expected CNS effects are therefore drowsiness, lethargy, and coma, although extrapyramidal symptoms and hallucinations have also been observed.[67,68]

Although drowsiness during clinical use of the drug does occur infrequently, increased irritability and the other more significant CNS effects are associated with high serum concentrations of the drug (greater than 100 $\mu g/ml$). Since naloxone may be a GABA antagonist,[69] Steiman and associates have suggested its use in valproate-induced depression.[70] They used naloxone to treat a 19-month-old boy who had ingested 200 mg/kg of valproic acid. The child, who had been unconscious with pinpoint, poorly reactive pupils, responded within minutes and became alert and conversant, and the pupils were reactive to light.

The most lethal effects of valproic acid are the hepatotoxic reactions that occur occasionally with chronic use. Although elevations in serum SGOT, SGPT, and alkaline phosphatase may be transient and may return to normal with continued dosing, they may also herald acute hepatic failure and death. The mechanism of liver damage is not understood, but it undoubtedly parallels hepatotoxicity due to other short-chain fatty acids and hypoglycin.[71,72] Although an acute valproic acid ingestion has not been clearly associated with hepatotoxicity, biochemical measures of liver function should be obtained.

The absorption of orally administered sodium valproate occurs rapidly, with peak levels in 0.5 to 4 hours. Although drug metabolism and elimination are generally rapid (serum half-life: 8 to 10 hours), several instances of a prolonged half-life (30 hours) after an acute ingestion have been noted, due to either saturation of metabolizing enzymes[73] or hepatotoxicity.[71,72] Little drug is eliminated unchanged in the urine, but the duration of the anticonvulsant action of valproic acid in rodents is prolonged by bilateral nephrectomy.[66] Enterohepatic circulation may occur to a limited extent, and little drug is excreted fecally.

Drug interactions are numerous for valproic acid and may pose a problem following multiple drug ingestion. Phenobarbital serum levels consistently increase after addition of valproic acid to the drug regimen. However, Van der Kleijn and associates saw no change in the rate of elimination of phenobarbital after a valproate-phenobarbital ingestion.[73]

Valproic acid is highly bound to plasma proteins (90%) and may therefore compete with other highly bound drugs (i.e., phenytoin), leading to alterations in elimination rates of the compounds. In the case of competitive protein binding, serum concentrations of the drugs may not accurately reflect the amount of free drug and the ultimate pharmacologic/toxicologic effect of the compound. Mutual inhibition between the elimination rates of ethanol and valproic acid may occur, indicating interference with alcohol dehydrogenase enzyme.

In conclusion, the acute toxicity of valproic acid has been reported to be low in both animals and humans. Recovery after an ingestion of up to 36 g has been uneventful following conservative management. Standard methods of emesis, lavage, and catharsis should be employed. Supportive therapy for generalized CNS depression should be undertaken, and a trial of naloxone may be used if necessary. Drug elimination may be prolonged and drug interactions are likely to occur in multiple drug ingestions. Biochemical methods of assessing potential hepato-toxicity should be monitored.

Primidone and other barbiturates. Barbiturate intoxications are discussed in Chapter 4. The fact that several of the anticonvulsant barbiturates convert to active metabolites may lead to confusion, however. For example, metharbital (Gemonil) is metabolized by the liver via N-demethylation to form barbital, so that treatment should be implemented as for barbital ingestions. Mephobarbital (Mebaral) is converted primarily to phenobarbital. Primidone (Mysoline) has two active metabolites: phenylethyl-malonamide (PEMA) and phenobarbital.

Although primidone ingestions have proven lethal in some cases, alkaline diuresis may aid in removing the parent compound before its conversion to phenobarbital.[74] Ingestions of 400 mg/kg of body weight have been managed adequately with supportive therapy and forced diuresis.[75] One distinguishing feature of primidone intoxication is the resultant crystalluria, identified as crystals of primidone,[76] occurring at serum concentrations of greater than 80 μg/ml. The treatment plan must include consideration of the metabolites phenobarbital and PEMA, which are potentially more toxic than the parent compound.

Carbamazepine. Carbamazepine (Tegretol) is chemically a member of the tricyclic antidepressant group of drugs, which are presented in Chapter 7. Carbamazepine undoubtedly exerts the same type of cardiac effects, as suggested by Herzberg,[77] and CNS-depressant effects. Salcman and associates reported a case of a 16-year-old who ingested 116 mg/kg of carbamazepine and was stuporous for 2 days with only supportive care.[78] One unique feature of this drug is that it can induce, on chronic administration, hypo-natremia and inappropriate antidiuretic hormone secretion. This particular effect may be blocked by phenytoin.[79]

The response of a carbamazepine over-dose to therapeutic measures such as the administration of physostigmine is presently unknown, but should parallel results seen with other tricyclic antidepressant intoxications.

Clonazepam. Benzodiazepine overdose and treatment is presented and discussed in Chapter 5. Little information is available on intoxications with the products used exclusively as anticonvulsants. Welch, Rumack, and Hammond have reported a 4-year-old child who ingested an unknown quantity of clonazepam (Clonopin), and who passed from periods of alert agitation to unresponsive coma several times.[80] The child was given supportive therapy and was alert 36 hours after ingestion, a time period compatible with the long elimination half-life of the drug. Bladin also reported a 2½-year-old child who ingested 60 mg of clonazepam, responded after 12 hours, and simply remained ataxic for 72 hours afterwards.[81] There is, therefore, a large margin of safety in acute clonazepam overdose.

Succinimides. The succinimides, including ethosuximide (Zarontin), meth-suximide (Celontin), and phensuximide (Milontin), have been in use in the treatment of absence epilepsy since the early 1950s. Although a large number of adverse effects are associated with this group of drugs, many are not dose related, and few reports of acute intoxication can be found. Dose-related adverse effects commonly associated with these drugs include nausea, vomiting, lethargy, and dizziness.

The succinimides are primarily converted to several major metabolites. Only 10% to 20% of these drugs appears unchanged in the urine. The metabolites may possess pharmacologic activity and may play a role in the acute intoxication. Karch reported an 18-year-old patient who ingested nearly 10 g of methsuximide.[82] The girl initially could be easily aroused, but lapsed into a coma 9 hours postingestion. She was treated symptomatically and finally awoke 80 hours postingestion. Although blood levels of the parent compound decreased quickly, levels of the metabolite (2-methyl-2-phenylsuccinimide) remained high 60 hours postingestion. The continued presence of the metabolite may implicate it in the persistence of toxic symptoms.

Therapy for intoxication with this group of compounds remains symptomatic. Although the benefits are still speculative, a forced diuresis, unless contraindicated, may aid in removing the more polar metabolites contributing to the toxicity of these drugs.

REFERENCES

1. Lehtovaara R: Post-rotational nystagmus. An unreliable sign of diphenylhydantoin toxicity. *Epilepsia*, 14:447–449, 1973.
2. Buchthal F, Svensmark O, and Schiller PJ: Clinical and elctroencephalographic correlation with serum levels of diphenylhydantoin. *Arch Neurol*, 2:624–630, 1960.
3. Friedman HM, Fishman RA, and Yahr MD: Determinations of plasma and cerebrospinal fluid levels of Dilantin in the human. *Trans Am Neurol Assoc*, 85:166–170, 1960.
4. Patel H, and Crichton JU: The neurologic hazards of diphenylhydantoin in childhood. *J Pediatr*, 73:676–684, 1968.
5. Levy LL, and Fenichel GM: Diphenylhydantoin activated seizures. *Neurology*, 15:716–722, 1965.
6. Iivananinen I, et al: Electroencephalography and phenytoin toxicity in mentally retarded epileptic patients. *J Neurol Neurosurg Psychiatry*, 41:272–277, 1978.
7. Fariss BL, and Lutcher CL: Diphenylhydantoin-induced hyperglycemia and impaired insulin release: effects of dosage. *Diabetes*, 30:177–181, 1976.
8. Klein JP: Diphenylhydantoin intoxication associated with hyperglycemia. *J Pediatr*, 69:463–465, 1966.
9. Holcomb R, et al: Intoxication with 5,5-diphenylhydantoin (Dilantin). *J Pediatr*, 80:627–632, 1972.
10. Mauguiere F, et al: Transient hyperkinesia after a single intravenous perfusion of diphenylhydantoin. *Eur Neurol*, 18:116–123, 1979.
11. Murphy MJ, and Goldstein MN: Diphenylhydantoin-induced asterixis. *JAMA*, 229:538–540, 1974.
12. Findler, G, and Lavy S: Transient hemiparesis: A rare manifestation of diphenylhydantoin toxicity. *J Neurosurg*, 50:685–687, 1979.
13. Zinsmeisters S, and Marks R: Acute athetosis as a result of phenytoin toxicity in a child. *Am J Dis Child*, 130:75–76, 1976.
14. Jan JE, and Kliman MR: Extrapyramidal disturbances and vascular changes during diphenylhydantoin intoxication. *Can Med Assoc J*, 111:636–637, 1974.
15. Rosenblum E, Rodichok L, and Hansen PA: Movement disorder as a manifestation of diphenylhydantoin toxicity. *Pediatrics*, 54:364–366, 1974.
16. Ahmad S, et al: Involuntary movements caused by phenytoin intoxication in epileptic patients. *J Neurol Neurosurg Psychiatry*, 38:225–231, 1975.
17. Shuttleworth E, Wise G, and Paulson G: Choreoathetosis and diphenylhydantoin intoxication. *JAMA*, 230:1170–1171, 1974.
18. Kooiker JC, and Sumi SM: Movement disorder as a manifestation of diphenylhydantoin intoxication. *Neurology*, 24:68–71, 1974.
19. Joubert P, and Vorster B: Incomplete right bundle-branch block associated with diphenylhydantoin toxicity. *S Afr Med J*, 49:2149, 1975.
20. Parker WA, and Gumnit RJ: Diphenylhydantoin toxicity: Dose-dependent blood dyscrasia. *Neurology*, 24:1178–1180, 1974.
21. Wilson JT, Höjer B, and Rane A: Loading and conventional dose therapy with phenytoin in children. Kinetic profile of parent drug and main metabolite in plasma. *Clin Pharmacol Ther*, 20:48–50, 1976.
22. Wilson JT, et al: High incidence of a concentration-dependent skin reaction in children treated with phenytoin. *Br Med J*, 1:1583–1586, 1978.
23. Wand M, and Mather JA: Diphenylhydantoin intoxication mimicking botulism. *N Engl J Med*, 286:88, 1972.
24. Frantzen E, et al: Phenytoin (Dilantin) intoxication. *Acta Neurol Scand*, 43:440–446, 1967.
25. Vallarta JM, Bell DB, and Reichert A: Progressive encephalopathy due to chronic hydantoin intoxication. *Am J Dis Child*, 128:27–34, 1974.
26. Kutt H, et al: Diphenylhydantoin and phenobarbital toxicity. *Arch Neurol*, 11:649–656, 1964.
27. Karlin JM, and Kutt H: Acute diphenylhydantoin intoxication following halothane anesthesia. *J Pediatr*, 76:941–944, 1970.
28. Rogers HJ, et al: Phenytoin intoxication during concurrent diazepam therapy. *J Neurol Neurosurg Psychiatry*, 40:890–895, 1977.
29. Richens A, and Houghton HW: Phenytoin intoxication caused by sulthiame. *Lancet*, 2:1442, 1973.
30. Vincent FM, Mills L, and Sullivan JK: Chloramphenicol-induced phenytoin intoxication. *Ann Neurol*, 3:469, 1978.
31. Rose JQ, et al: Intoxication caused by interaction of chloramphenicol and phenytoin. *JAMA*, 237:2630–2631, 1977.
32. Harper JM, et al: Phenytoin-chloramphenicol interaction. *Drug Intell Clin Pharm*, 13:425–429, 1979.
33. Kutt H, et al: Diphenylhydantoin intoxication: a complication of isoniazid therapy. *Am Rev Respir Dis*, 101:377–384, 1970.

34. Brennan RW, et al: Diphenylhydantoin intoxication attendent to slow inactivation of isoniazid. *Neurology*, 20:687–693, 1970.

35. Albani M: An unusual case of phenytoin intoxication. *Neuropaediatrie*, 9:185–188, 1978.

36. Bochner F, et al: Factors involved in an outbreak of phenytoin intoxication. *J Neurol Sci*, 16:481–487, 1972.

37. Cates W, and Silsly HD: Diphenylhydantoin intoxication in a group of military aviators: A case report. *Toxicology*, 1:377–382, 1973.

38. Fichman MP, Kleeman CR, and Bethune JE: Inhibition of antidiuretic hormone secretion by diphenylhydantoin. *Arch Neurol*, 22:45–53, 1970.

39. Tanay A, Yust I, Peresecenschi G, et al: Long-term treatment of the syndrome of inappropriate antidiuretic hormone secretion with phenytoin. *Ann Intern Med*, 90:50–52, 1979.

40. Garrettson LK, and Jusko WJ: Diphenylhydantoin kinetics in overdosed children. *Clin Pharmacol Ther*, 17:481–491, 1975.

41. Pruitt AW, et al: A complex pattern of disposition of phenytoin in severe intoxication. *Clin Pharmcaol Ther*, 18:112–120, 1975.

42. Wilder BJ, Buchanan RA, and Serrano EE: Correlation of acute diphenylhydantoin intoxication with plasma levels and metabolite excretion. *Neurology*, 23:1329–1332, 1973.

43. Gill MA, et al: Phenytoin overdose kinetics. *West J Med*, 128:246–248, 1978.

44. Atkinson AJ, and Shaw JM: Pharmacokinetic study of a patient with diphenylhydantoin toxicity. *Clin Pharmacol Ther*, 14:521–528, 1973.

45. Arnold K, and Gerber N: The rate of decline of diphenylhydantoin in human plasma. *Clin Pharmacol Ther*, 11:121–134, 1970.

46. Wilder BJ et al: Efficacy of intravenous phenytoin in the treatment of status epilepticus: Kinetics of central nervous system penetration. *Ann Neurol*, 1:511–518, 1977.

47. Ang MK, Guiang R, and Berger AR: Diphenylhydantoin (Dilantin) neurotoxicity—A deceptive syndrome. *J Am Geriatr Soc*, 17:1102–1107, 1969.

48. Boston Collaborative Study Group: Diphenylhydantoin side effects and serum albumin levels. *Clin Pharmacol Ther*, 14:529–532, 1973.

49. Schmidt D, and Kupferberg HJ: Diphenylhydantoin, phenobarbital and primidone in saliva, plasma, and cerebrospinal fluid. *Epilepsia*, 16:735–741, 1975.

50. McAuliffe JJ, et al: Salivary levels of anticonvulsants: A practical approach to drug monitoring. *Neurology*, 27: 409–413, 1977.

51. Svensmark C, and Kristensen P: Determination of diphenylhydantoin and phenobarbital in small amounts of serum. *J Lab Clin Med*, 61:501–507, 1963.

52. Jones MD, and Helfer RE: A teething lotion resulting in the misdiagnosis of diphenylhydantoin administration. *Am J Dis Child*, 122:259–260, 1971.

53. Laubscher FA: Fatal diphenylhydantoin poisoning: A case report. *JAMA*, 198:1120–1121, 1966.

54. Neuvonen PJ, Elfving SM, and Elonen E: Reduction of absorption of digoxin, phenytoin and aspirin by activated charcoal. *Eur J Clin Pharmacol*, 13:213–218, 1978.

55. Tenckhoff H, et al: Acute diphenylhydantoin intoxication. *Am J Dis Child*, 116:422–425, 1968.

56. Blair AAD, et al: Acute diphenylhydantoin and primidone poisoning treated by peritoneal dialysis. *J Neurol Neurosurg Psychiatry*, 31:520–523, 1968.

57. Wilson JT, Huff JG, and Kilroy AW: Prolonged toxicity following acute phenytoin overdose in a child. *J Pediatr*, 95:135–138, 1979.

58. Thiel GB, et al: Acute Dilantin poisoning. *Neurology*, 11:138–142, 1961.

59. Schreiner GE: The role of hemodialysis (artificial kidney) in acute poisoning. *Arch Intern Med*, 102:896–913, 1958.

60. Martin E, et al: Removal of phenytoin by hemodialysis in uremic patients. *JAMA*, 234:1750–1751, 1977.

61. Schmeisser M: Todliche vergiftung mit Zentrophil beim kind. *Kinderarztl Prax*, 20:158–161, 1952.

62. Tichner JP, and Enselberg CD: Suicidal Dilantin (sodium diphenylhydantoin) poisoning. A case report. *N Engl J Med*, 245:723–725, 1951.

63. Coutselinia A, Dimopoulos G and Varsami P: Fatal intoxication with diphenylhydantoin: Report of two cases. *Forensic Sci*, 6:131–133, 1975.

64. Utterbach RA: Parenchymatous cerebellar degeneration complicating diphenylhydantoin (Dilantin) therapy. *Arch Neurol Psychiatry*, 80:180–181, 1958.

65. Hofman WW: Cerebellar lesions after parenteral Dilantin administration. *Neurology*, 8:210–214, 1958.

66. Pinder RM, et al: Sodium valproate: A review of its pharmacological and therapeutic efficacy in epilepsy. *Drugs*, 13:81–123, 1977.

67. Lautin A, et al: Extrapyramidal syndrome with sodium valproate. *Br Med J*, 2:1035–1036, 1979.

68. Chadwick DW, et al: Acute intoxication with sodium valproate. *Ann Neurol*, 6:552–553, 1979.

69. Brueker E, Dingledine R, and Iverson LL: Evidence for naloxone and opiates as GABA antagonists. *Br J Pharmacol*, 58:458P, 1976.

70. Steiman GS, Woerpel RW, and Sherard ES: Treatment of accidental sodium valproate overdose with an opiate antagonist. *Ann Neurol*, 6:274, 1979.

71. Suchy FJ, et al: Acute hepatic failure associated with the use of sodium-valproate. *N Engl J Med*, 300:962–965, 1979.

72. Gerber N, et al: Reye-like syndrome associated with valproic acid therapy. *J Pediatr*, 95:142–144, 1979.

73. Van der Kleijn E, et al: Clinical pharmacokinetics of benzodiazepine, barbiturates and short chain fatty acids. In *Clinical Pharmacokinetics: A Symposium*. Washington, D.C., American Pharmaceutical Association, 1974, p. 94.

74. Lagenstein I, et al: Intoxication with primidone: Continuous monitoring of serum primidone and

its metabolites during forced diuresis. *Neuropaediatrie*, 8:190–195, 1977.

75. Kappy MS, and Buckley J: Primidone intoxication in a child. *Arch Dis Child*, 44:282–284, 1969.

76. Bailey DN, and Jatlow PI: Chemical analysis of massive crystalluria following primidone overdose. *Am J Clin Path*, 58:583–589, 1972.

77. Herzberg L: Carbamazepine and bradycardia (letter). *Lancet*, 1:1097–1098, 1978.

78. Salcman M, and Pippenger CE: Acute carbamazepine encephalopathy (letter). *JAMA*, 213:915, 1975.

79. Sordillo P, et al: Carbamazepine-induced syndrome of inappropriate antidiuretic hormone secretion. *Arch Intern Med*, 138:299–301, 1978.

80. Welch TR, Rumack BH, and Hammond K: Clonazepam overdose resulting in cyclic coma. *Clin Toxicol*, 10:433–436, 1977.

81. Bladin PF: The use of clonazepam as an anticonvulsant—Clinical evaluation. *Med J Aust*, 1:683–688, 1973.

82. Karch SB: Methsuximide overdose. *JAMA*, 223:1463–1465, 1973.

Chapter 11

Central Nervous System Stimulants

Gary M. Oderda
Wendy Klein-Schwartz

Amphetamine, or phenylisopropylamine, is the prototype of a class of drugs producing CNS stimulation (Figure 11–1). Since amphetamine is the name of a specific chemical, it is inappropriate to refer to these compounds as amphetamines.[1] Technically, it would be more appropriate to refer to these agents as "amphetamine-like." However, for simplicity, throughout this article the more common term "amphetamines" will be used.

Amphetamine was introduced originally to be used via inhalation as a bronchodilator and nasal mucosal constrictor. Amphetamines (Table 11–1) subsequently have been used as CNS and respiratory stimulants (e.g., for barbiturate intoxications), as anorectics, as antidepressants, and for the treatment of narcolepsy and hyperkinesis in children. Many of these uses have been abandoned. Of particular interest to toxicologists is the current feeling that CNS and respiratory stimulants (such as nikethamide and doxapram) have no place in the treatment of intoxicated patients. Although some feel that amphetamines are useful in promoting weight loss, their efficacy for this purpose is highly doubtful, and the potential risks outweigh the benefits. Currently, only narcolepsy and treatment of hyperkinesis in children are well-recognized indications for the clinical use of amphetamines.

Abuse of amphetamines is a significant problem. Use of these agents by civilian and military employees to combat battle fatigue, improve production, and for similar purposes was common during World War II. In the postwar period, amphetamines were available on a nonprescription basis

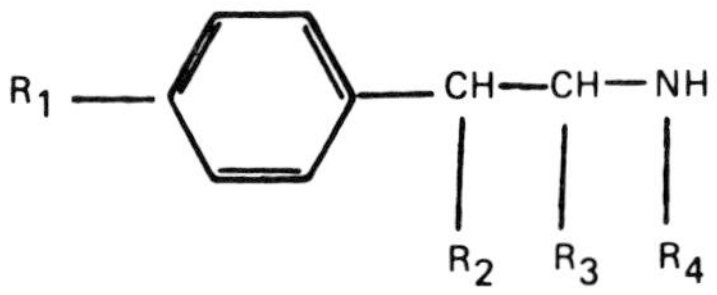

		R$_1$	R$_2$	R$_3$	R$_4$
Examples:	Amphetamine	H	H	CH$_3$	H
	Methamphetamine	H	H	CH$_3$	CH$_3$
	Fenfluramine	m-CF$_3$	H	CH$_3$	C$_2$H$_5$

Fig. 11–1. Chemical structure of amphetamines.

in Japan. In 1954, when controls were instituted, it was estimated that there were 200,000 amphetamine addicts in Japan.[2] Prior to the institution of production controls in the U.S., it had been estimated that 5,000,000,000 to 8,000,000,000 therapeutic doses of amphetamines were produced annually; one half of this amount was thought to be diverted into illicit channels.[3]

Production quotas for 1979, for example, were as follows: amphetamine, 2715 kg; phenmetrazine, 1123 kg; and methamphetamine, 190 kg.[4] If it is assumed that the therapeutic dose is 10 mg for amphetamine, 25 mg for phenmetrazine, and 5 mg for methamphetamine, these production figures would allow 271,500,000 dosage units for amphetamine, 44,920,000 for phenmetrazine, and 38,000,000 for methamphetamine. This is only a small percentage of previous estimates.

However, it must be remembered that these quotas do not include drugs pro-

Table 11–1.   Common Amphetamine Products

GENERIC NAME	TRADE NAME	USUAL DAILY THERAPEUTIC DOSE
Amphetamine	Benzedrine Biphetamine and others	2.5–10 mg 1–3×
Benzephetamine HCl	Didrex	25–50 mg 1× to a maximum of 50 mg 3×
Chlorphentermine HCl	Pre-Sate	65 mg 1×
Clortermine	Voranil	50 mg 1×
Dextroamphetamine	Dexamyl Dexedrine and others	2.5–5 mg 1–3×
Diethylpropion HCl	Tenuate Tepanil Dospan Ten-tab	25 mg 3× or 75 mg extended-release 1×
Fenfluramine HCl	Pondimin	20 mg 3× to a maximum of 40 mg 3×
Methamphetamine HCl	Desoxyn Fefamine etc.	2.5–5 mg 1–3× or 5–15 mg of extended-release 1×
Phendimetrazine tartrate	Plegine	35 mg 2–3× Maximum = 70 mg 3×
Phenmetrazine HCl	Preludin	25 mg 2–3× Maximum of 25 mg 3× or 75 mg of extended-release 1×
Phentermine	Ionamin	8 mg 3× or 15–30 mg of resin complex 1×

duced illicitly. It is estimated that 8% of the total population of the U.S. has used stimulants (except cocaine) for nonmedical purposes, and that 1% are current users (defined as having used the drug at least once in the past month). Usage is highest in the 18–25-year-old age group, with 21% having used a stimulant at least once and 3% being current users.[5]

Intoxications commonly are the results of accidental ingestions in children and drug abuse or suicide attempts in adolescents and adults. During 1977, 1151 ingestions of "amphetamine-type" preparations were reported to the National Clearinghouse for Poison Control Centers. Of these reported ingestions, 526 were prescription preparations that were either amphetamines or amphetamine-like drugs. The age distribution of these 526 reported cases was: 41.4%, under 5 years old; 42.0%, 5 years and older, and 16.5%, age unspecified.

CASE REPORT

A 17-year-old white male was brought to the emergency room by ambulance, 2 hours after ingestion of an unknown number of tablets thought to be prescription "diet pills." On arrival in the ER, the patient was excited and agitated. He paced up and down the room complaining of bugs crawling on the walls and on his skin. When approached by hospital staff, he became extremely hostile, screaming that they were "out to get me." He became combative to the point where he had to be physically restrained.

The vital signs at this time were blood pressure, 160/95; pulse, 140/min and regular; rectal temperature, 40°C; and respirations, 24/min. He was noted to be flushed and sweating, with excoriations on his arms and legs. Mucous membranes appeared dry. On physical examination, there was no evidence of trauma or head injury. Pupils were dilated and sluggishly reactive to light. Chest, cardiac and abdominal examination results were within normal limits. Reflexes were 4+ bilaterally.

CLINICAL ASSESSMENT AND MANAGEMENT OF THE PATIENT

In an assessment of CNS-stimulant intoxication, the following must be considered: (1) substances capable of producing this syndrome, (2) laboratory data that will help in the evaluation of this patient, (3) manifestations and mechanisms of an overdosage of CNS stimulants, (4) appropriate therapy, (5) the possible complications, (6) the endpoints of therapy, (7) prognosis.

MAJOR DIAGNOSTIC CONSIDERATIONS

In this case, we were presented with a patient exhibiting signs of CNS stimulation. In addition, the patient was tachycardic, hypertensive, hyperthermic, and mydriatic. The identity of the ingested agent was not clear and the amount ingested was also unknown.

Although this information is not necessary for development of the initial management scheme, identification of the ingested agent is useful in the prediction of complications that may arise during the course of the intoxication. Certain treatment measures, such as those aimed at enhancing renal elimination of the drug, that are beneficial for certain agents may be ineffective and potentially harmful in other situations. Therefore, eventual identification of the agent ingested or of the class of drugs to which the ingested agent belongs is essential.

SUBSTANCES CAPABLE OF PRODUCING CNS STIMULATION

On the basis of the CNS and cardiovascular effects this patient exhibited, as well as his history of ingestion of prescription diet pills, the CNS-stimulant class of drugs was considered.

A large number of natural and synthetic compounds can produce CNS stimulation, either by blocking inhibitory influences, as in the case of strychnine and picrotoxin, or by enhancing excitation, either directly or via endogenous neurotransmitters.[6] There is a large number of sympathomimetic and sympathomimetic-like agents on the market. Although relative potencies are different, in general the acute toxic effects of these products are the same as those of amphetamines (Table 11–2).

Fenfluramine (Pondimin), although structurally similar to amphetamine, produces CNS depression rather than stimulation.[7,8] This effect may be evident in therapeutic as well as toxic doses. However, signs of CNS stimulation such as agitation and seizures have been reported in intoxicated patients, with toxic doses ranging from 300 to 2000 mg.[8]

Methylphenidate (Ritalin) and pemoline (Cylert) are indicated for the treatment of

hyperactive syndrome of childhood, and in large doses will produce symptoms of CNS stimulation that are qualitatively similar to those of amphetamines. Initial management of patients intoxicated with these drugs would be similar to the initial management of an amphetamine overdose. Mazindol (Sanorex), an anorectic agent chemically unrelated to amphetamines, has pharmacologic activity similar to that of amphetamines, and the spectrum of symptoms in an intoxicated patient would be expected to be similar.

Caffeine, theophylline, and theobromine are methylated xanthines, which stimulate the CNS and heart, relax smooth muscle, and produce diuresis. Large doses can produce convulsions and death. Doses of caffeine 50 to 250 mg will affect the cortex only, whereas doses of 250 to 500 mg will affect the medulla as well. At doses greater than 1000 mg, the spinal cord is affected.[9,10]

Caffeine is found in coffee, tea, and colas. The average cup of coffee contains 100 to 150 mg of caffeine, compared with 60 to 75 mg per cup of tea and 40 to 60 mg per glass of cola. Caffeine is found in over-the counter (OTC) stimulants such as No Doz and Caffedrine, which contain 100 and 250 mg respectively.[10] Caffeine is also commonly found in OTC analgesic products such as Anacin.

Caffeine has been identified in many street drugs that are misrepresented as "speed." Toxicity may be expected at doses greater than 1 g, especially in children, and 5 to 10 g is a potentially lethal dose in adults.[9,12] A 3-g dose was fatal in a 5-year-old child.[13] Another source states that the lethal intravenous dose has been reported to be 3.2 g, whereas the oral lethal doses range from 18–50 g.[10]

Agents other than CNS stimulants of the amphetamine type also had to be considered in the patient presented. Anticholinergic agents produce both central and peripheral signs and symptoms similar to those exhibited by this patient.

Table 11–2.   Symptomatic Assessment of the Severity of Amphetamine Poisoning. (Reprinted, by permission of The New England Journal of Medicine, *278*:1361, 1968.)

SYMPTOMS	SEVERITY
Restlessness, irritability, insomnia Tremor, hyperreflexia Sweating, mydriasis, flushing	1+
Hyperactivity, confusion Hypertension, tachypnea, tachycardia, extrasystoles Fever (mild) Sweating, etc.	2+
Delirium, mania, self-injury Marked hypertension, tachycardia, arrhythmias Hyperpyrexia	3+
Above plus: Convulsions and coma Circulatory collapse and death	4+

Central toxic effects include agitation, delirium, hallucinations, and seizures. Acute brain syndrome and toxic psychosis also have been reported.[14-16] Peripheral toxicity includes tachycardia, hyperpyrexia, mydriasis, urinary retention, decreased GI motility, and decreased secretions.

Agents capable of producing the anticholinergic syndrome include antihistamines, antipsychotics, tricyclic antidepressants, antiparkinsonian agents, antispasmodics, and belladonna alkaloids.[17] Acute overdosage with tricyclic antidepressants is characterized by CNS stimulation, cardiovascular abnormalities, and atropine-like effects.[17-18] Patients initially demonstrate CNS stimulation such as agitation, delirium, hallucinations, and convulsions, followed by coma. Arrhythmias, especially sinus tachycardia, and conduction disturbances are commonly seen. Other manifestations include hypo- or hyperpyrexia, hypotension, myoclonus, and choreoathetosis.

Low doses of phencyclidine (PCP) may produce an acute confusional state characterized by agitation, combativeness, dysarthria, disorientation, and fearfulness.[19,20] Because symptoms often closely resemble those of an acute schizophrenic episode, this is a common misdiagnosis. Phencyclidine-induced psychosis may take weeks to resolve. Other clinical findings vary depending on the dose ingested, and may include ataxia, muscle rigidity, blank stare appearance, nystagmus, diaphoresis, hypersalivation, flushing, fever, hypertension, repetitive motor movements, myoclonus, coma, and convulsions.

Lysergic acid diethylamide (LSD) produces changes in perception, thought, mood, and activity.[21] Visual, auditory, and tactile hallucinations occur, and orientation is fragmented. A person experiencing a "bad trip" may have feelings of loneliness, anxiety, fear, and panic, as well as notions of persecution. Suicidal and prolonged psychotic states have been induced. Clinical findings include mydriasis, hypertension, tachycardia, hyperactive reflexes, and tremor. The effects, both psychic and physiologic, of other hallucinogens, such as MDA, DMT, DOM (STP), and mescaline, closely resemble those of LSD.

Cocaine produces a condition of hyperstimulation characterized by overalertness, euphoria, and feelings of great power.[22,23] An unpleasant tension associated with paranoid thinking may occur. Hallucinations, delusions, and violent behavior have also been reported frequently. Physiologic symptoms include arrhythmias, dilation of pupils, tremors, convulsions, and delirium. With high doses, CNS stimulation is followed by CNS depression, with death resulting from either cardiovascular collapse or respiratory failure. Cocaine has been reported to produce a syndrome of paranoid psychosis with chronic high dose administration, which may be diagnostically difficult to distinguish from paranoid schizophrenia.[24] For further discussion of cocaine, see Chapter 12.

Patients undergoing withdrawal from alcohol, barbiturates, and other sedative-hypnotics may also exhibit signs of CNS stimulation, as well as some of the physiologic effects demonstrated by this patient. A more complete history of prior drug use may help to rule out this possibility. Although alcohols, barbiturates, and sedative-hypnotics are not found in prescripton diet pills, histories are often unreliable and therefore cannot be the sole basis for the ruling out of suspected agents.

LABORATORY DATA HELPFUL IN EVALUATION

A general toxicology screen of the blood and urine may help rule out some of the agents discussed in the previous section. Of the drugs being considered, the following may be screened for, depending on the laboratory: amphetamines, cocaine, tricyclic antidepressants, caffeine, some anticholinergic drugs (e.g., chlorpheniramine, diphenhydramine, and phenothiazines), and phencyclidine.

In the present case, urine and blood samples were sent for a toxicology screen, and the urine sample results were positive for amphetamines. Quantitative analysis was not performed. Treatment decisions in patients who have ingested amphetamines are little influenced by quantitative levels. The treatment is primarily determined by the clinical status of the patient. Identification of amphetamines obviously is needed to confirm the clinical impression and allows one to consider the possibility of acid diuresis in severe ingestions.

Blood amphetamine is difficult to quantitate unless large amounts are present.[25] Several well-documented fatalities have occurred in patients with amphetamine blood levels as low as 40 μg/dl.[26] Therapeutic blood levels of amphetamine are in the range of 5 to 10 μg/dl.[25] Blood levels of fenfluramine, 2800 μg/dl,[8] and phenmetrazine, 400 μg/dl,[27] have also been measured in fatal cases. In many areas, quantitative blood amphetamine levels are not readily available, and it is customary to perform urine screening for amphetamine. Also, amphetamine levels can be determined quantitatively in urine samples as well.

MANIFESTATIONS AND MECHANISMS OF CNS-STIMULANT OVERDOSE

Central Nervous System Effects

The agitation and combativeness seen in the patient presented were most likely effects of amphetamines to produce CNS stimulation. One commonly sees a spectrum of symptoms that, depending on the dose ingested, may range from restlessness, irritability, and insomnia to hyperactivity, confusion, and convulsions.[25,28] A severity rating scale has been developed by Espelin and Done (Table 11–2).[27]

Four theories have been proposed to explain the mechanism of action of amphetamines: (1) direct effect (mimicking of the effect of catecholamines at the receptor site), (2) inhibition of monoamine oxidase (MAO), (3) impairment of catecholamine reuptake, and (4) direct release of catecholamines into the synaptic cleft. Currently, the theories most widely accepted are direct synaptic release of catecholamines and inhibition of reuptake, both of which would increase the amount of catecholamines available for receptor stimulation.[29]

It has been shown that *d*-amphetamine (dextroamphetamine) is 10 times more potent in inhibiting reuptake of norepinephrine than *l*-amphetamine (levamphetamine). Interestingly, *d*- and *l*-amphetamine are equipotent in inhibiting reuptake by dopamine neurons.[29]

Locomotor activity is thought to mirror the central stimulation seen in man. Since *d*-amphetamine is 10 times more potent than *l*-amphetamine in enhancing locomotor activity in rats, it is felt that this effect, and perhaps central stimulation in man, might involve brain norepinephrine.[29]

Stereotypic behavior (e.g., purposeless searching and grooming) is commonly reported in animals following amphetamine administration, and similar activity is seen in human amphetamine abusers. Since *d*-amphetamine is only twice as potent as *l*-amphetamine in eliciting stereotypic behavior, it is felt that dopamine is the catecholamine of major importance. Since the activity of the isomers is not equivalent, norepinephrine may play some role.[29–31]

In humans, it appears that the central stimulatory properties involve the reticular activating system and the medial forebrain bundle, or the reward system.[32,33]

Stimulation of the latter produces pleasurable feelings; thus, this may account for the euphoria reported, as well as for the abuse potential.

Amphetamine psychosis most frequently is seen following chronic abuse and develops gradually.[34] Psychosis has been reported following a single acute dose when the patient previously had experienced an amphetamine psychosis.[35] Acute single large doses also can produce a hallucinatory paranoid panic state, as was described in this patient.[34] Hallucinations are usually visual in patients who become acutely psychotic after a single large dose, whereas auditory hallucinations are more common in patients whose psychoses develop gradually with frequent dosage.[29] Tactile hallucinations, as seen in this patient, have also been described in amphetamine psychosis.

Symptoms of amphetamine psychosis were described by Bell in his report of 14 patients admitted to psychiatric units because of psychoses that developed during amphetamine intoxications.[30] Within this group, hallucinations were present in 13 of the 14 patients. All 13 had auditory hallucinations, and 5 had visual hallucinations. Delusions of persecution were present in all patients and delusions of influence in 5. Disturbances of affect were common, as were euphoria and depression. Of the 14 patients, 3 developed schizophrenia, and their psychotic symptoms continued for many months following discontinuation of amphetamine exposure. In general, psychotic symptoms tend to begin to dissipate within 2 to 3 days after amphetamine is stopped, and usually symptoms are gone totally within 10 days.[34] Some feel that an extended psychosis is seen in those patients who are "prepsychotic," "psychosis prone," or "vulnerable" individuals.[2] Compulsive behavior may occur, and is considered to be a human manifestation of stereotypic behavior in animals.[36]

Griffith studied amphetamine psychosis in a group of volunteers who were heavy amphetamine users.[37] Each subject was of normal intelligence, had not experienced an amphetamine psychosis previously, was not schizophrenic, and did not have schizophrenic tendencies. Each subject received orally 10 mg/hr of *d*-amphetamine sulfate night and day. Psychosis was noted in each subject between 2 and 5 days following a dose of 120 to 700 mg of the drug. In this group, the psychosis dissipated within 8 hours in three subjects and continued for 3 days in the remaining subject.

Amphetamine-induced psychosis is due to an excess of dopamine at specific receptor sites in the CNS. Therefore, dopamine antagonists such as chlorpromazine and haloperidol are effective in reversing amphetamine psychosis.[29,38] Doses commonly employed are 25 to 30 mg of chlorpromazine given IM or orally, or 5 mg of haloperidol given IM or orally. Improvement may be noted in 1 hour: however, complete resolution of psychosis may require 7 to 10 days.

Temperature

Hyperthermia is commonly encountered in significant amphetamine ingestions. In the case reported, rectal temperature was 40°C (104°F). Temperatures as high as 43°C (109.4°F) have been reported in human ingestions. Although there has been some question whether hyperpyrexia is a peripheral or a central effect, recent evidence presented by Bareggi and associates suggests that it is a peripheral effect.[30] In mice, hypothermia is produced following intraventricular administration of amphetamine, whereas hyperthermia is seen when amphetamine is administered peripherally. Stimulation of central dopaminergic neurons may produce hypothermia, whereas stimulation of the peripheral norepinephrine system may produce hyperthermia.

Temperature and plasma amphetamine levels follow a similar time course, both peaking at approximately 1½ hours post-ingestion and declining in a similar fashion. Askew has shown that in animals given amphetamines experimentally, those with temperatures lower than 41.7°C usually survived, whereas those with temperatures higher than 42.4°C usually died.[40] In those cases that end fatally, hyperpyrexia is commonly reported. Those patients with temperatures above 40°C have poor prognoses.[25]

Respiratory Rate

Hyperpnea is commonly seen in acute amphetamine ingestions. In the case reported, the respiratory rate was 24/min. Although in man, therapeutic doses of amphetamine do not affect respiratory rate, large doses produce stimulation of the respiratory center and thus increase the respiratory rate.[33]

Pupil Reaction

This patient's pupils were widely dilated and sluggishly reactive to light. Pupillary response is secondary to alpha-adrenergic stimulation of the radial muscle of the iris, producing mydriasis.

Cardiovascular Effects

Acute hypertension and tachycardia are observed. Both alpha- and beta-adrenergic effects are seen, including an increase in diastolic and systolic blood pressure,[33] as in the case reported. Other sympathomimetic effects commonly seen include flushing and diaphoresis.

INDICATED THERAPEUTIC MEASURES

The first step in the management of an amphetamine overdose is to evaluate the patient clinically and to assess the severity of the intoxication. Initial therapy must be aimed at the treatment and prevention of life-threatening symptoms. Once the patient is stable, attention can be turned to minimization of absorption of the amphetamine from the GI tract and elimination of the drug from the body. Subsequent therapy mainly consists of supportive and symptomatic care.

Correction of Life-Threatening Symptoms

The major life-threatening complications of acute amphetamine intoxication include convulsions, hyperthermia, hypertension, and cardiovascular collapse. Therefore, initial treatment of these patients should be aimed at assessment of these complications and controlling of those that might develop. In the case presented, the patient was agitated and combative, as well as hyperthermic and mildly hypertensive. Since these symptoms were potentially life threatening, treatment was instituted immediately.

Agitation and combativeness are signs of CNS stimulation, which may precede the onset of convulsions. Phenothiazines are generally recommended to antagonize the CNS effects of amphetamines. Espelin and Done found adequate sedation and uniform termination of both CNS excitation and sympathomimetic effects of amphetamines following administration of chlorpromazine. Within a few minutes of intramuscular administration of chlorpromazine, the CNS effects subsided, whereas sympathomimetic effects such as hypertension responded more slowly, requiring 2 to 3 hours to subside. In contrast, patients were found to respond poorly to barbiturates, even when large doses were given parenterally.[28]

Espelin and Done recommend 1 mg/kg of chlorpromazine in a pure amphetamine overdose, based on their experience. This dose causes adequate reversal of symptoms in most patients, without producing serious depression. The dose may be repeated every 30 minutes as needed. In patients who have ingested a combination of an amphetamine and sedative, 0.5 mg/kg of chlorpromazine is recommended in order to avoid excessive CNS depression.

Butyrophenones such as haloperidol and droperidol also have been used successfully in the management of amphetamine overdose. In one case, a patient who had been intoxicated with methamphetamine became quiescent and indifferent to environmental stimuli, with minimal hypnotic effect, within 10 minutes of an intravenous administration of droperidol.[41] Gary and Saidi feel that butyrophenones have an advantage over chlorpromazine in that they cause less respiratory depression and produce a less sustained hypotension and reflex tachycardia.[41]

Animal studies have demonstrated that chlorpromazine and haloperidol are capable of protecting against the lethal effects of amphetamines. One study in rats demonstrated a high degree of benefit against lethality of *d*-amphetamine when haloperidol was given 15 minutes after the amphetamine. A dose of 0.5 to 1.0 mg/kg of haloperidol was found to be equivalent to 10 to 15 mg/kg of chlorpromazine in protection against lethality. As association between the antidotal effects and the hyperthermia-blocking action was suggested.[42] In amphetamine-intoxicated dogs, haloperidol blocked the hyperthermia induced by amphetamine, as well as the cardiovascular and metabolic effects.[43] This was felt to be consistent with the antidopaminergic activity of haloperidol.

Lemberger and co-workers found that, in rats, haloperidol would be superior to chlorpromazine in the treatment of amphetamine toxicity.[44] Chlorpromazine increased the half-life of ^{3}H-amphetamine in the rat brain and in the whole animal, slowing the disappearance of ^{3}H-amphetamine from the rat brain. In contrast, haloperidol did not produce these effects. Both drugs were effective in blocking amphetamine-induced stereotypic behavior. However, these findings cannot be extrapolated to man because of differences in the metabolic fate of amphetamine in man and rat.

Diazepam has also been used successfully in the treatment of agitation and other signs of CNS stimulation following amphetamine overdose.[45] Since chlorpromazine and haloperidol lower the seizure threshold and thereby may predispose the patient to seizures, diazepam may have an advantage over these agents. However, chlorpromazine and haloperidol are direct antagonists of amphetamine effects and therefore may be beneficial in the treatment of other manifestations of amphetamine poisoning, such as hypertension and hyperthermia.

On the basis of these studies of the effects of phenothiazines, butyrophenones, and diazepam on amphetamine-induced CNS toxicity, the following recommentations can be made. In a mildly symptomatic patient (severity rating = 1+) (Table 11–2), diazepam should be administered initially, either orally or IV, at a dose of 10 mg in an adult or 0.1 to 0.3 mg/kg in a child. In a more severely poisoned patient (severity rating = 2+ to 3+) or in one who did not respond to diazepam initially, chlorpromazine or haloperidol should be administered orally or IM, and the patient should be monitored closely for precipitation of seizures. In a pure amphetamine overdose in children, 1 mg/kg of chlorpromazine should be administered, whereas the usual dose in adults is 25 to 50 mg. The adult dose of haloperidol is 2.5 to 5 mg. In a combined amphetamine-sedative overdose, the initial dose of these drugs should be halved. In the present case, chlorpromazine (50 mg) was administered IM. Within 1 hour after administration, the patient appeared calm and was no longer combative or agitated.

Hyperthermia, which was present in this patient, is frequently associated with amphetamine overdoses. In both animals and humans, hyperthermia appears to be closely linked with morbidity and lethality of an amphetamine intoxication. Since the hyperthermic response is related to metabolism in hyperactive skeletal muscle, factors that increase body metabolism will increase amphetamine toxicity, whereas those that decrease body metabolism will decrease amphetamine toxicity.[46]

In animals, curarization has been found to prevent hyperthermia. Environmental temperature and physical exertion may greatly potentiate the rise in temperature induced by amphetamines. Since convulsions often are associated with a hyperthermic condition, hyperthermia must be treated vigorously, especially if the temperature exceeds 39°C (102°F).[34]

The following measures should be undertaken to lower the body temperature. The patient should be placed in a cool room. Physical activity should be minimized. Administration of a tranquilizer may be necessary to decrease combativeness and the associated increased physical activity. A hypothermic blanket should be used to return body temperature to normal.

Chlorpromazine may be required to control shivering. Body temperature should be monitored every 15 minutes until it is stabilized at a temperature below 39°C (102°F), at which time it may be monitored at longer intervals. In the present case, the patient was placed in a cool air-conditioned room, and a hypothermic blanket was used to reduce his temperature. Within 1½ hours, his temperature decreased to 38°C (100.4°F).

Hypertension is another common complication of amphetamine poisoning, and may require immediate therapy to decrease the blood pressure in order to prevent other sequelae, such as subarachnoid hemorrhage. In some cases, chlorpromazine alone may be sufficient to lower the blood pressure to an acceptable level. However, if hypertension is severe, an alpha blocking agent such as phenoxybenzamine or phentolamine may be indicated.[25] In hypertensive emergencies, sodium nitroprusside or diazoxide should be considered.

In the present case, the patient's blood pressure decreased to 140/85 2 hours after administration of chlorpromazine (50 mg IM) for agitation. It was not necessary to administer other drugs to lower the blood pressure.

Prevention of Further Absorption

One of the first steps in the definitive treatment of an amphetamine overdose is to minimize absorption of drug from the GI tract. Procedures that should be considered are emesis or lavage, activated charcoal, and a saline cathartic. In the determination of which of these procedures is indicated, the following parameters must be evaluated: symptoms, dose of amphetamine, time since ingestion, and dosage form.

Symptoms. The first consideration is the clinical condition of the patient. Emesis and lavage cannot be performed in a patient who is undergoing seizures. Since amphetamines lower the seizure threshold to various stimuli, some sources recommend that emesis be performed rather than lavage.[47] However, both procedures may be sufficient stimuli to precipitate seizures. Medications used to treat agitation and seizures may cause CNS depression, in which case emesis is contraindicated. Phenothiazines have antiemetic properties and may therefore represent a relative contraindication to the use of an emetic. However, several studies have shown that most patients will vomit in spite of the prior administration or ingestion of a phenothiazine.[48,49]

On the basis of these considerations, the following general recommendations can be made. Evacuation of the stomach contents should be performed if the ingestion has occurred within the past 4 hours. If the patient is alert, syrup of ipecac should be administered. If the patient is lethargic or comatose, lavage should be performed following intubation with a cuffed endotracheal tube. If the ingestion has occurred more than 4 hours ago and the product ingested is a slow-release preparation, activated charcoal and a saline cathartic should be administered; however, at this point, emesis or lavage will probably not be beneficial. Since fecal excretion of amphetamines is minimal and amphetamines would not be expected to be excreted in the bile,[50,51] repeated administration of activated charcoal and cathartics is not expected to be of any additional benefit.

In the case presented, following the administration of chlorpromazine to diminish agitation and combativeness, the patient was given 15 ml of syrup of ipecac followed by 12 oz of water. He vomited approximately 20 minutes later. No tablets or capsules were noted in the vomitus. Activated charcoal, 60 g in a water slurry, was administered orally, followed by 250 mg/kg of magnesium sulfate. The activated charcoal was administered to adsorb amphetamine remaining in the GI tract after emesis, and the saline cathartics were administered to facilitate the removal of the charcoal-amphetamine mass by hastening intestinal transit. The patient had a charcoal stool 3½ hours later, indicating that the charcoal-drug complex had passed through the GI tract.

Dose. It is difficult to determine the toxic dose of an amphetamine, since there is a wide range of individual susceptibility to these drugs, and tolerance to large doses can develop with chronic abuse. Another problem in the assessment of the potential for toxicity is the unreliability of historical information. The lethal dose of *d*-amphetamine in animals varies from 10 to 85 mg/kg.[52] In adults, the acute lethal dose has been reported as 20 to 25 mg/kg, whereas in children, the low dose of 5 mg/kg is often quoted as toxic and potentially fatal.[39,52] Adding to the confusion is a case report of death in a 23-year-old male following ingestion of 1.5 mg/kg of methamphetamine.[39] In view of the wide range of potentially toxic doses, any overdose should be treated vigorously and

aggressively with measures to prevent further absorption of the amphetamine, until sufficient time has elapsed to evaluate the development of symptoms.

Time. The time since ingestion is important in the assessment of whether or not any drug would be expected to remain in the GI tract. After oral administration, amphetamines are rapidly absorbed from the GI tract, as evidenced by the rapid onset of symptoms. CNS effects usually appear within 30 minutes to 1 hour after ingestion.[41,50]

It has been demonstrated that amphetamines increase gastric emptying time,[53] and decrease the propulsive motility of the small intestine via a peripheral mechanism.[54] Although gastric emptying time may be delayed by as much as 40%, this results in an increase of less than 1 hour, with gastric emptying occurring at 2¾ hours after ingestion of a therapeutic dose, compared with the 2 hours required for complete gastric emptying without amphetamine. Therefore, for emesis or lavage to be effective, it should be performed as soon as possible after the ingestion and probably will not be of value after 4 hours postingestion.

Dosage Forms. Drugs intended for oral administration are available in a variety of forms, including tablets, capsules, and liquids. Currently there is a large number of amphetamine products on the market in the form of elixirs, solutions, tablets, and capsules, as well as resin complex capsules (e.g., Biphetamine) and partly sustained-release capsules (e.g., Dexamyl Spansules). Amphetamines may also be found in combination with other centrally acting drugs. Both of these factors are important in the determination of the symptoms and their time of onset, as well as how long procedures designed to minimize GI absorption, will be beneficial. Studies of the rate of absorption of soluble amphetamine salts compared with resin complexes have demonstrated that absorption is significantly slower following ingestion of the resinate.[55] With this in mind, one would expect the onset of symptoms to be delayed with the resinate or with a sustained-release capsule and would expect significant benefit to be derived from administration of activated charcoal and a cathartic for as long as 10 to 12 hours after ingestion of a slow-release product.

Facilitation of Removal of Absorbed Amphetamines

Amphetamines are widely distributed in the body. In contrast to catecholamines, which cross the blood-brain barrier with difficulty, amphetamines readily enter the brain and are found there in high concentrations.[33,50] Only a small percentage of the ingested dose is found in the plasma,[41] and the volume of distribution is three to five times the total body volume.[41,55] Amphetamines are detoxified by the liver, and the metabolites and unchanged drug are excreted renally. Highly polar compounds such as ephedrine are principally excreted unchanged.[51] As the lipid solubility of the compound increases, the amount of drug eliminated unchanged drops. Amphetamines are metabolized by several pathways, with deamination predominating in man. Deamination of amphetamine is followed by oxidation, resulting in the formation of hippuric acid, which is excreted renally.[56]

Other factors that affect the proportion of the dose excreted unchanged, besides lipid solubility, include urine volume and urine pH. Gunne and Anggard investigated the effect of urine volume on renal clearance of amphetamines.[57] In the pH range of 5.2 to 6.0, at a low urine output (less than 30 ml/hr), the clearance of amphetamine was about half that observed during conditions of average urine production (30 to 125 ml/hr). During water diuresis (greater than 125 ml/hr), the clearance of amphetamine was further increased. From these findings, it is evident that forced diuresis can be employed to increase the excretion of amphetamines

through an increase in urine volume and urine flow in the renal tubules, and thus a decrease in reabsorption.

The rate of excretion of amphetamine is pH dependent, since it is a weak base with a pKa of 9.93. As urine pH increases, the ratio of nonionized to ionized drug in the intraluminal fluid of the tubules increases relative to that in the plasma, which results in an increase in drug reabsorption and a reduced excretion rate.[58] Conversely, as urine pH decreases, the ratio of nonionized to ionized drug in the tubules decreases, which results in a decrease in drug reabsorption and an enhanced excretion rate.

Many studies in animals and man demonstrate the effect of acidification of the urine on amphetamine clearance. Beckett and co-workers found that at a urine pH of 5, 54.5% of the dose of d-amphetamine was excreted over a 16-hour period, compared with 2.9% at a pH of 8.[58] Davis and associates administered amphetamine to four healthy adults to examine the effect of urinary pH on the rate of disappearance of amphetamine from plasma and on the metabolic fate of this drug.[56] Under conditions of acid urine production (pH 5.5 to 6.0), 70% of the administered dose was excreted in the first 24 hours, with a half-life of 8 to 10.5 hours. Excretion of unchanged amphetamine was approximately four times as great as excretion of deaminated metabolites. Under alkaline urine conditions (pH 7.5 to 8.0), 45% of the administered dose was excreted in the first 24 hours, with a half-life of 16 to 31 hours. Excretion of the deaminated metabolites was almost equal to that of unchanged amphetamine. Therefore, when urine pH is acidic, amphetamine is largely excreted unchanged by the kidney, whereas under alkaline conditions, amphetamine is metabolized to a greater extent. The longer amphetamine remains in the blood, the more it is metabolized.

Similarly, Anggard et al found a half-life of 7 to 14 hours and rapid clearing of psychotic symptoms with acidic urine, compared with a half-life of 18 to 34 hours under alkaline urine conditions.[59] Gunne and Anggard found that for every unit increase in urinary pH, there was an increase in plasma half-life of approximately 7 hours.[57] Thus at a urinary pH of 5.0, the half-life was 5 hours, compared with 21 hours at a urine pH of 7.3.

On the basis of these studies, forced acidic diuresis is indicated in amphetamine overdose to enhance the renal elimination of amphetamine, thereby shortening the half-life of the drug in the body and the duration of clinical effects. Forced diuresis cannot be performed in a patient with impaired renal function and should not be initiated until an adequate urine flow has been established.

Forced fluid administration can also be hazardous in the face of an elevated blood pressure; this parameter must be measured and brought under control before this procedure is initiated. Fluids are administered intravenously, along with a diuretic such as mannitol or furosemide. The goal is a urine flow of 3 to 6 ml/kg/hr in children and 2 to 4 ml/kg/hr in adults. The urine is acidified with ammonium chloride or ascorbic acid, administered either orally or intravenously. The goal is a urine pH of 5.5 or lower.

In the case presented, furosemide in a dose of 40 mg was administered intravenously and 5% dextrose in normal saline solution was infused at the rate of 350 ml/hr. Ascorbic acid, 1 g every 6 hours administered orally, resulted in a urine pH of 5.5. Urine pH initially was monitored every 2 hours.

In an attempt to further increase the rate of removal of amphetamines from the body, peritoneal dialysis or hemodialysis may be employed. These measures are indicated following a significant ingestion in which the patient does not improve with more conservative means of therapy, such as forced acidic diuresis.

There are several case reports that illustrate the effectiveness of dialysis. Zalis and Parmley removed 24.8 mg of amphetamine sulfate with 3½ hours of peritoneal dialysis.[39] However, their patient did not survive, as dialysis was not initiated until 5 days postingestion. They recommmend that dialysis be utilized early in the treatment of acute amphetamine poisoning associated with severe systemic manifestations, and particularly in the presence of renal or hepatic damage. Wallace and co-workers successfully dialyzed a 1 year-old child, removing 66.66 mg of methamphetamine in 17 exhanges, totaling approximately 8 L of dialysate.[60] Five hours into the procedure, the child began to improve clinically.

Hemoperfusion, a relatively new procedure available for removal of poisons from the body, has not been employed in amphetamine overdoses. Further investigation into this form of therapy is needed.

In the management of a patient who has been intoxicated with an amphetamine, the recommended treatment of choice is forced acidic diuresis and intensive supportive therapy. However, dialysis should be instituted in the case of a severely poisoned patient who does not respond with forced acidic diuresis and whose condition is deteriorating, or a severely poisoned patient with renal damage. Hemodialysis is more efficient than peritoneal dialysis, requiring significantly less time to remove a given quantity of the dialyzable substance.[60,61] However, it is less readily available than peritoneal dialysis. On the other hand, peritoneal dialysis is relatively safe and usually can be instituted more rapidly than hemodialysis. It is available in any hospital, since highly specialized equipment is unnecessary, and medical personnel are readily trained in the technique. The choice will depend on the age of the patient and the availability of equipment and personnel. The patient presented in this case did not require either of these procedures.

Symptomatic and Supportive Care

Following correction of life-threatening symptoms and institution of measures to minimize absorption and enhance elimination, supportive therapy is essential. The patient should be placed in a quiet, cool, and darkened room. Since the stimulatory effects of amphetamines are aggravated by external stimuli, the patient should be kept as undisturbed as possible, and manipulations should be kept at a minimum.

Measures should be instituted to protect the patient from self-injury, such as restraints or padded bed rails. Seizure precautions should be maintained, with a padded tongue blade and diazepam easily accessible. Vital signs should be monitored frequently, the interval depending on the severity of the intoxication. Equipment for intubation and resuscitation should be available. Close observation of fluid balance is essential.

POSSIBLE COMPLICATIONS

Cardiovascular System

Peripherally, amphetamines produce their effects via indirect adrenergic stimulation. Both alpha and beta effects are seen. As mentioned previously, tachycardia and hypertension are produced. Amphetamines may also produce arrhythmias. A tachyarrhythmia of 150/min has been reported in a 14-year-old female following a large acute dose of diethylpropion.[62] The EKG revealed wide and varying QRS complexes with indefinite P-waves. The patient responded to propranolol but not to carotid massage.

In a case reported by Veltri and Temple, a 17-year-old died 3 hours after a fenfluramine ingestion.[8] Terminal events included convulsions, cardiac arrhythmia, and a cardiopulmonary arrest. Sinus tachycardia may deteriorate to a ventricular flutter,[62] or fibrillation. In a review of reported fatalities, Kalant and Kalant state that in six cases, electrocardiographic, pathologic or circumstantial evidence suggests ventricular fibrillation as the cause of death.[63]

Tachyarrhythmias may be treated with propranolol, in intravenous doses of 1 to 2 mg. Other antiarrhythmics should be considered, depending on the response to propranolol or the type of arrhythmia present.

Hypotension and circulatory collapse have been reported.[25,33,39,64] These effects commonly occur late in the course and in severe ingestions.[50] Hypotension should be treated with fluid administration and by placement of the patient in the Trendelenberg position. Vasopressors may be used if these measures are insufficient.

Significant complications secondary to hypertension have been reported. Cerebral hemorrhage was seen in a long-term amphetamine abuser.[65] Margolis and Newton reported several young amphetamine abusers with angiographic evidence of intracerebral hematomas and multiple infarctions.[66] Zalis and Pauley report a fatal ingestion of oral methamphetamine that showed diffuse petechial hemorrhages, cerebral edema, tubular degenerations, and centrilobular hepatic necrosis at autopsy.[39] Similar effects have been reported by others.[64,65]

Central Nervous System

Convulsions are frequently seen in severe intoxications and are part of a continuum of CNS-stimulatory effects beginning with restlessness and hyperactivity.[28] Convulsions are frequently associated with hyperpyrexia.[34] CNS depression, including coma, may follow the stimulatory phase, making treatment of the CNS stimulation with sedatives somewhat difficult, particularly if a combination amphetamine-sedative product has been ingested.

If the patient is convulsing, he should be protected from injury and a clear airway ensured. A soft object should be placed between the teeth to protect the tongue. Intravenous diazepam should be administered to control seizures, at a dose of 10 mg in an adult and 0.1 to 0.3 mg/kg in a child. If the seizure is refractory to diazepam, phenobarbital should be given intravenously. If a coma is present, an adequate airway should be maintained and respirations supported. The patient should be intubated with a cuffed endotracheal tube.

Depression may be seen in amphetamine abusers. This is particularly true in patients who chronically take large doses. During a ''speed run,'' amphetamines are injected as often as every 2 hours for periods of up to 12 days, during which time the individual is continuously awake.[35] Following the ''speed run,'' the patient sleeps. The length of sleep is related to the length of the run and may last as long as 5 days.[35] Upon awakening, patients may continue to be lethargic and depressed. It is at this point that another speed run may be begun. Medical therapy for this depression is usually not necessary.

ENDPOINTS OF THERAPY

Successful management of an amphetamine overdose requires close attention to the following areas: (1) Control of seizures, severe agitation, and behavioral changes, (2) management of hypertension and arrhythmias, (3) lowering of fever, (4) minimization of drug absorption, and (5) enhancement of drug elimination from the body.

PROGNOSIS

The prognosis for an amphetamine ingestion is difficult to predict on the basis of the dose ingested because of the large range of reported toxic and lethal doses. Although the course of an intoxication varies from one individual to the next, severe hyperthermia appears to be a factor associated with a poor prognosis. Temperatures greater than 40°C must be treated aggressively in order to minimize the morbidity and mortality rates of amphetamine intoxication. As is true with other intoxications, factors such as cardiovascular collapse and cardiorespiratory arrest indicate an unfavorable course.

REFERENCES

1. Shulgin AT: Abuse of the term amphetamines. *Clin Toxicol, 9*:351–352, 1976.
2. Schick JFE, Smith DE, and Wesson DR: An analysis of amphetamine toxicity and patterns of use. *J Psychedelic Drugs, 5*:113, 1972.
3. Edison GR: Amphetamine: A dangerous illusion. *Ann Intern Med, 74*:605–610, 1971.
4. Personal Communication, Drug Enforcement Administration.
5. *Natl Inst Drug Abuse Capsule,* March 17, 1978.
6. Franz DN: Central nervous system stimulants. In *The Pharmacological Basis of Therapeutics.* 5th Ed. Edited by LS Goodman and A Gilman. New York, Macmillan, 1975, pp. 359–366.
7. Huff BB (ed): *Physicians' Desk Reference.* 32nd Ed. Oradell, New Jersey, Medical Economics Co., 1978, pp. 1365–1366.
8. Veltri JC, and Temple AR: Fenfluramine poisoning. *J Pediatr, 87*:119–121, 1975.
9. Ritchie JM: Central nervous system stimulants (cont). In *The Pharmacological Basis for Therapeutics.* 5th Ed. Edited by LS Goodman and A Gilman. New York, Macmillan, 1975, pp. 367–368.
10. Walker CA: Stimulant products. In *Handbook of Nonprescription Drugs.* 5th Ed. Washington, D.C., American Pharmaceutical Association, 1975, pp. 191–193.
11. Van Tyle WK: Internal analgesic products. In *Handbook of Nonprescription Drugs.* 5th Ed. Washington, D.C., American Pharmaceutical Association, 1975. pp. 121–123.
12. Rumack BH (ed): Caffeine management. *Poisindex.* Denver, Colorado, Micromedex, Inc., May 1979.
13. Reilly MJ (ed): Respiratory and cerebral stimulants. In *American Hospital Formulary Service.* Washington, D.C., American Society of Hospital Pharmacists, 28:20, 1978.
14. Granacher RP, Baldessarini RJ, and Messner E: Physostigmine treatment of delirium induced by anticholinergics. *Am Fam Physician, 13(5)*:99–103, 1976.
15. Muller DJ: Unpublicized hallucinogens: The dangerous belladonna alkaloids. *JAMA, 202*:650–651, 1967.
16. Baile WF, DePaulo JR, and Schmitz CW: Emergency room management of organic brain syndrome caused by over-the-counter hypnotics. *Md State Med J, 26*:61–63, 1977.

17. Skoutakis VA: Management of acute tricyclic antidepressant poisonings. *Clin Toxicol Consultant*, 1:15–23, 1979.

18. Burks JS, et al: Tricyclic antidepressant poisoning. *JAMA, 230*:1405–1407, 1974.

19. Burns RS, and Lerner SE: Perspectives: Acute phencyclidine intoxication. *Clin Toxicol, 9*:477–501, 1976.

20. Aronow R, and Done AK: Phencyclidine overdose; An emerging concept of management. *JACEP, 7*:56–59, 1978.

21. Hofmann FG: Hallucinogens: LSD and other agents having similar effects. In *A Handbook on Drugs and Alcohol Abuse*. New York, Oxford University Press, 1975, pp. 223–243.

22. Cohen S: Cocaine, *JAMA, 231*:74–75, 1975.

23. Hofmann FG: Central nervous system stimulants. In *A Handbook on Drugs and Alcohol Abuse*. New York, Oxford University Press, 1975, pp. 223-243.

24. Post RM: Comparative psychopharmacology of cocaine and amphetamine. *Psychopharmacol Bull, 12(4)*:39–41, 1976.

25. Rumack BH (ed): Amphetamine management. *Poisindex*. Denver, Colorado, Micromedex, Inc., May, 1979.

26. Holmgren P, and Lindquist O: Lethal intoxication with centrally stimulating amines in Sweden 1966–1973. *Z Rechtsmedizin, 75*:265–279, 1975.

27. Norheim G: A fatal case of phenmetrazine poisoning. *J Forensic Sci Soc, 13*: 287–289, 1973.

28. Espelin DE, and Done AK: Amphetamine poisoning: Effectiveness of chlorpromazine. *N Engl J Med, 278*:1361–1365, 1968.

29. Snyder SH: Catecholamines in the brain as mediators of amphetamine psychosis. *Arch Gen Psychiatry, 27*:169–179, 1972.

30. Bareggi SP., Gonemi R, and Becker RE: Stereotyped behavior and hyperthermia in dogs: Correlation with the levels of amphetamine and p-hydroxyamphetamine in plasma and CSF. *Psychopharmacology, 58*:89-94, 1978.

31. Hart JB, and Wallace J: The adverse effects of amphetamines. *Clin Toxicol, 8*:179–190, 1975.

32. Executive Office of the President, Washington, D.C.: Amphetamines. *Natl Clgh Drug Abuse Inf, 28*:1, 1974.

33. Innes IR, and Nickerson M: Norepinephrine, epinephrine and the sympathomimetic amines. In *The Pharmacological Basis of Therapeutics*. 5th Ed. Edited by LS Goodman and A Gilman. New York, Macmillan, 1975, pp. 447–513.

34. Ellinwood EH: Treatment of reactions to amphetamine-type stimulants. *Curr Psychiatr Ther, 15*:163–169, 1975.

35. Kramer JC, Fischman VS, and Littlefield DC: Amphetamine abuse. *JAMA, 201*:305–309, 1967.

36. Kramer JC: Introduction to amphetamine abuse. *J Psychedelic Drugs, 2*:8–13, 1969.

37. Griffith JD, et al: Experimental psychosis induced by administration of *d*-amphetamine. In *Amphetamines and Related Compounds*. Edited by E Costa and S Gratini. New York, Raven Press, 1970, pp. 897–904.

38. Perry PJ, and Juhly RP: Amphetamine psychosis. *Am J Hosp Pharm, 34*:883–885, 1977.

39. Zalis EG, and Parmley LF: Fatal amphetamine poisoning. *Arch Intern Med, 112*:822–826, 1963.

40. Askew BM: Hyperpyrexia as a contributory factor in the toxicity of amphetamine to aggregated mice. *Br J Pharmacol, 19*:245–257, 1962.

41. Gary NE, and Saidi P: Methamphetamine intoxication: A speedy new treatment. *Am J Med, 64*:537–540, 1978.

42. David WM, Logston DG, and Hickenbottom JP: Antagonism of acute amphetamine intoxication by haloperidol and propranolol. *Toxicol Appl Pharmacol, 29*:387–403, 1974.

43. Catravas JD, et al: The effects of haloperidol, chlorpromazine and propranolol on acute amphetamine poisoning in the conscious dog. *J Pharmacol Exp Ther, 202*:230–243, 1977.

44. Lemberger L, et al: The effects of haloperidol and chlorpromazine on amphetamine metabolism and amphetamine stereotype behavior in the rat. *J Pharmacol Exp Ther, 174*:428–433, 1970.

45. Darmady JM: Diazepam for fenfluramine intoxication *Arch Dis Child, 49*:328–330, 1974.

46. Zalis EG, Lundberg GD, and Knutson RA: The pathophysiology of acute amphetamine poisoning with pathologic correlation. *J Pharmacol Exp Ther, 158*:115–127, 1967.

47. Simpson H, and McKinlay I: Poisoning with slow release fenfluramine. *Br Med J, 1*:462–463, 1975.

48. Thoman ME, and Verhulst HL: Ipecac syrup in antiemetic ingestion. *JAMA, 196*:433–435, 1966.

49. Manoguerra AS, and Krenzelok EP: Rapid emesis from high-dose ipecac syrup in adults and children intoxicated with antiemetics or other drugs. *Am J Hosp Pharm, 35*:1360–1362, 1978.

50. Cassarett MG: Social poison. In *Toxicology: The Basic Science of Poisons*. 1st Ed. Edited by LJ Cassarett and JD Doull. New York, Macmillan, 1975, pp. 627–654.

51. Caldwell J: The metabolism of amphetamines in mammals. *Drug Metab Rev, 5*:219–280, 1976.

52. Baldessarini RJ: Pharmacology of the amphetamines. *Pediatrics, 49*:694–701, 1972.

53. Northup DW, and Van Liere EJ: Effect of isomers of amphetamine and desoxyephedrine on gastric emptying in man. *J Pharmacol Exp Ther, 109*:358–360, 1953.

54. Van Liere EJ, Stickney JC, Northup DW, and Bell RO: Effect of dl-amphetamine sulfate and its isomers on intestinal motility. *J Pharmacol Exp Ther, 103*:187–189, 1951.

55. Hinsvark ON, et al: The oral bioavailability and pharmacokinetics of soluble and resin-bound forms of amphetamine and phentermine in man. *J Pharmacokinet Biopharm, 1*:319–328, 1973.

56. Davis JM, et al: Effects of urinary pH on amphetamine metabolism. *Ann NY Acad Sci, 179*:493–501, 1971.

57. Gunne LM, and Anggard E: Pharmacokinetic studies with amphetamines—relationship to neuropsychiatric disorders. *J Pharmacokinet Biopharm, 1*:481–495, 1973.

58. Beckett AH, Rowland M, and Tutner P: Influence of urinary pH on excretion of amphetamine. *Lancet*, 1:303, 1965.

59. Anggard E, et al: Amphetamine metabolism in amphetamine psychosis. *Clin Pharmacol Ther*, 14:870–880, 1973.

60. Wallace HE, Neumayer F, and Gutch CF: Amphetamine poisoning and peritoneal dialysis. *Am J Dis Child*, 108:657–661, 1964.

61. Simon NM, and Krumlovsky FA: The role of dialysis in the treatment of poisoning. *Ration Drug Ther*, 5:1–7, 1971.

62. Goldfinger P: Tachyarrhythmia induced by sympathomimetic drug overdose: A case treated with propranolol. *Milit Med, 139*:550–551, 1974.

63. Kalant H, and Kalant OJ: Death in amphetamine users: Causes and rates. *Can Med Assoc J*, 112:229–304, 1975.

64. Harvey JK, Todd CW, and Howard JW: Fatality associated with Benzadrine ingestion. *Del State Med J, 21*:111–115, 1949.

65. Dinnen A: Cerebral hemorrhage due to stimulants. *Med J Aust*, 2:101–102, 1971.

66. Margolis MT, and Newton TH: Methamphetamine ("speed") arteritis. *Neuroradiology*, 2:179–183, 1971.

Chapter 12

Cocaine

Gary M. Oderda
Wendy Klein-Schwartz

Cocaine, or benzoylmethylecgonine, is an alkaloid obtained from the leaves of Erythroxylon coca, a plant found in western South America, particularly in Bolivia and Peru. Although other erythroxylon species contain trace amounts of cocaine, Erythroxylon coca is the major source,[1] its leaves containing approximately 0.5% to 1% of this alkaloid (Fig. 12–1).

The use of coca leaves dates back to around the sixth century A.D. The reader is referred to several articles that review the history of cocaine use in detail.[2,3,4] Cocaine has remained popular throughout the ages, and beginning in the early 1970s, another upsurge in its popularity occurred.[5] From 1974 to 1979, cocaine-related injuries have tripled, as have cocaine-related deaths.[6,7]

In 1979, almost 817,000 kg of coca leaves were imported by Stepan Chemical Company, the sole legitimate importer of coca leaves in the United States.[7,8] From the imported coca leaves, pharmaceutical cocaine is extracted and sold to Merck, Inc. or exported to Europe. Merck is the primary distributor of cocaine, allocating the drug to Eli Lilly & Co., Mallinckrodt, Inc. and other distribution houses. It is believed that diversion of cocaine from legitimate sources is minimal. The "de-cocainized" resin extract is used to produce Coca-Cola.

Cocaine is also brought into this country illicitly from South America. Peru and Bolivia are the major cultivators of Erythroxylon coca; Colombia and, to a lesser extent, Ecuador are the focal points for refining and international trafficking of cocaine.[7,9,10] The Drug Enforcement Administration (DEA) estimates that in 1978, approximately 60 to 65 metric tons of

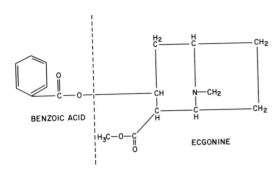

Fig. 12–1. Structure of cocaine.

cocaine were available for the worldwide market. Of this amount, approximately 19 to 25 metric tons were imported illicitly into the United States, with an estimated retail value of $12,350,000,000 to $16,250,000,000.[11] This compares to 19 to 23 metric tons in 1977 at an estimated retail value of $12,160,000,000 to $14,720,000,000, and 14 to 19 metric tons imported in 1976.[9,11]

Cocaine trafficking is less structured than heroin trafficking, and the routes of entry into the United States are broken down as follows: 45% by air, 30% by sea, and 25% overland through Mexico.[11] Cocaine enters the United States in the form of the hydrochloride salt and is relatively pure (80% to 95%).[1] Cocaine hydrochloride is obtained from coca leaves by a process involving extraction to form coca paste, which is converted to cocaine base and then prepared as the hydrochloride salt.[9] The cocaine is then divided many times and is often cut or "stepped on" with mannitol, lactose, glucose, cornstarch, and inositol.[1,7] Other common adulterants include lidocaine, procaine, tetracaine, caffeine, amphetamine, and quinine. Heroin may be added and the mixture sold as a "speedball."

Cocaine is known by a variety of slang names including Snow, Flake, Girl, Her, Lady, Blow, She, Jam, Happy Trails, Rock, Nose-Candy, Star-Spangled Powder, Dama Blanca, Rich Man's Drug, Pimp's Drug, Gold Dust, Bernice, C, and others.[4,12]

According to the DEA, the street-level purity of cocaine in 1979 averaged about 12% nationally.[7] However, there is probably significant variation in purity from one area of the country to the next. For example, in 1979 the purity of an ounce of cocaine in the Chicago area was estimated to be between 30% and 60%, whereas in California in 1976 it was an average of 53% to 63%.[13,14] The current price of an ounce of cocaine is $1200 to $1400, and 1 g sells for between $75 and $100.[15] Because it is so expensive, cocaine is considered the "champagne of drugs."[4] Enormous profits are obtained by almost all of the individuals involved in cocaine distribution.[7] The DEA estimates that the South American farmer sells 500 kilos of coca leaves for about $250. This is processed into 1 kg of cocaine hydrochloride, which when smuggled into the United States sells for $38,000 to $40,000. When cut down to an average of 12% purity, it sells for about $800,000. In contrast to these figures, pure wholesale of cocaine for medical use costs about $33.00 per ounce.[16]

According to the National Institute on Drug Abuse (NIDA), approximately 6,500,000 Americans used cocaine at least monthly in 1978.[11] The most common route of abuse is intranasal, or "snorting" of the drug. Cocaine is usually arranged into lines approximately ⅛ inch wide by 1 inch long, which is then inhaled into the nostrils with a straw or a large denomination bill.[12,14] One gram of cocaine produces 30 to 40 lines. Cocaine may be snorted from a "cokespoon" which holds about 5 to 10 mg of powder. The user inhales one "cokespoon" per nostril. The usual practice in one group of users was to snort cocaine on an average of three times per night at 15- to 30-minute intervals.[14] Some users will snort every 10 to 20 minutes.[12] When cocaine is snorted, the onset of action is usually reported as 5 to 10 minutes, and has a duration of 30 minutes to 1 hour.[5]

Another mode of administration is the intravenous route, for which the onset is immediate, producing an intense "rush".[5,12] Cocaine hydrochloride has also been mixed with marihuana or tobacco and smoked.[14,17] More recently, cocaine base, known as "free base," has become popular. This is an intermediate compound in the preparation of the hydrochloride salt from coca leaf extracts and is less susceptible to decomposition on heating than the hydrochloride salt. It can be reobtained from street cocaine via simple extraction kits available in paraphernalia shops. Users report greater effects from "free base" than with the hydrochloride salt.

Oral administration is not usually used to achieve a "high" with cocaine. Most cases of oral ingestion involve patients who swallow cocaine-condoms to smuggle the drug into the country,[15,18] or who swallow large amounts to avoid detection by police.[19] Occasionally, cocaine is used topically on the oral or genital mucosa, or is mixed with liquor to make a "liquid lady."[19]

Laws restricting cocaine availability in the United States date back to the early 1900s. Although some state legislation was passed prior to 1914, the Harrison Narcotics Act of 1914 was the first major federal legislation restricting the availability of cocaine and coca.[2] This law required registration with the Internal Revenue Service of those parties involved in importation, manufacture, distribution, or dispensing of opium, coca, or their derivatives, and that careful records of their transfers be kept. The Comprehensive Drug Abuse Prevention and Control Act of 1970 replaced the earlier legislation, and placed cocaine into Schedule II, which means that cocaine has an acceptable medical use but also a high potential for abuse. The only currently accepted medical use for cocaine is as a topical local anesthetic and vasoconstrictor for the nose, throat, larynx, and lower respiratory passages.[20,21]

Determination of fatal and toxic doses of cocaine is difficult, since this information is routinely obtained by history and in-volves the ingestion of street cocaine. The amount taken is only an estimate and the purity is unknown. Although chronic cocaine abusers have been reported to take up to 10 g per day,[22] 1200 mg is usually considered to be a fatal dose in adults, and severe toxic effects have been reported with as little as 20 mg.[4,23] In one instance a fatality was reported following the oral ingestion of 2 to 3 g,[24] whereas recovery was seen in a patient in whom a condom containing approximately 5 g of cocaine had ruptured in the stomach.[15] After examination of a group of 24 deaths from cocaine alone, it was felt that in all cases of death after oral ingestion, the amount swallowed or released into the gastrointestinal tract was 1 g or more.[19]

CASE REPORT

A 23-year-old male was brought to the emergency room by ambulance 3 hours after he had ingested cocaine orally to avoid arrest. His friends reported that 1½ hours after the ingestion, he became nervous and disoriented. He vomited several times and began shaking and trembling. At this point an ambulance was called. On examination, the paramedics described an extremely agitated man with a pulse of 150/min and a blood pressure of 180/100 mm Hg. En route to the emergency room, the patient had several tonic-clonic convulsions and was treated with diazepam and phenobarbital. On arrival in the ER, the patient was unconscious and unresponsive to painful stimuli. His respirations were shallow and in a Cheyne-Stokes pattern. Systolic blood pressure was 50 mm Hg, and pulse was 140/min and regular. Rectal temperature was 39°C. Physical examination revealed dilated pupils that were unreactive to light, dry mucous membranes, hyperemia of nasal vasculature, hypoactive reflexes, and peripheral cyanosis. Initial arterial blood gases were pH, 7.20; Po_2, 50 mm Hg; Pco_2, 34 mm Hg; and HCO_3^-, 16 mEq/L.

CLINICAL ASSESSMENT AND MANAGEMENT OF THE PATIENT

Initial evaluation of this patient's condition revealed several potentially life-threatening symptoms, which required immediate therapeutic intervention. Prompt assessment of the respiratory, cardiovascular, and CNS status, as well as institution of appropriate supportive measures to maintain adequate respirations, blood pressure, and to control the seizures, are critical for the survival of this patient. In proper assessment and treatment of this patient, the following must be considered: (1) manifestations and mechanisms of acute cocaine overdosage, (2) role of the toxicology laboratory in the evaluation of this patient, (3) indicated therapeutic measures, (4) effects seen with chronic cocaine abuse, and (5) prognosis.

MANIFESTATIONS AND MECHANISMS OF COCAINE OVERDOSAGE

There is a large number of reports on the pharmacologic effects of cocaine. Although some of the information on the effects of cocaine has been determined in studies under controlled conditions in man, much of the information is based on uncontrolled clinical observations, case reports, animal studies, street knowledge, and myths.[25] Therefore, many of the effects attributed to cocaine have not been confirmed in man. Ideally, an effect should be demonstrated in controlled experimental situations in a number of independent laboratories as well as consistently observed in nonlaboratory situations.[25] Byck and Van Dyke have categorized the reported effects of cocaine by the type and reliability of the evidence and the reader is referred to this excellent review of the subject.[25]

The toxicologic manifestations of cocaine intoxication are mainly observed in the CNS, autonomic nervous system, respiratory system, and cardiovascular system.

Central Nervous System Effects

Cocaine is a potent CNS stimulant and local anesthetic. The anesthetic effect is due to its blocking action on nerve conduction. The mechanism of the CNS-stimulant action is not known, but it is believed to be due either to the effect of cocaine on catecholamines or to a depression of the inhibitory pathways of the brain.[12,26] The stimulant effect is initially cortical, moving downward through the brain. With small doses, there is an increase in motor activity, and the effects are characterized by euphoria, excitement, restlessness, confusion, apprehension, anxiety, and delirium.[4,21,23] As the dose increases, CNS stimulation progresses from the cortex to the lower motor centers,[23] resulting in tremors and convulsive movements. The patient may also complain of dizziness, headaches, nausea, and vomiting. Twitching of small muscles such as those of the face and fingers may occur. The early stimulation is then followed by advanced stimulation, and is characterized by tonic-clonic convulsions and hyperreflexia.

In a retrospective analysis of cocaine-related deaths, it was noted that patients developed convulsions approximately 30 to 60 minutes after an oral cocaine ingestion, and within a few minutes to an hour after cocaine snorting.[19] In this series of patients, however, users who ingested the drug intravenously did not develop convulsions, and some investigators speculate that when the cocaine blood level rises rapidly, the stimulatory effects may be fleeting or may not even occur, and that the cardiovascular system effects predominate[19,21] Other investigators, however, have reported convulsions with the intravenous use of cocaine.[5]

Subsequent to the advanced CNS stimu-

Table 12–1.   The "Caine" Reaction. (Reprinted from Gay, GR, et al: Cocaine: History, epidemiology, human pharmacology, and treatment. A perspective on a new debut from an old girl. Clin Toxicol (RT Rappolt, ed.), 8:149–178, 1978, by courtesy of Marcel Dekker, Inc.)

PHASE	CENTRAL NERVOUS SYSTEM	CIRCULATORY SYSTEM	RESPIRATORY SYSTEM
Early stimulation	Excitement, apprehension; other symptoms of emotional instability. Sudden headache. Nausea, vomiting. "Twitchings" of small muscles, particularly of face, fingers.	Pulse varies; probably will slow. Elevation (usual) in blood pressure may occur. Fall in blood pressure may occur. Pallor of skin.	Increased respiratory rate and depth.
Advanced stimulation	Convulsions (tonic and clonic) resemble grand mal seizure.	Increase in both pulse rate and blood pressure.	Cyanosis, dyspnea, rapid (gasping) or irregular respiration.
Depression	Paralysis of muscles. Loss of reflexes. Unconsciousness. Loss of vital functions. Death.	Circulatory failure. No palpable pulse. Death.	Respiratory failure. Ashen gray cyanosis. Death.

lation, depression of the CNS occurs, characterized by hyporeflexia, respiratory and cardiovascular depression, and coma. The highest centers are the first to be depressed, followed by the lower motor centers. Death is usually secondary to respiratory or circulatory depression and arrest. This biphasic response, characterized by an initial stimulation and then followed by abrupt, generalized CNS depression, has been termed the "caine" reaction by Gay and associates (Table 12–1).

The patient presented in this case exhibited all of the toxicologic effects described above as a result of the oral cocaine ingestion. Initially, the patient experienced CNS stimulation, which rapidly progressed from nervousness, disorientation, and trembling to tonic-clonic convulsions. Subsequently, profound CNS depression developed, with coma, respiratory depression, hypotension, and hyporeflexia.

Autonomic Nervous System Effects

Cocaine produces both central and peripheral sympathetic nervous system ef-

fects, potentiating the responses of sympathetically innervated organs to epinephrine, norepinephrine, and sympathetic nerve stimulation.[23] The exact mechanism by which cocaine exerts its effect on the sympathetic system is not clearly understood.[21] At one point, cocaine was believed to prevent the degradation of norepinephrine.[21] At present, the following explanations of cocaine's action are accepted. (1) Cocaine inhibits the reuptake of catecholamines at the receptor site.[21,23,26] This action may be interrelated, in that the blockade of catecholamine reuptake gives rise to the state of catecholamine supersensitivity.[21,27] (2) Cocaine may also promote the release as well as centrally block the neuronal reuptake of dopamine.[28–30] This action may play a role in the CNS effects of cocaine. (3) An effect on serotonin activity and content has also been suggested.[31]

The effects of cocaine on the sympathetic nervous system play a role in the CNS and cardiovascular effects of cocaine, as well as in the vasoconstricting actions, pupillary changes, and body temperature alterations which occur in acute intoxications and which were seen in the case presented.

Respiratory Effects

Cocaine produces an initial increase in the respiratory rate and depth of respiration. With large doses, this is followed by rapid shallow breathing, which may deteriorate to a Cheyne-Stokes pattern. Progressive respiratory depression resulting in cyanosis and respiratory failure may occur. The mechanism of these actions is initial stimulation and then depression of the respiratory center in the medulla.[4,23,28,32,33] Cocaine may also have some effect on the lungs, because autopsies in animals and humans have demonstrated pulmonary congestion, edema, and hemorrhage.[28,34]

Although most sources report respiratory depression as the cause of death in cocaine overdose, one study in dogs suggests that cardiac arrest plays a more significant role in fatalities than respiratory depression.[28] In the case presented, the patient exhibited shallow respirations in a Cheyne-Stokes pattern and peripheral cyanosis.

Cardiovascular Effects

Cocaine produces significant cardiovascular effects. Small doses of cocaine may slow the heart secondary to central vagal stimulation,[23,27] whereas with moderate doses, cocaine produces a dose-related increase in heart rate and blood pressure.[35-37] Catravas and associates observed powerful inotropic, chronotropic, and hypertensive responses to cocaine in dogs given the drug by IV infusion.[28] They noted an immediate significant increase in systolic blood pressure. Diastolic pressure and mean arterial pressure rose over 10 minutes, after which diastolic blood pressure declined toward the control level. Cardiac output, left ventricular pressure, and heart rate increased, while right atrial pressure remained unchanged. Approximately 1 to 2 minutes before death, the blood pressure declined rapidly, and death was attributed to cardiac arrest. In human volunteers, lower doses (e.g., 10 mg IV) have resulted in increases in systolic blood pressure, whereas slightly larger doses (25 mg IV) increase both systolic and diastolic pressures.[35]

Arrhythmias have been reported with the medical use of cocaine, as well as with cocaine abuse and overdose. Sinus tachycardia is probably the most common rhythm disturbance, although ventricular dysrhythmias such as bigeminy and PVCs have been described therapeutically.[18] Benchimol and associates describe a patient in whom an accelerated ventricular rhythm, which correlated with a subjective sensation of palpitations, developed as a consequence of cocaine abuse.[27] With large doses, ventricular fibrillation and cardiac standstill may occur.[4,39] Following the initial increase in blood pressure, a decrease in blood pressure may occur and cardiac depression ensues.[21]

The cardiovascular effects of cocaine are probably related to the central and peripheral sympathomimetic effects of the drug.[23] The cardiovascular responses could result also from central actions of cocaine via direct or indirect stimulation of mesencephalic or other areas that are usually associated with control of cardiovascular function.[28] Cocaine is also believed to have a direct action on the heart.[27] Therefore, extremely large doses may be directly cardiotoxic producing cardiac depression and arrest.[4,27] The anesthetic properties of cocaine may contribute to this decrease in electrical excitability, conduction rate, and force of contraction of the myocardium.[4,5,23] Hypoxia secondary to convulsions or respiratory depression may sensitize the heart to the sympathomimetic actions of cocaine, resulting in an arrhythmia. Acidemia with increased blood lactate may also adversely affect cardiac function.

The patient in the case presented exhibited the biphasic circulatory system response, characterized by an initial increase in both pulse and blood pressure, and a subsequent decrease in blood pressure.

Temperature

Although relatively low doses of cocaine administered intravenously to volunteers result in no change in body temperature,[37] large doses produce hyperpyrexia in animals and man.[4,23,28,33,39] In dogs given cocaine by IV infusion, temperatures peaked at 41.3 ± 0.5°C.[28] Severe hyperthermia is a factor that is believed to contribute to a lethal outcome.[28,39] The mechanisms of increased body temperature include (1) greatly increased muscular activity, (2) vasoconstriction, resulting in decreased heat loss, and (3) a direct central effect on the heat-regulating center in the hypothalamus.[4,23,33] In the case presented, the patient had an elevated body temperature of 39°C.

Pupil Reaction

Mydriasis is seen with acute cocaine intoxication, as well as with chronic cocaine abuse. It is the result of potentiation of tonic sympathetic nerve discharge to the radial muscle of the iris.[4,40] The patient's pupils in the case presented were dilated and unreactive to light.

Other Effects

Nausea and vomiting are often reported with cocaine intoxications, as were present in this patient, and are due to cocaine's stimulation of the vomiting center in the medulla.[23,33] Diarrhea may also occur, and is secondary to spasms of the smooth muscle of the gastrointestinal tract as a result of the sympathomimetic effect of the drug. In dogs, cocaine has been observed to increase plasma glucose and whole blood lactate levels, and to produce a linear decrease in arterial pH.[28]

ROLE OF THE TOXICOLOGY LABORATORY

Qualitative and quantitative analytic procedures are available for identification of cocaine powder and cocaine in biologic fluids. A "street" qualitative procedure has been described by Samuels,[41] which involves the application of several drops of commercial hypochlorite-containing bleach on a flat glass surface. A small amount of the "cocaine" is added to the bleach, and if cocaine is present, a fluffy white precipitate is seen. Other agents tested for that are commonly sold as cocaine or used as cocaine diluents either did not react or produced a different color than cocaine.

Svensson, in reproducing Samuel's work, tested benzocaine, which had not been tested by Samuels, and found that initially it would be difficult to distinguish between cocaine and benzocaine samples.[42] However, while standing, the benzocaine mixture turned yellowish orange, whereas the cocaine retained the same color. Since benzocaine is a local anesthetic, one might expect it to be a possible cocaine contaminant. However, it has not appeared as a common contaminant on the street.

The usefulness of quantitative analytic procedures for cocaine in the clinical setting is limited because of the wide range of effects seen in different patients with the same blood levels and degrees of intoxication, as well as the time required to obtain the results from a blood assay.

Oral or intranasal doses of 2 mg/kg of cocaine result in peak blood levels of approximately 0.01 to 0.04 mg/dl.[43] However, large intersubject variability has been noted, with as high as a five-fold difference in peak levels in patients given the same dose of cocaine by the same route. Several papers have examined blood levels measured at autopsy. In 2 patients, blood levels of 0.75 to 0.82 mg/dl were present.[34] In a group of 3 patients, the blood levels ranged from 0.11 to 0.75 mg/dl,[5] whereas in 13 patients, an average blood level of 0.60 mg/dl was found (lidocaine was present, but was not analyzed for, in some of these patients).[19]

The Wetli study noted that the average blood cocaine concentration level was highest (0.92 mg/dl) following oral administration, intermediate (0.44 mg/dl) after snorting, and lowest (0.30 mg/dl) after IV use.[19] In a multicentered series of 23 fatalities in patients in whom blood cocaine levels were measured and cocaine alone was present, 70% of the deaths occurred at levels below 0.9 mg/dl, whereas approximately 30% were 0.1 mg/dl or lower.[44]

One must interpret these low levels with caution, since sensitivity limits are generally in the range of 0.1 to 0.2 mg/dl.[44] Alternatively, survival has been reported in a patient with a blood level of 0.11 mg/dl, and in a patient who developed severe symptoms when a condom containing cocaine ruptured in his stomach and produced a blood level of 0.36 mg/dl at the onset of symptoms, and 0.52 mg/dl the next evening.[15]

Most clinical toxicology laboratories do not perform quantitative cocaine blood level analysis, but will perform a qualitative urine test to determine if benzoylecgonine, a metabolite of cocaine, is present. This qualitative urine test is also part of most toxicology screens. In this patient, blood and urine were sent for a general toxicology screen to rule out the ingestion of other agents. The blood was negative for all agents tested for except diazepam and long-acting barbiturates. The urine was positive for barbiturates, diazepam, and cocaine. The diazepam and barbiturate levels were in the therapeutic range, as one would expect, from the doses given to treat seizures in the ambulance.

INDICATED THERAPEUTIC MEASURES

Correction of Life-Threatening Symptoms

The symptoms seen with acute cocaine ingestions depend on the phase of the intoxication, e.g., early stimulation, advanced stimulation, or depression. The major life-threatening symptoms include respiratory depression and failure, hypertension, arrhythmias, hypotension, and circulatory collapse. Initial treatment of these patients should be aimed at assessment and treatment of those complications that are present, and anticipation and treatment of those that might develop.

Respiratory support may be necessary during the depression phase. Initial assessment of the patient must include evaluation of the potency of the airway and adequacy of respiration. Whereas some patients may require oxygen given solely by venturi mask or nasal prongs, other patients may require mouth-to-mouth resuscitation and/or a manual resuscitation bag, followed by endotracheal intubation and artificial ventilation. The modality of therapy will depend on the severity of symptoms and the treatment site.

This patient was intubated and placed on a ventilator at a rate of 18 with a fraction of inspired oxygen (FIO_2) of 28% based on the presence of cyanosis, Cheynes-Stokes respiration, and poor arterial blood gases. Shortly thereafter, the cyanosis resolved and arterial blood gas values were pH, 7.32; Po_2, 95 mm Hg; Pco_2, 40 mm Hg; and HCO_3^- (bicarbonate) of 22 mEq/L.

Convulsions usually occur during the advanced stimulation phase. The drug of choice for control of convulsions is diazepam administered IV in a dose of 0.1 to 0.3 mg/kg in children and up to 10 mg in adults. If inadequate response is obtained with diazepam, phenobarbital should be administered IV at a dose of 5 mg/kg in children and 60 to 100 mg in adults. Beyond the initial convulsions that occurred in the ambulance while en route to the ER, this patient had no further convulsions, and thus no additional treatment was required.

Cardiovascular effects are prominent in cocaine-intoxicated patients and may include hypertension and arrhythmias followed by hypotension. During the advanced stimulation phase, an increase in blood pressure and heart rate is common. Propranolol has been shown to reverse hypertension and tachycardia, which develop following both medical and non-medical use of cocaine.[4,29,38,45]

Rappolt and associates recommend the IV administration of propranolol at a dose of 1 mg every minute as needed, up to a total of 8 mg.[45] Heart rate and blood pressure generally return to normal in 1 to 3 minutes. This protocol is somewhat controversial, however, since these cardiac effects are often short-lived and most patients are not in "danger of a cerebro-vascular accident, (malignant) cardiac arrhythmias and high output heart failure."[36] Therefore, in most patients, therapeutic intervention is not indicated or necessary. However, if medical intervention is required, propranolol is the drug of choice. Since this patient was not hypertensive, and a life-threatening arrhythmia was not present on his arrival in the ER, propranolol was not administered.

Hypotension is seen during the depression phase and is usually treated with positioning of the patient, administration of fluids, and if necessary, administration of vasopressors such as dopamine. This patient was admitted to the intensive care unit and placed on a cardiac monitor. Since hypotension was significant, he was placed in a Trendelenburg position, and IV fluids were administered. When this did not adequately raise the patient's blood pressure, dopamine was infused at an initial rate of 5 μg/kg/min. However, when this therapeutic approach also did not produce the desired response, the dosage of dopamine was raised incrementally to 12 μg/kg/min, at which time a blood pressure of 100/60 was obtained.

Elevated body temperature also can be a major problem requiring emergency medical treatment. Depending on the severity of the hyperpyrexia, the following treatment modalities may be considered: (1) placement of the patient in a cool room, (2) minimization of physical activity, (3) sponging of the patient with tepid or cool water, and (4) placement of the patient in a hypothermic blanket. Since his elevation of temperature was not severe, this patient was placed in a cool, well-ventilated room. Temperature was monitored frequently, and no further treatment was required.

Prevention of Further Absorption

Since most cocaine exposures occur either through the intravenous or intranasal route, attempts at prevention of absorption are not warranted. Following intranasal application of a cocaine solution, Van Dyke and associates demonstrated measurable cocaine levels at 15 minutes and peak levels at 60 to 120 minutes.[46] In contrast, Javaid and associates reported earlier peak levels between 30 to 60 minutes following snorting of cocaine powder.[47] Although cocaine has been demonstrated on nasal mucosa 3 hours after intranasal application,[46] some clinicians feel that the flushing of mucosal surfaces may in fact increase absorption and is not recommended.[22]

When cocaine is ingested orally, one must consider whether emptying of the GI tract is warranted. Although it is commonly felt that orally cocaine is ineffective, millions of South Americans currently chew coca leaves, a practice which began thousands of years ago. Recently, Van Dyke and associates studied the absorption of cocaine orally administered in gelatin capsules.[43] Following a dose of 2 mg/kg in healthy male volunteers, cocaine was detected in the plasma 30 minutes after ingestion; it increased gradually over the next 30 minutes, and reached a peak at 50 to 90 minutes at a level of approximately 0.1 to 0.4 mg/dl, and then decreased gradually over the next 4½ to 5 hours. Interestingly, the peak "high" seen in Van Dyke's study was statistically higher following oral administration than following intranasal administration, although peak highs occurred earlier following intranasal administration. In looking at data of Van Dyke and associates,[46] Mayersohn and Perrier have calculated that 20% of an oral dose of cocaine is absorbed and reaches the systemic circulation unchanged.[48]

Several cases have been reported in which patients had swallowed cocaine-containing condoms or balloons to smuggle the drug into the United States. One patient ingested six condoms, each containing 5 g of cocaine.[15] An attempt was made to remove one of the condoms by endoscopy. Unfortunately, the condom ruptured during this attempt. Severe toxicity developed, and because of the concern that the remaining five condoms might rupture, they were removed by gastrostomy. The authors concluded that surgical removal is the method of choice, since emetics and cathartics are unreliable and endoscopy could be dangerous.[15]

In patients who have ingested large amounts of the cocaine powder, attempts to empty the stomach are warranted up to about 4 hours postingestion. If the patient is showing signs of advanced stimulation or CNS depression, an emetic is contraindicated and lavage should be performed. Information as to whether activated charcoal and cathartics are effective for oral cocaine exposure is unavailable. However, with a seriously intoxicated patient, these modalities of therapy should be administered.

Since our patient had orally ingested an unknown amount of cocaine within the past 4 hours, lavage was initiated after the patient had been intubated with a cuffed endotracheal tube to prevent aspiration of the stomach contents. After lavage, 60 g of activated charcoal was administered through the lavage tube, followed by 15 g of magnesium sulfate. The lavage tube was then pulled.

Facilitation of Cocaine Excretion

Before the different therapeutic approaches (e.g., forced diuresis, acidifica-

tion of urine, dialysis) indicated for the acceleration of cocaine excretion are discussed, the pharmacokinetic properties of cocaine must be examined.

Cocaine is readily absorbed from all mucous membranes. The rate of absorption is slow, however, because of the local vasoconstriction cocaine produces. Despite this fact, in acute intoxications, the rate of absorption can exceed the rate of detoxification and excretion. As a result, cocaine can be highly toxic. After absorption, cocaine is detoxified by the liver, though small amounts may be excreted unchanged in the urine. The mean half-life of cocaine has been reported to be from 0.9 to 2.8 hours.[43,46]

The metabolic pathways for the degradation of cocaine are shown in Figure 12–2, and metabolites include norcocaine, benzoylecgonine, ecgonine methyl ester, and ecgonine. Norcocaine has been shown to be equal in activity to cocaine in inhibiting the uptake of norepinephrine by synaptosomes prepared from rat brain,[49] and more active than cocaine as a local anesthetic.[50] Norcocaine is formed by N-demethylation primarily in the liver, by the mixed-function oxidase system, and accounts for the excretion of 2.6% to 6.2% of the administered dose of cocaine.[50]

Benzoylecgonine is another major metabolite, representing 29% to 45% of an administered dose. Stewart and associates have demonstrated that benzoylecgonine is not formed by the action of plasma esterases, as previously thought; most, if not all, is believed to be formed by a nonenzymatic hydrolysis of cocaine.[51]

Ecgonine methyl ester, another major metabolite, accounts for 32% to 49% of an administered dose in the urine during the first 28 hours, and is produced largely by plasma cholinesterase.[49] Inaba and associates have demonstrated that in a patient with low plasma cholinesterase activity, less ecgonine methyl ester and more norcocaine were seen in the urine than in a subject with normal cholinesterase activ-

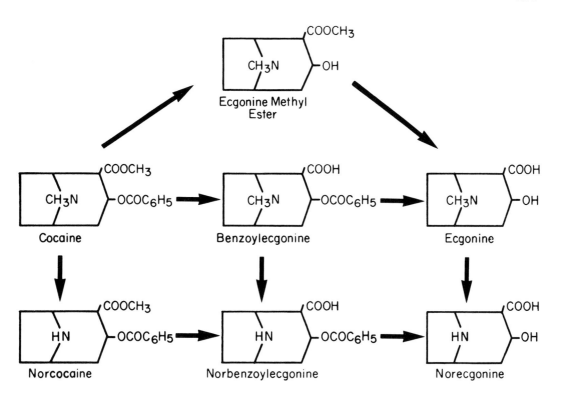

Fig. 12–2. Cocaine metabolism.

ity.[50] Stewart has also shown that liver esterase may be responsible for some production of ecgonine methyl ester.[51] From 1% to 3% of an administered dose of cocaine is excreted in the urine as ecgonine. The production of ecgonine is thought to occur either by hydrolysis of benzoylecgonine by plasma cholinesterase or by nonenzymatic hydrolysis of ecgonine methyl ester.

A small portion of administered cocaine, however, is excreted renally unchanged.[53] A 23-year-old male, who was dependent on IV cocaine and diacetylmorphine, and who had received 15 to 25 doses of cocaine, excreted from 0.4% to 5.7% of the administered dose as unchanged cocaine in the urine over a period of several days. Although the percentage of cocaine excreted unchanged was dependent on the pH of the urine, with the maximum percentage being excreted dur-ing the day on which the average urinary pH was the lowest, this was offset by a decrease in the percentage excreted as benzoylecgonine.[53] Therefore, since only a small percentage of cocaine is excreted unchanged regardless of the urinary pH, acidification of the urine would not enhance renal elimination significantly, and acidosis may worsen the cardiotoxicity of cocaine. In addition, because of the pharmacokinetic properties of cocaine, forced diuresis, dialysis, or charcoal hemoperfusion are ineffective in significantly enhancing the excretion of cocaine.

EFFECTS OF CHRONIC COCAINE ABUSE

Cocaine is abused for its CNS stimulant effect. The first recognizable effects are the cortical effects, manifested in animals by increased motor activity.[4,23] Euphoria, excitement, restlessness, and hyperstimulation, as well as a heightened sense of self-confidence and well-being, are reported.[23,32,45] The cocaine user imagines improved intellectual and physical capabilities, with a lessened sense of fatigue. Cocaine seems to enlarge and glorify the world, producing feelings of great power. Along with this elevation in mood and sense of increased energy and alertness, task performance is often improved.[21]

Some cocaine users experience extreme restlessness, headache, hypervigilance, and an unpleasant tension associated with paranoid thinking.[32] With chronic heavy use, the drug produces insomnia, anorexia, anxiety reactions, oversuspiciousness, and paranoid thinking with hallucinations and delusions. Siegel examined hallucinations in a group of contemporary cocaine users, in which 37 of the 85 subjects experienced some perceptual phenomena, mainly increased sensitivity to light, halos around bright lights, and difficulty in focusing.[40] However, many had chronic mydriasis.

Approximately 18% of this group had hallucinatory experiences, which were first noticed after 6 months of cocaine use. Visual phenomena were the first to be noticed, followed immediately by tactile hallucinations, and shortly thereafter by olfactory, auditory, and then gustatory phenomena. The occurrence of "cocaine bugs" (sensation of bugs crawling under the skin) or "Magnan's sign" was classified in this series as a pseudohallucination, since none of the subjects saw the bugs or really thought bugs were there. However, other investigators have reported that patients have imagined seeing the bugs. Magnan and Saury,[25] as reported by Siegel,[40] observed cocaine bugs to be the first hallucinatory phenomenon to develop, followed by hallucinations of sight, hearing, and smell.

Although hallucinations are usually associated with chronic use, they have also been reported with large acute ingestions.

Siegel hypothesizes that the mechanism of cocaine hallucinations may be related to cocaine's stimulant effects, including cortical arousal, seizure-type electrical discharges in the temporal lobe, and increased activity in the reticular activating system.[40] These effects, coupled with possible selective depression of inhibitory areas of the brain, would allow for release of perceptions (hallucinations) that were previously suppressed.

The chronic cocaine user may be prone to violence.[32,33,54] In fact, the stereotype of the crazed, homicidal "dope fiend" is the cocaine addict.[32] Increasing nervousness, inability to concentrate, irrational thinking, and delusions of persecution and grandeur have been reported. A syndrome of schizophrenic-like, paranoid psychosis may ensue. Several animal studies have attempted to elucidate why the acute effects of a stimulant such as cocaine on mood (e.g., euphoria), with chronic administration, progress to effects that produce a psychotic process.[55–58] Monkeys, following repetitive administration of cocaine, began to demonstrate an increased severity of motor inhibition, catalepsy, bizarre visual tracking and staring behavior, dyskinesias, and increased frequency of seizures, after an initial period of excitation manifested by hyperactivity and stereotypy.[56,58] The concept of kindling has been proposed to interpret these findings. Kindling refers to repetitive electrical stimulation of limbic system structures, particularly the amygdalae, which eventually results in the production of major motor seizures in response to a stimulation that was previously subthreshold.[56] Cocaine may act in part by "pharmacologic kindling" of the limbic system, associated with increased behavior effects and possibly convulsions.

A kindling-like mechanism, in combination with the effects of cocaine on the reuptake and release of catecholamines, may help explain the development of psychosis. Perhaps the chronic administration of cocaine results in a "reverse tolerance" to the drug.[55] Of interest is the fact that lithium has been shown to increase thresholds of after-discharges in the limbic system, which Post and Kopanda suggest may affect a kindling-like mechanism.[58] Cronson and Flemenbaum describe five cases in which patients receiving lithium could not obtain a "high" from cocaine.[59] Although these authors speculate that lithium improves a masked affective disorder in these patients, perhaps there is a relationship between these findings and Post and Kopanda's speculations.[58]

Tolerance to and physical dependence on cocaine have not been demonstrated, although psychic dependence probably develops.[4,39] Although there is no physical withdrawal syndrome per se, when the drug is withdrawn, depression and somnolence occur. A postulated mechanism relates this phenomenon to depletion of norepinephrine and/or other biogenic amine stores in the CNS.[2,32]

Cocaine and amphetamine produce similar effects in man and animals.[21,37,57] In fact, they are often considered in the same drug class, with amphetamine as the prototype. The toxic effects are similar, including behavior changes and paranoid psychosis with chronic administration, as well as CNS and cardiovascular symptoms during acute ingestions.

Cocaine is used clinically by otolaryngologists as a local anesthetic because of its ability to block the transmission of painful stimuli, and it is the only anesthetic that produces vasoconstriction. When cocaine is applied topically, the vasoconstriction is a local effect probably related to the sympathomimetic action of the drug, whereas when cocaine is administered systemically, the vasoconstriction may be the result of central vasomotor stimulation.[23]

When snorted, cocaine produces constriction of the small vessels of the nasal mucosa. Chronic cocaine snorters may suffer from a chronic stuffy nose secondary to reactive hyperemia, and are prone to infection of the nasal mucosa and upper respiratory tract as a result of chronic local irritation.[33] The intense and repeated local vasoconstriction may result in ulceration or perforation of the nasal septum;[32,33] however, this is rare.[5] Cocaine delays ejaculation and orgasm and is claimed by users to be an aphrodisiac.[32]

PROGNOSIS

Generally, fatalities from cocaine occur soon after exposure. In a retrospective study of cocaine deaths, Finkle and associates have shown that one third of the victims die within the first hour of ingestion, and an additional one third in less than 5 hours.[44] It is felt that the first 3 hours following ingestion are the most critical and that survival beyond that time indicates an improved prognosis.

In this case, the patient regained consciousness approximately 6 hours postadmission. He extubated himself and required no further respiratory therapy. At this point, the dopamine dose was gradually tapered and discontinued. At 24 hours postadmission the patient was transferred out of the intensive care unit to a medical floor, and recovered uneventfully

REFERENCES

1. Hawks R: Cocaine: The material. In *Cocaine 1977, NIDA Res Monogr Series.* Edited by RC Petersen and RC Stillman. 13:47–61, 1977.
2. Petersen RC: History of cocaine. In *Cocaine 1977, NIDA Res Monogr Series.* Edited by RC Petersen and RC Stillman. 13:17–34, 1977.
3. Carroll E: Coca: The plant and its use. In *Cocaine 1977, NIDA Res Monogr Series.* Edited by RC Petersen and RC Stillman. 13:35–45, 1977.
4. Gay GR, et al: Cocaine: History, epidemiology, human pharmacology, and treatment. A perspective on a new debut for an old girl. *Clin Toxicol* (RT Rappolt, ed.), 8:149–178. New York, Marcel Dekker, Inc., 1975.
5. DiMaio VJM, and Garriott JC: Four deaths due to intravenous injection of cocaine. *Forensic Sci,* 12:119–125, 1978.

6. Bensinger PB: Statement before the Subcommittee on Criminal Justice, Committee on the Judiciary, U.S. Senate, Sept. 11, 1979.

7. Bensinger PB: Statement before the Select Committee on Narcotics Abuse and Control, U.S. House of Representatives, July 24, 1979.

8. Personal Communication, Drug Enforcement Administration, Jan. 18, 1980.

9. Anon: The flow of illicit drugs into the United States and its enonomic significance. Drug Enforcement Administration, 1977.

10. Anon: Federal strategy for drug abuse and drug traffic prevention. Strategy Council on Drug Abuse, 1979.

11. Bensinger PB: Statement before the Permanent Subcommittee on Investigation, U.S. Senate, Dec. 7, 1979.

12. Wesson DR, and Smith DE: Cocaine: Its use for central nervous system stimulation including recreational and medical uses. In *Cocaine 1977, NIDA Res Monogr Series.* Edited by RC Petersen and RC Stillman. *13*:137–152, 1977.

13. O'Grady JE: Hub of the midwest traffic. *Drug Enforcement, 6*:20–21, 1979.

14. Siegel RK: Cocaine: Recreational use and intoxication. In *Cocaine 1977, NIDA Res Monogr Series.* Edited by RC Petersen and RC Stillman. *13*:119–136, 1977.

15. Suarex CA, Arango A, and Lester JL: Cocaine-condom ingestion. *JAMA, 238*:1391–1392, 1977.

16. Microspace Pharmacy System Rx, Spectro Industries, Dec. 21, 1979.

17. Siegel RK: Cocaine smoking. *N Engl J Med, 300*:373, 1979.

18. Fainsinger MH: Unusual foreign bodies in bowel. *JAMA, 237*:2225–2226, 1977.

19. Wetli CV, and Wright RK: Death caused by recreational cocaine use. *JAMA, 241*:2519–2522, 1979.

20. Barash PG: Cocaine in clinical medicine. In *Cocaine 1977, NIDA Res Monogr Series.* Edited by RC Petersen and RC Stillman. *13*:193–200, 1977.

21. Naraghi M, and Adriani J: Clinical uses of cocaine. *Psychopharmacol Bull, 12*:48–49, 1976.

22. Rumack BH (ed): Cocaine management. *Poisindex.* Denver, Colorado, Micromedex, Inc., Feb, 1980.

23. Ritchie JM, and Cohen PJ: Cocaine, procaine and other synthetic local anesthetics. In *The Pharmacological Basis of Therapeutics.* 5th Ed. Edited by LS Goodman and A Gilman. New York, Macmillan, 1975, pp. 379–403.

24. Price KR: Fatal cocaine poisoning. *J Forensic Sci Soc, 14*:329–333, 1974.

25. Byck R, and Van Dyke C: What are the effects of cocaine in man? In *Cocaine 1977, NIDA Res Monogr Series.* Edited by RC Petersen and RC Stillman. *13*:97–117, 1977.

26. Kalsner S, and Nickerson M: Mechanism of cocaine potentiation of responses to amines. *Br J Pharmacol, 35*:428–439, 1969.

27. Benchimol A, Bartall H, and Desser KB: Accelerated ventricular rhythm and cocaine abuse. *Ann Intern Med, 88*:519–520, 1978.

28. Catravas JD, et al: Acute cocaine intoxication in the conscious dog: Pathophysiologic profile of acute lethality. *Arch Int Pharmacodyn Ther, 235*:328–340, 1978.

29. Rappolt RT, et al: Use of Inderal (propranol-Ayerst) in I-a (early stimulative) and I-b (advanced stimulative) classification of cocaine and other sympathomimetic reactions. *Clin Toxicol, 13*:325–332, 1978.

30. Rappolt RT, Gay GR, and Inaba DS: Propranolol in the treatment of cardiopressor effects of cocaine. *N. Engl J Med, 295*:448, 1976.

31. Blum K: Depressive states induced by drugs of abuse: Clinical evidence, theoretical mechanisms and proposed treatment. *J Psychedelic Drugs, 8*:235–262, 1976.

32. Cohen S: Cocaine. *JAMA, 231*:74–75, 1975.

33. Gay GR, et al: "An ho, ho baby, take a whiff on me." La Dama Blanca cocaine in current perspective. *Anesth Analg Curr Res, 55*:582–587, 1976.

34. Lundberg GD, et al: Cocaine-related death. *J Forensic Sci, 22*:402–408, 1977.

35. Resnick RB, Kestenbaum RS, and Schwartz LK: Acute systemic effects of cocaine in man: A controlled study by intranasal and intravenous routes. *Psychopharmacol Bull, 12*:44–47, 1976.

36. Fennell WH, et al: Cardiovascular effects of cocaine. *New Engl J Med, 295*:960–961, 1976.

37. Fischman MW, et al: Cardiovascular and subjective effects of intravenous cocaine administration in humans. *Arch Gen Psychiatry, 33*:983–989, 1976.

38. Orr D, and Joine I: Anaesthesia for laryngoscopy: A comparison of the cardiovascular effects of cocaine and lignocaine. *Anaesthesiology, 23*:194–202, 1968.

39. Anon: Cocaine. *Med Lett Drugs Ther, 21*:18–19, 1979.

40. Siegel RK: Cocaine hallucinations. *Am J Psychiatry, 135*:309–314, 1978.

41. Samuels RW: Evaluation of sodium hypochlorite as a screening reagent for the identification of cocaine. *Clin Toxicol, 12*:543–550, 1978.

42. Svensson CK: Sodium hypochlorite as a screening agent for cocaine. *Pharm Alert, 10*:2–3, 1979.

43. Van Dyke C, et al: Oral cocaine: Plasma concentrations and central effects. *Science, 200*:211–213, 1978.

44. Finkle BS, and McCloskey KL: The forensic toxicology of cocaine. In *Cocaine 1977, NIDA Res Monogr Series.* Edited by RC Petersen and RC Stillman. *13*:153–192, 1977.

45. Rappolt RT, et al: Propranolol in cocaine toxicity. *Lancet, 2*:640–641, 1976.

46. Van Dyke C, et al: Cocaine: Plasma concentrations after intranasal application in man. *Science, 191*:859–861, 1976.

47. Javaid JI, et al: Cocaine plasma concentration: Relation to physiological and subjective effects in humans. *Science, 202*:227–228, 1978.

48. Mayersohn M, and Perrier D: Kinetics of pharmacologic response to cocaine. *Res Commun Chem Pathol Pharmacol 22*:465–474, 1978.

49. Hawks RL, et al: Norcocaine: A pharmacologi-

cally active metabolite of cocaine found in brain. *Life Sci, 15*:2189–2195, 1974.

50. Inaba T, Stewart DJ, and Kalow W: Metabolism of cocaine in man. *Clin Pharmacol Ther, 23*:547–552, 1978.

51. Stewart DJ, et al: Cocaine metabolism: Cocaine and norcocaine hydrolysis by liver and serum esterases. *Clin Pharmacol Ther, 25*:464–468, 1979.

52. Kogan MJ, et al: Quantitative determination of benzoylecgonine and cocaine in human biofluids by gas-liquid chromatography. *Anal Chem, 49*:1965–1969, 1977.

53. Fish F, and Wilson WDC: Excretion of cocaine and its metabolites in man. *J Pharm Pharmacol (Suppl), 21*:135S–138S, 1969.

54. Anon: Cocaine "snorting" for fun. *Med J Aust, 2*:40, 1976.

55. Ellinwood EH, and Striplins JS: Behavioral and electrophysiological effects of chronic cocaine intoxication. *Psychopharmacol Bull, 12*:38–39, 1976.

56. Post RM Comparative psychopharmacology of cocaine and amphetamine. *Psychopharmacol Bull, 12*:39–41, 1976.

57. Altshuler HL, and Burch NR: The effects of cocaine on the EEG of the monkey: Behavioral and pharmacological correlates. *Psychopharmacol Bull, 12*:41–42, 1976.

58. Post RM, and Kopanda RT: Cocaine, kindling, and psychosis. *Am J Psychiatry, 133*:627–634, 1976.

59. Cronson AJ, and Flemenbaum A: Antagonism of cocaine highs by lithium. *Am J Psychiatry, 135*:856–857, 1978.

Chapter 13

Phencyclidine (PCP)

Leo J. Sioris
Vasilios A. Skoutakis

Phencyclidine (PCP) was initially synthesized in 1957 by Parke-Davis and Company (Fig. 13–1). In 1958, it was made available for experimental use in humans as a general anesthetic under the trade name Sernyl. Although it proved generally effective as an anesthetic, and in fact superior to many anesthetics because it did not depress respiration, it also produced many adverse side effects. Patients emerging from anesthesia developed extreme agitation, disorientation, delirium, and hallucinations.[1] Consequently, it was not long before experimental use in humans was discontinued. In 1967, PCP again became commercially available under the name Sernylan, "for veterinary use only," as an anesthetic for primates. Bioceutic Labs, Inc., the veterinary division of Philips Roxane Laboratories, Inc., acquired the production rights to Sernylan in 1969 and is currently the sole legitimate source of PCP.

The illicit use of PCP first began to appear in the Haight-Ashbury district of San Francisco in 1967, under the name of "Peace Pill." Early abusers found the drug's effects to be unlike any other "drug trip" previously experienced. Soon thereafter, it became apparent that "bad trips" frequently occurred, and as a result, PCP had vanished from the illicit drug scene in the Bay area by early 1968.[2,3] In the summer of 1968, a new drug called "Hog" appeared briefly on the illicit market on the East Coast and later was identified as PCP. It too quickly fell into disfavor.[4]

PCP returned to the illicit drug market in the early 1970s and, because of its unfavorable reputation, was commonly disguised or misrepresented as

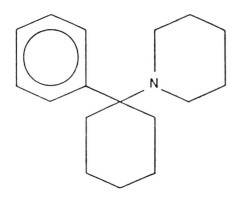

Fig. 13–1. Structure of phencyclidine (PCP).

other glamorous, expensive agents such as tetrahydrocannabinol (THC), lysergide (LSD), mescaline, psilocybin, and cocaine. In one study conducted at the University of Southern California, for example, only 3% of the drug samples analyzed that contained PCP were actually sold as such.[3] Misrepresentation allowed and continues to allow clandestine laboratories to enjoy large margins of profit, since PCP can be synthesized easily with few inexpensive, readily available reagents.[5] The cost of producing a pound of PCP is approximately $75. The profit that can be gained from the sale of this pound may be as much as $20,000.[4]

PCP continues to appear nationally in the illicit drug market, and although many people use PCP unknowingly, conscious use represents the main part of current abuse. A profile of its use in the New York City area indicates that PCP has grown immensely in popularity, without misrepresentation, in many young drug users in both black and white communities.[6] Another survey in Detroit indicates that PCP was the most commonly encountered drug in a series of 1000 cases of drug intoxication from which blood and urine samples were submitted to an emergency toxicology service.[7]

PCP is known by a variety of slang or street names, such as Angel Dust, Dust, Crystal, Crystal Joints, Peace, Weed, Supergrass, Superweed, Rocket Fuel, Elephant Tranquilizer, Horse Trank, Cadillac, Cyclones, Soma, Mist, Goon, CJ, J, and others.[8] It can be found on the street in a variety of sizes and shapes (e.g., powder, tablets, capsules, leaf mixture, and 1-g "rock" crystal forms). The crystalline powder form is found most frequently and is contained in capsules.[9] PCP also can be found on parsley, mint, or other leaves, and is usually in the form of a "joint."[10] It can be taken by mouth, by smoking (inhalation), by snorting (insufflation), and rarely by the intravenous route.[11]

Presently, PCP, has become an important drug of abuse, and it is the most commonly encountered illicit psychotropic drug seen in patients admitted to hospital emergency rooms. The increase in ER admissions is related not only to misrepresentation and the increased popularity of PCP, but to the inconsistencies in the concentration of illicit dosage forms as well.[9,12]

Because of PCP's widespread use and availability and the increased hospital admissions of patients due to accidental and suicidal ingestions from PCP, clinicians should become familiar with the clinical diagnostic considerations, the mechanisms of the toxicologic manifestations, required laboratory tests, and therapeutic modalities available for the successful management of these patients.

CASE REPORT

A 4½-year-old girl was taken to the emergency room approximately 45 minutes after she had ingested a white powder, which had been bought on the street by friends of the patient's parents as "Angel Dust." The patient became lethargic within 15 to 20 minutes after ingestion and was comatose on arrival at the ER. She was intubated, given two doses of naloxone hydrochloride (Narcan) each 0.2 mg (IV) and was transported to the University of Tennessee Medical Center.

On arrival at the Medical Center, the patient was unconscious, with pinpoint pupils, and hyperactive deep tendon reflexes. She was not responsive to deep pain, but the gag reflex was present. Her vital signs at this time were heart rate, 127 beats/min with a regular sinus rhythm; respirations, 24/min and shallow and regular; blood pressure, 160/105 mm Hg; and rectal temperature, 101°F. Diffuse rhonchi were heard over both lung fields, and excessive secretions were present in the oropharynx. The EKG revealed nonspecific ST-segment and T-wave changes.

ASSESSMENT AND TREATMENT OF THE PATIENT

In order for the clinician to assess and treat the PCP intoxicated patient effectively, the following should be considered: (1) clinical manifestations of PCP intoxication, (2) the proposed mechanism of PCP-induced toxic effects, (3) the key diagnostic indicators, (4) the significance of urine and serum level determinations, (5) appropriate therapy, (6) possible tolerance or dependence developing from the use of PCP, (7) the general prognosis.

CLINICAL MANIFESTATIONS OF PCP INTOXICATION

The clinical presentation of PCP-intoxicated patients is characterized most commonly by dose-dependent symptoms and is conveniently classified into three groups: low dose, 5 to 10 mg; moderate dose, 10 to 20 mg; and high dose, more that 20 mg.[3,4,13] It should be pointed out, however, that because of the development

of tolerance, these dose ranges are arbitrary.

Low dose (5 to 10 mg). Patients on low doses usually ingest the drug by smoking it with marihuana or other materials. The onset of the syndrome is rapid (2 to 3 minutes), but manifestations may last for hours. Blood pressure or pulse rate will be slightly elevated or normal. The pupils will be midsized or constricted and will react to light. Nystagmus, both horizontal and vertical, is usually present. There may be analgesia to pinprick, and vomiting may occur. Ataxia and muscle rigidity are present, and deep tendon relexes are hyperactive. The patient often is uncommunicative and may refuse to speak.[3,4,13,14] A blank stare under ptotic lids also is often present, along with anxiety, disorientation, and acute confusion resembling paranoid schizophrenia, making immediate differentiation from psychosis difficult.[15]

Moderate dose (10 to 20 mg). Moderate doses may be consumed by the frequent smoker, but nasal insufflation is the most common route of administration. The onset of action is again rapid. The moderate state is marked by coma or stupor, and the coma may last for more than 1 to 2 hours and may require intensive supportive care. Several days may be required for complete recovery, marked by alternate periods of sleeping and wakefulness, with confusion and anxiety.

Observation of blood pressure, pulse, and eye movements reveals a resemblance to the low-dose findings. Frequently, vomiting and hypersalivation are part of the picture. Neurologic dysfunction is severe, with purposeless movements ranging from facial grimacing and dystonic posturing to myoclonic jerks. Profound muscular rigidity will be present. Although comatose, the patient may appear awake, with open eyes and normal respiration, but will respond only to deep pain.[3,4,13,14]

High dose (>20 mg). Most patients with a high-dose intoxication have attempted suicide or have accidentally ingested a large oral dose of PCP. The onset of this syndrome may be delayed for 30 to 60 minutes after an oral dose. Such patients may be comatose for days, and recovery may require a week.[1,3,4,13] Domino and associates reported that one patient remained comatose for 10 days,[16] and we have observed a patient who remained comatose for 6 days. Therefore, the most characteristic feature of intoxication with high or massive doses of PCP is prolonged coma. In addition, the eyes may remain open, with nystagmus appearing at rest.

Blood pressure elevations are greater than those associated with low- and moderate-dose intoxications and may be sustained for several days. Hypertensive crises have also been reported to occur 3 days postingestion.[17] Body temperature and respiratory rate commonly are increased. Tremors, increased deep tendon reflexes, muscle rigidity, and excessive secretions also are manifested in greater frequency than in low and moderate-dose intoxications. Seizures, opisthotonos, acute dystonias, cardiac arrhythmias, acute renal failure, and status epilepticus have aslo been reported to occur in these patients.[1,3,4,13,18–21]

The recovery period is marked by those symptoms seen with low-dose intoxication (e.g., confusion, disorientation, agitation), along with intermittent relapse into stupor. This recovery phase or postingestion psychosis has been termed "phencyclidine psychosis."[22] Deaths attributed to PCP intoxication are usually the result of accidents related to the psychotic delirium of these patients rather than to a direct effect of the drug (e.g., drownings, jumping off cliffs, automobile accidents, inability to flee from fires, street fights, or other dangers).[23] Therefore, during the recovery phase, these patients should be followed and monitored closely.

PROPOSED MECHANISM OF PCP-INDUCED TOXIC EFFECTS

Presently, the neuropsychiatric disturbances seen in PCP-intoxicated patients are believed to be related to PCP's alteration of synaptic transmission in the brain.[24] Several studies have demonstrated altered concentrations of central neurohumoral transmitters after administration of PCP.[25,26] Areas of the CNS where PCP is believed to act include the sensory cortex, thalamus, midbrain, and spinal cord.[27]

With regards to other physiologic manifestations of PCP intoxication, specifically the elevation of blood pressure, Ilett and associates have suggested that the site of PCP action is the alpha-adrenergic receptor.[19] These investigators have demonstrated experimentally that phenoxybenzamine (Dibenzyline) and phentolamine (Regitine), two alpha-adrenergic blocking agents, reduce or completely block the pressor response to PCP. In addition, PCP also has been reported to potentiate the pressor response to epinephrine, norepinephrine, and serotonin.[27]

Hitner and associates suggest that PCP's potentiation of catecholamines may be cocaine-like in inhibiting the neuronal uptake of these transmitters.[28] The elevated blood pressure in these patients does not appear to be the result of increased cardiac output, since PCP has been found to be a direct myocardial depressant, causing a reduction in the force of contraction and a decrease in the rate of contraction in isolated cardiac muscle.[19] Tachyphylaxis to the pressor effects of PCP has also been reported to develop rapidly.[28] This explains the sinus tachycardia and occasional arrhythmias, bradycardia, and hypotension that have been reported to occur with PCP intoxications.[26,29]

PCP also has been shown experimentally to possess anticholinergic actions.[30,31] The anticholinergic effects are of rapid onset and short duration; they are dose related and considerably less potent than those of atropine. Therefore, mydriasis is not commonly seen in PCP-intoxicated patients. Changes in body temperature, however, are seen in PCP intoxications, as in the case presented. The anticholinergic action of PCP is believed to occur by comparative antagonism through specific binding at the receptor site.[30,31]

The cause of acute renal failure reported in PCP-intoxicated patients has been shown to be secondary to the development of hypotension and myoglobinuria rather than a direct effect of the drug.[32] Cogen and asssociates recently reported development of rhabdomyolysis and myoglobinuria resulting from dystonic motor activity accompanied by isometric muscle contraction in two patients.[20]

The mechanism of PCP's action on the respiratory system cannot be explained with certainty at this time. Initial pharmacologic research reveals the drug to be a CNS depressant with CNS-stimulant properties.[33] A later report by this same group of investigators concluded that PCP acts primarily as a CNS depressant.[34] Clinical findings during PCP intoxications, however, indicate that in low- to moderate-dose intoxications, respiration is either unaffected or stimulated, whereas in high-dose intoxication, respiratory depression, Cheyne-Stokes respiration, apnea, and respiratory arrest commonly occur.[1,35]

In the case presented, the patient exhibited the majority of symptoms seen in high-dose intoxications (e.g., increased heart rate, temperature, blood pressure, excessive secretions, and hyperactive deep tendon reflexes). Shortly after admission, and once emergency measures and supportive therapy were instituted (see section on treatment) and blood was obtained for biochemical, hematologic, and drug level determinations, the patient had two short seizures, consisting of an opisthotonic position with tonic extension of the arms and legs. These episodes were

controlled with the intravenous administration of diazepam (Valium), 2.0 mg, at each occasion.

KEY DIAGNOSTIC INDICATORS

Unlike most other psychedelic drugs (e.g., mescaline, marihuana, LSD, psilocybin), PCP offers specific clues that can lead the clinician to a diagnosis in the case of intoxication of unknown origin.

The low-dose state is frequently interpreted by many clinicians as secondary to an unknown psychedelic drug. However, the absence of mydriasis and the presence of gross ataxia and horizontal and vertical nystagmus are diagnostic indicators of a PCP intoxication.

The moderate state may be interpreted initially as a sedative-hypnotic overdose. However, the presence of hypertension and hyperreflexia (deep tendon reflexes) and the absence of prominent respiratory depression differentiate PCP-intoxication from a sedative-hypnotic overdose.

When a patient arrives in the ER in the high-dose state, the differentiation from causes other than PCP intoxication may be difficult. Again, if hypertension is present, and if there is no significant depression of respiration, a sedative-hypnotic overdose can be ruled out. In addition, if opisthotonic posturing is present in a child or seizure activity in an adult, a PCP intoxication should be suspected. If the patient is in status epilepticus or a postictal state, however, the underlying cause may be difficult to assess. In such cases, the EEG findings and the toxicology laboratory (see following section) may assist in the diagnosis.

Stockard and associates described specific EEG findings characterized by rhythmic theta activity, which is sometimes interrupted by periodic slow- or sharp-wave complexes,[36] whereas Meyer and associates described disappearance of alpha and beta activity, with diffuse slowing in occipital, temporal, and parietal areas.[37] The characteristic prolonged recovery phase is also diagnostic of PCP intoxication.

SIGNIFICANCE OF URINE AND SERUM LEVEL DETERMINATIONS

Although urinary and serum PCP determinations are helpful in the overall assessment of the intoxicated patient, and particularly in cases of unknown intoxications, a definite relationship between PCP urine or serum levels and symptoms (e.g., degree of respiratory depression, seizure activity, cardiovascular or renal involvement) has yet to be documented. Urine concentrations of PCP have ranged from 0.4 to 23 μg/ml in patients with low- to moderate-dose intoxication, and from 0.91 to 151.9 μg/ml in comatose patients.[38-40] Serum levels have ranged from 0.049 to 3.70 μg/ml in comatose patients, whereas those exhibiting symptoms of low- to moderate-dose intoxication have had serum levels varying from 0.051 to 0.19 μg/ml.[38,39,41]

When a fatality has been related directly to PCP ingestion or use, the serum levels have ranged from 0.3 to 7.0 μg/ml.[21,40] Again, a considerable degree of overlap exists, and definitive correlations of urine or serum levels with clinical condition cannot be made at this time. In addition, the patient's clinical status during the recovery phase and the acute intoxication stage have not been correlated with half-life of PCP. In humans, half-life determinations have been reported to vary from 11 to 80 hours.[41,42]

In the case presented, initial PCP serum and urine levels were reported from the toxicology laboratory 2 hours postadmission to be 1.3 μg/ml and 2.3 μg/ml, respectively. These results are consistent with those reported in other PCP-comatose patients. However, during the patient's hospitalization, no correlation between the serum or urine levels and the patient's clinical condition while in the acute in-

toxication phase or recovery phase was demonstrated. The fluctuation of the PCP serum and urine levels noted in this patient was probably due to the distribution and binding of PCP throughout body tissues, and particularly in the CNS.[27] The half-life of PCP in this patient was calculated to be 17.8 hours.

INDICATED THERAPEUTIC MEASURES

Presently, there is no known agent available that is specifically antagonistic to the toxic effects of PCP. Therefore, as with most other intoxications, standard emergency procedures and specific therapeutic interventions should be carried out, depending on the severity of the intoxication.

Emergency Procedures

Low dose. The key to management of a patient intoxicated with a low-dose of PCP is to place the patient under observation in an isolated, warm, nonthreatening environment. Protection from self-harm may also be necessary. Attempts to "talk down" the patient have been reported to worsen the psychiatric symptoms.[43] Our own observation, however, is that supportive conversation with the disturbed patient is beneficial. Most patients may be released to their family members or friends within 3 to 4 hours postadmission.

Moderate dose. In a patient who has a moderate-dose intoxication, monitoring of vital signs and close observation for clonic movements or muscle rigidity, which usually precede seizure activity, are essential. As with the low-dose intoxication, sensory stimulation should be controlled and minimized. Furthermore, during the recovery phase from coma or stupor, the patient should be protected from self-harm for the entire recovery phase.

If psychotic episodes develop, the intravenous administration of diazepam (Valium), in a dose of 0.1 mg/kg in children or

10 mg in adults, is indicated, and the patient's respiratory rate should be closely monitored. Haloperidol, with its low incidence of side effects, may also prove useful. Its effectiveness for the treatment of the acutely psychotic patient has been well documented.[44]

The use of phenothiazines is contraindicated in PCP intoxications because there is no evidence that their administration shortens the recovery phase or antagonizes the behavioral effects of PCP. In addition, hypotension has been reported to occur in some PCP-intoxicated patients treated with chlorpromazine.[38] Phenothiazines also are thought to lower the seizure threshold and to provoke seizures in the already predisposed patient.[45] Chlorpromazine may be helpful, however, in controlling the "phencyclidine psychosis" that may persist following the acute intoxication phase.[22,46]

High dose. The general principles for the management of the intoxicated comatose patient would apply to high-dose acute PCP intoxication. Respiratory status, blood pressure, cardiac rate and rhythm, muscle tone and movement, and renal function should be monitored. Intubation of the PCP-intoxicated patient can be difficult because of the intact pharyngeal and laryngeal reflexes, as well as muscle hypertonicity. The use of succinylcholine chloride may prove beneficial in easing a difficult intubation. These patients should also be kept well hydrated, because excessive secretions increase fluid loss. In addition, frequent suctioning may help prevent aspiration of secretions.

Blood pressure elevations usually are not high enough to require treatment with antihypertensive agents. However, diazoxide (Hyperstat) and hydralazine hydrochloride (Apresoline) have been used with success to treat hypertensive crises.[17] Experience in animals has shown that adrenergic blocking agents are not effective.[33] In addition, sympathomimetic agents should be avoided or used with extreme caution in the treatment of shock in these patients, since such drugs may enhance the toxic cardiovascular effects of PCP, which is thought to sensitize the heart to epinephrine and levarterenol.

For the treatment of PCP-induced seizures, the administration of diazepam (Valium) or phenytoin (Dilantin) has proved effective.[35,38]

Specific Therapeutic Interventions

Prior to a discussion of the specific therapeutic interventions (e.g., lavage, charcoal, laxatives, forced diuresis, acidification of urine), a brief review of the clinical pharmacology of PCP is warranted. PCP is a lipid-soluble compound; it readily traverses biomembranes and is distributed throughout body tissues, particularly in the CNS.[27] The onset of action after smoking or insufflation occurs in 3 to 5 minutes, but may be delayed for 30 to 60 minutes after oral ingestion. Effects occur seconds after an intravenous administration. Plasma PCP concentrations vary widely, and values between 40 and 200 μg/ml have been reported in overdose cases.[16] In addition, the urine concentration exceeds plasma concentration 10- to 20-fold in such cases, and part of the ingested drug may be excreted unchanged. Metabolic studies of PCP in animals have suggested that rapid oxidative hydroxylation is the major metabolic pathway.[48,49] Domino has reported that the drug is excreted in man as the mono-4-hydroxypiperidine conjugate.[50] A subsequent study by Lin and associates detected two monohydroxyl metabolites in patients intoxicated with PCP.[39] There is no evidence that these metabolites are pharmacologically active. PCP behaves as an organic base, and the pKa is approximately 8 or 9.

Based on the pharmacologic properties of PCP, evacuation of the stomach by gastric lavage, followed by the administration of activated charcoal and a saline cathartic, is indicated. Furthermore, forced diuresis and acidification of the urine would also promote the excretion of PCP and hence decrease its potential toxic effects.

Done and associates have introduced a new therapeutic approach to the management of the PCP-intoxicated patient, based on the pharmacologic properties of the drug.[42,51] Their studies indicated that extensive amounts of PCP are secreted into the gastric lumen. Concentrations of PCP in the gastric drainage were found to be 30 to 50 times those in the serum. With a pKa of 8.5, PCP becomes ionized in the stomach, but potentially may be reabsorbed in the alkaline intestine. This iontrapping scheme provides the basis for the recommendation of constant gastric suctioning to enhance PCP elimination.

This same group of investigators also studied the degree to which acidification of the urine may effect a change in PCP clearance rates.[42,51] Acidification of the urine with ammonium chloride produced a 10-fold increase in the clearance of PCP at a urine pH of 6.5, and a 100-fold increase at a urine pH less than 5.5. Additionally, forced diuresis with furosemide doubled the clearance rates. Without urine acidification, forced diuresis produced little, if any, additional change. In their conclusion, these authors went so far as to claim "success"—without serious complications—in all patients in whom these modes of therapy were applied.

In the case presented, after the initial emergency measures were implemented and the vital functions were adequately controlled, lavage was initiated with normal saline solution used as the lavage fluid. Thereafter, 1 g/kg of activated charcoal and 250 mg/kg of magnesium sulfate were administered to the patient through the nasogastric tube. At the same time, 1 mg/kg of furosemide (Lasix) and 75 mg/kg of ammonium chloride were administered IV.

The endpoint of these therapeutic interventions was to remove or promote the excretion of PCP from the body. A charcoal-laden stool was passed by the patient 3 hours after the administration of charcoal and magnesium sulfate. Besides the two episodes of seizures that occurred 1 hour postadmission and that were controlled by the administration of diazepam (discussed in the section on toxic manifestations), no other seizure episodes developed. All biochemical and hematologic results, including those of urinalysis, EKG, and x-ray examination, were reported to be within normal limits approximately 2 hours postadmission. The patient was responsive to her mother 8 hours postadmission. She was still hyperreflexic 16 hours postadmission, but was alert and responsive to her environment. A reevaluation of the biochemical and hematologic indices, including urinalysis, EKG, and x-ray examination results, at this time revealed no abnormalities. The tube was removed without difficulty, and the patient maintained her respiratory rate. She was discharged 72 hours postadmission in her usual state of health.

POSSIBLE TOLERANCE OR DEPENDENCE

Few data are available regarding the development of tolerance to and physical dependence on PCP. Studies in laboratory animals have suggested that mild tolerance can develop to the behavioral effects of PCP.[52,53] Lerner and associates have also reported the occurrence of tolerance to the psychic effects, as well as the development of chronic toxicity from long periods of regular use of PCP.[3]

Problems with memory and speech appear to be the most consistently reported changes. Recent memory lapses and difficulty with thinking are the primary complaints associated with memory. Speech difficulties include stuttering, inability to speak or speech blocking, and difficulty with articulation. These problems have persisted for as long as 6 months to 1 year following the chronic use of PCP. Other complaints include anxiety and nervousness, personality changes, social withdrawal, and social isolation. Chronic users of PCP have also been reported to develop "craving" or psychological dependence, but no withdrawal symptoms.[3] Cross tolerance between PCP and other drugs has not been demonstrated or reported.

GENERAL PROGNOSIS

The most characteristic feature of PCP intoxication is prolonged coma. The duration of coma and the recovery phase depends on the amount of PCP ingested, route of administration, and the patient's state of health. Most acutely confused patients are usually communicative 1 to 2 hours after admission to the ER, and alert and oriented within 3 to 4 hours. Once the patient is alert and oriented, the clinician should monitor the patient's state of consciousness for at least 2 to 3 hours. If the patient remains oriented and alert, he or she may be discharged.

If a patient remains stuporous or comatose, and responds only to deep pain for more than 3 hours, an observation period of at least 24 to 48 hours is recommended. The recovery phase may vary from 24 hours to several days, depending on the dose ingested and the route of administration.

Suicide has been reported to occur during the recovery or "come-down" phase in some patients. Therefore, prior to discharge, patients and clinicians should be warned about the depression, irritability, and nervousness that may occur during this period. For hospitalized patients who have ingested large amounts of PCP, close monitoring is indicated for at least 72 hours postadmission, or until toxicologic manifestations are no longer evident.

Deaths attributed to PCP intoxication are usually the result of accidents or are due to the behavioral toxicity of the drug. Coordination difficulties, muscle rigidity, and sensory disturbances may severely hamper the patient's ability to swim, drive, or sense imminent danger. As a result, deaths resulting from drowsiness, jumping off cliffs, automobile accidents, and the inability to flee from fires far outnumber those occurring as a direct result of PCP ingestion during the acute intoxication phase.

REFERENCES

1. Greifenstein FE, et al: A study of l-aryl cyclohexyl amine for anesthesia. *Anesth Analg*, 37:283–294, 1958.
2. Meyers F, Rose A, and Smith D: Incidents involving the Haight-Ashbury population and some uncommonly used drugs. *J Psychedelic Drugs*, 1:139–146, 1967–1968.
3. Lerner SE, and Burns RS: Phencyclidine use among youth: History, epidemiology, and acute and chronic intoxication. *Natl Inst Drug Abuse Res Monogr Ser*, 21:66–118, 1978.
4. Morgan JP, and Solomon JL: Phencyclidine: Clinical pharmacology and toxicology. *NY State J Med*, 78:2035–2038, 1978.
5. Shulgin AT, and MacLean DE: Illicit synthesis of phencyclidine (PCP) and several of its analogs. *Clin Toxicol*, 9:553–560, 1976.
6. Young RP: Angel dust fever. *Village Voice*, 22:1 (Dec. 12), 1977.
7. Horwitz JP, et al: Adjunct hospital emergency toxicology service. A model for a metropolitan area. *JAMA*, 235:1708–1712, 1976.
8. Sioris LJ, and Krenzelok EP: Phencyclidine intoxication: A literature review. *Am J Hosp Pharm*, 35:1362–1367, 1978.
9. Lundberg GC, Gupta RC, and Montgomery SH. Phencyclidine: Patterns seen in street drug analysis. *Clin Toxicol*, 9:503–511, 1976.
10. Perry DC: PCP revisited. *Pharm Chem Newsletter*, 4 (9), 1975
11. Burns RS, and Lerner SE: Street PCP use: Clinical studies of acute and chronic intoxication. Paper presented to the California Association of Toxicologists, San Jose, California, August 2, 1975.
12. Schlueter W: Clearing the dust on phencyclidine. *Minneapolis Health Dept Bull*, April 1977.
13. Burns SR, Lerner SE, and Corrado R: Phencyclidine—States of acute intoxication and fatalities. *West J Med*, 123:345–349, 1975.
14. Herskowitz J, and Oppenheimer EY: More about poisoning with phencyclidine ("PCP," "Angel Dust"). *N Engl J Med*, 297:1405, 1977.
15. Cohen BD, et al: Comparison of phencyclidine with other drugs. *Arch Gen Psychiatry*, 6:395–401, 1962.
16. Domino EF, and Wilson AE: Effects of urine acidification on plasma and urine phencyclidine levels in overdosage. *Clin Pharmacol Ther*, 23:421–424, 1978.

17. Eastman JW, and Cohen SN: Hypertensive crises and death associated with phencyclidine poisoning. *JAMA, 231*:1270–1271, 1975.

18. Dorand RD: Phencyclidine ingestion: Therapy review. *South Med J, 70*:117–119, 1977.

19. Ilett KF, et al: Mechanism of cardiovascular actions of 1-1-phenylcyclohexylpiperidine hydrochloride (phencyclidine). *Br J Pharmacol Chemother, 28*:73–83, 1966.

20. Cogen FC, et al: Phencyclidine-associated acute rhabdomyolosis. *Ann Intern Med, 88*:210–212, 1978.

21. Kessler FG, et al: Phencyclidine and fatal status epilepticus (letter). *N Engl J Med, 291*:979, 1974.

22. Luisanda RV, and Brown BI: Clinical management of the phencyclidine psychosis. *Clin Toxicol, 9*:539–545, 1976.

23. Burns RS, and Lerner SE: Phencyclidine deaths. *JACEP, 7*:135–141, 1978.

24. Leonard BE: Hallucinogenic drugs and central transmitter substances. *Int J Neurosci, 4*:35–43, 1972.

25. Leonard BE, and Tonge SR: Some effects of a hallucinogenic drug (phencyclidine) on neurohumoral substances. *Life Sci, 9*:1142–1152, 1970.

26. Hitzerman RJ, Loh HH, and Domino EF: Effect of phencyclidine on the accumulation of ^{14}C-catecholamines formed from ^{14}C-tyrosine. *Arch Int Pharmacodyn, 202*:252–258, 1973.

27. Domino EF: Neurobiology of phencyclidine (Sernyl), a drug with unusual spectrum of pharmacological activity. *Int Rev Neurobiol, 6*:303–347, 1964.

28. Hitner H, and DiGregorio GJ: Preliminary investigation of the peripheral effects of phencyclidine. *Arch Int Pharmacodyn, 212*:36–42, 1974.

29. Johnstone M, Evans V, and Baigel S: Sernyl (C1–395) in clinical anesthesia. *Br J Anesth, 31*:433–439, 1959.

30. Mayani S, et al: Psychotomimetic drugs as anticholinergic agents—I. *Biochem Pharmacol, 23*:1263–1281, 1974.

31. Mayani S, et al: Acetycholine-like arrangement in psychomimetic anticholinergic drugs. *Proc Natl Acad Sci USA, 70*:3103–3107, 1973.

32. Dandauino R, et al: Un cas d'intoxication aigue à la phencyclidine avec atteinte musculaire importante et insufficance renale aigue. *Union Med Can, 104*:56–60, 1975.

33. Chen G, et al: The pharmacology of 1-(1-phenylcyclohexyl) piperidine HCl. *J Pharmacol Exp Ther, 127*:241–250, 1959.

34. Chen G: Evaluation of phencyclidine cataleptic activity. *Arch Int Pharmacodyn, 157*:193–201, 1965.

35. Liden CB, Lovejoy FH, and Costello CE: Phencyclidine: Nine cases of poisoning. *JAMA, 234*:513–516, 1975.

36. Stockard JJ, et al: Electroencephalographic findings in phencyclidine intoxication. *Arch Neurol, 33*:200–203, 1976.

37. Meyer JS, Griefenstein F, and DeVault M: A new drug causing symptoms of sensory deprivation: Neurological, electroencephalographic and pharmacological effects of Sernyl. *J Nerv Ment Dis, 129*:54–61, 1959.

38. Burns RS, and Lerner SE: Perspectives: Acute phencyclidine intoxication. *Clin Toxicol, 9*:477–501, 1976.

39. Lin DCK, et al: Quantitation of phencyclidine in body fluids by gas chromatography, chemical ionization mass spectrometry and identification of two metabolites. *Biomed Mass Spectrom, 2*:206–214, 1975.

40. Reynolds PC: Clinical and forensic experiences with phencyclidine. *Clin Toxicol, 9*:547–552, 1976.

41. Marcham JA, Ramsey MP, and Sellers EM: Quantification of phencyclidine in biological fluids and application to human overdose. *Forensic Appl Pharmacol, 35*:129–136, 1976.

42. Done AK, et al: Pharmacokinetic observations in the treatment of phencyclidine poisoning—a preliminary report. In *Management of the Poisoned Patient*. Edited by BH Rumack and AR Temple. Princeton, Science Press, 1977, pp. 79–95.

43. Stein JI: Phencyclidine induced psychosis: The need to avoid unnecessary influx. *Milit Med, 138*:590–591, 1973.

44. Fox SM: Haloperidol in the treatment of phencyclidine intoxication (letter). *Am J Hosp Pharm, 36*:452, 1979.

45. Byck R: Drugs and the treatment of psychiatric disorders. In *The Pharmacological Basis of Therapeutics*. 5th Ed. Edited by LS Goodman and A Gilman. New York, Macmillan, 1975, p. 159.

46. Rainey JM, and Growder MK: Prolonged psychosis attributed to phencyclidine: Report of three cases. *Am J Psychiatry, 132*:1076–1078, 1975.

47. Anon: *Poisindex*. Denver, Colorado, Micromedex, Inc., 1977.

48. Ober RE, et al: Metabolism of 1-(1-phenylcyclohexyl)piperidine (Sernyl®). *Fed Proc, 22*:539, 1963.

49. Wong LK, and Biemann K: Metabolites of phencyclidine. *Clin Toxicol, 9*:583–591, 1976.

50. Domino EF: Neurobiology of phencyclidine. In *International Review of Neurobiolgy*. Edited by CC Pfeiffer and JR Smythies. New York, Academic Press, 1964, pp. 79–95.

51. Aronow R, and Done AK: Phencyclidine overdose: An emerging concept of management. *JACEP, 7*:56–59, 1978.

52. Balster RI, and Chait LD: The behavioral pharmacology of phencyclidine. *Clin Toxicol, 9*:513–528, 1976.

53. Martin DP, et al: Methods of anesthesia in nonhuman primates. *Lab Anim Sci, 22*:837-843, 1972.

Chapter 14

Salicylates

Joseph C. Veltri
Marietta I.B. Thompson

Historically, salicylates have been recognized as the pre-eminent agents responsible for accidental intoxications in children. In the past decade, however, a concerted effort to package many of the salicylate products in child-resistant containers has resulted in a significant decrease in the frequency of accidental salicylate intoxications in children.[1,2] Unfortunately, although the frequency has decreased, salicylates continue to be the most commonly reported agents responsible for acute ingestions in children under 5 years of age.[3]

The high incidence of these exposures is more understandable when one considers the availability and wide use of salicylates. Aspirin, for example, which is the most common formulation of the salicylates, is among the most widely used agents in medicine and is indiscriminately employed by both laymen and health professionals for a variety of ailments. Salicylate products are available for administration orally as tablets, capsules, solutions, suspensions, and powders, rectally as suppositories, and topically, as pastes and ointments.[4]

Fortunately, most acute accidental ingestions are mild and relatively inconsequential if treated appropriately. However, salicylate ingestions occasionally can result in serious complications and fatal outcomes when taken in large quantities acutely or when given to children in excessive doses over a period of days, because of the development of chronic salicylism. An understanding of the pathophysiology, diagnosis, and proper treatment of salicylate ingestions is essential for the appropriate diagnosis and management of the acutely or chronically intoxicated patient.

227

CASE REPORT

A 10-year-old female was referred to the University of Utah Medical Center (UUMC) by her family physician for possible meningitis. The history revealed that 3 days prior to admission, the child developed symptoms of an upper respiratory tract infection with a temperature of 38.4°C, nasal congestion, and general malaise. The child's mother began treatment with two adult aspirin tablets (325 mg each) every 4 to 6 hours. In addition, the child was given one Coricidin "D" (chlorpheniramine maleate, aspirin, phenylpropanolamine HCL) tablet every 4 to 6 hours for nasal congestion. On the following day, the child developed "funny breathing" as described by her mother, with nausea and vomiting. The patient's mother administered bismuth subsalicylate (Pepto-Bismol), 1 tablespoonful every 4 to 6 hours, for the nausea and vomiting. The patient continued to receive these drugs regularly until the day of admission. On the morning of the day of admission, the mother took the child to their family physician because her child's condition had worsened.

On examination by the family physician, the patient was noted to be hyperthermic, tachypneic, lethargic, and intermittently disoriented with regard to time and place. The child was referred to UUMC. Physical examination on admission revealed an ataxic, hyperpneic, and disoriented child, with a rectal temperature of 40°C. The blood pressure was 115/75 mm Hg; pulse, 85/min; and respirations, 38/min and irregular. Pertinent laboratory values on admission were sodium, 147 mEq/L; potassium, 3.1 mEq/L; chloride, 98 mEq/L; bicarbonate, 11 mEq/L; pH, 7.20; P_{CO_2}, 24 mm Hg; blood urea nitrogen (BUN), 27 mg/dl; base deficit, 19; hematocrit, 50 vol %; serum salicylate level, 80 mg/dl; and a cerebral spinal fluid salicylate level of 35 mg/dl.

One month prior to admission, the patient had been seen for a routine physical examination, at which time her weight was charted at 30 kg. On admission, the child's weight was 27 kg. The weight loss can be attributed to dehydration, which also was supported by other clinical findings, such as rapid pulse rate, poor skin turgor, dry lips and mouth membranes, and elevated BUN and hematocrit. At this time, the patient was thought to be suffering from chronic salicylism and was admitted to the pediatric intensive care unit. Thereafter, the patient was treated with decontamination (e.g., administration of activated charcoal and a saline cathartic) and general supportive measures, which included the administration of intravenous fluid and electrolyte therapy. Supportive and symptomatic therapy was continued for 3 days, and the remainder of the patient's hospital course was unremarkable. The patient was discharged on the fourth hospital day without complications.

CLINICAL ASSESSMENT AND MANAGEMENT OF THE PATIENT

In the vast majority of pediatric salicylate intoxication cases, the patient will be found either while ingesting the product or within a short time thereafter, usually before the symptoms are apparent. However, in cases of intentional ingestion or chronic salicylism, patients can be either asymptomatic or symptomatic at the initial presentation. Therefore, it is important in all cases for the clinician to obtain an adequate history, so that a rational decision can be made regarding an accurate diagnosis and proper management. In the absence of an obvious history of salicylate exposure, chronic salicylate poisoning may be overlooked by the clinician initially, and on occasion, the injury has been compounded by the administration of additional salicylates to treat salicylate-induced hyperthermia. The historical data base should include the age and weight of the patient, the product(s) ingested, an estimation of the amount ingested, the time of ingestion, the current status of the patient with regard to symptoms, and any previous salicylate therapy.

In the case presented, determination of the type and extent of previous therapy was critical because of the absence of an obvious history of an acute salicylate ingestion. However, a thorough history revealed the cause of the patient's salicylism. Each tablet of Coricidin "D" contains phenylpropanolamine and chlorpheniramine, plus 325 mg of aspirin. Each tablespoonful of Pepto-Bismol contains calcium carbonate, in addition to 130 mg of salicylate as a combination of methyl salicylate, bismuth subsalicylate, sodium salicylate, and salicylic acid. Initially, the patient was receiving 975 mg of salicylate every 4 to 6 hours, or about 4.8 g/day. By the second day of therapy, the child's mother was administering 1.1 g/dose, or about 5.5 g/day.

Following the establishment of an adequate historical data base, an initial estimation of the potential severity of the exposure can be made. Table 14–1 summarizes the protocol used by the staff of the Intermountain Regional Poison Control Center (IRPCC) to aid in determination of the potential danger of an acute

exposure to salicylates. It must be remembered that when a history is obtained, the total ingestion should be determined, including any salicylate taken therapeutically by the patient within the past 24 hours. In addition, the time since ingestion is an important factor in the assessment of the reliability of any symptoms that are or should be present. Symptoms often will provide the most meaningful clues to the severity of an intoxication, especially within 4 to 6 hours after ingestion.[5] If the reported ingestion is less than 150 mg/kg of body weight, and the patient is asymptomatic and remains so up to 4 hours after the call, it is unlikely that any significant toxic symptoms will occur. The majority of these cases can be managed by simple reassurance, demulcents, and follow-up to assure that the assessment was correct. Occasionally, acute ingestions of between 100 to 150 mg/kg of body weight will result in some nausea and vomiting secondary to the GI irritant effect of salicylates. These symptoms are usually of brief duration and should respond to demulcents.

When the reported ingestion is between 150 and 300 mg/kg of body weight, and it is reasonably certain that emesis can be induced within 4 hours of the ingestion, the patient can generally be managed at home by the induction of emesis with

Table 14–1. Protocol Used to Estimate the Severity of Salicylate Ingestions

History	Obtain an initial ingestion history, including substance ingested, amount ingested, time of ingestion, current symptoms, and any previous therapy.
Amount ingested	Calculate the ingested dose according to the following formula:

$$\frac{\text{No. tablets ingested} \times \text{mg ASA/tablet}}{\text{body weight in kg}} = \text{dose ingested in mg/kg}$$

1. *If no additional salicylates* have been ingested within the last 8 hours, calculate the dose as described above.
2. *If 2 or less doses* of salicylates have been ingested in the last 24 hours, with not more than 1 dose within the last 8 hours, add that amount to the total amount ingested acutely and calculate the dose as described above.
3. *If 1 or more doses* of salicylates have been ingested within the last 8 hours, and at least 4 doses within the last 24 hours, calculate the acutely ingested dose as described above and multiply the acutely ingested dose by 1.5. This dose will be your *adjusted acute dose.*

syrup of ipecac. Once emesis has occurred, the patient may remain at home, but periodic follow-up should continue for at least an additional 24 hours, to assure that an adequate amount of salicylate was removed from the stomach and the patient remains asymptomatic. In the absence of induced emesis, acute ingestions of greater than 150 mg/kg of body weight can be expected to produce objective symptoms, and the patient should be evaluated in a health care facility.

If the reported ingestion is greater than 300 mg/kg of body weight, it is unlikely that the patient can be managed at home even with the induction of emesis, since emesis will probably remove no more than about 50% of the ingested dose.[6] In these cases it may be appropriate to induce emesis prior to referral, if ipecac is on hand. However, the patient should be transferred and evaluated in a health care facility as soon as possible.

It should be emphasized, however, that the nonlinear elimination kinetics of salicylates make the determination of previous salicylate therapy important for a reasonable prediction of severity.[7] Patients who have received salicylate therapy prior to an acute ingestion are likely to develop objective symptoms as a consequence of relatively small acute ingestions if left untreated. Table 14–1 also recommends some general considerations if an acute ingestion occurs within 24 hours of previous salicylate therapy. If no more than two therapeutic doses of salicylate have been taken by the patient within 24 hours preceding the acute exposure, the amount of salicylate taken therapeutically should be added to the total amount ingested acutely. Calculations based upon this dose should provide a conservative approximation of the severity as if the exposure has occurred as a single acute ingestion.

If the patient has received more than two therapeutic doses of a salicylate product within 24 hours prior to the acute

ingestion, a conservative approximation of severity can be obtained by calculation of the acutely ingested dose and multiplication of that dose by 1.5. These recommendations are at best approximations, and the patient's clinical manifestations should be used as the primary indicator of severity.

Physician evaluation in a health care facility should be obtained for any patient with a history or symptoms suggesting moderate to severe salicylate toxicity. The evaluation should include a physical examination augmented by appropriate laboratory tests. A number of laboratory tests, such as arterial blood gases, electrolytes, glucose, BUN, serum creatinine, urine pH, specific gravity, osmolality, and serum salicylate levels are useful in the diagnosis of salicylate intoxications and are important factors in the determination of the level of care likely to be needed by the patient.

An arterial blood gas determination is useful in the assessment of the level of acid-base disturbance and the degree of "compensated respiratory alkalosis" present. In the case presented, the initial blood gas determination indicated that the patient had a mixed respiratory alkalosis and metabolic acidosis and an acidic pH. This clinical picture, when present in a 10-year-old child, indicates severe intoxication. Electrolytes are important determinants of the degree of electrolyte depletion and calculation of the anion gap, and BUN and hematocrit values provide an indication of the level of dehydration. A blood glucose level is important in view of the reports of severe hypoglycemia.[8–12]

A serum salicylate level is essential to the diagnosis. If the facility where the patient is treated is not equipped to measure serum salicylate levels, the sample should be sent to another institution for the determination. The time of the drawing of the blood sample for the initial salicylate level is critical for proper interpretation of the results. To allow for maximal absorption and distribution of the drug, at least 4 and preferably 6 hours should have elapsed between the time of ingestion and the first blood sample. To aid in the interpretation of the serum salicylate level, a nomogram has been developed by Done (Fig. 14–1), which has proven useful for the interpretation of serum salicylate levels following single acute ingestions.[5]

The nomogram, however, was developed by Done from retrospective clinical observations and bears no relationship to the elimination of salicylate. Thus, it is not useful in the prediction of the rate of elimination or future blood salicylate levels, since salicylates exhibit nonlinear elimination kinetics. The nomogram is also not useful in the evaluation of the severity of chronic salicylate intoxication. In these latter cases, the serum salicylate level bears little relationship to the severity of symptoms, and it becomes necessary to use other laboratory tests and objective

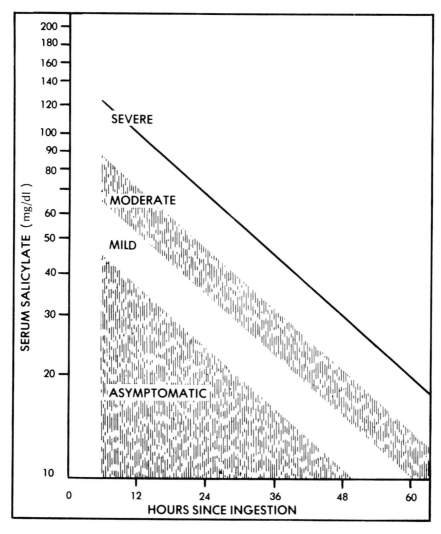

Fig. 14–1. Nomogram for estimating the severity of acute salicylate intoxication. (Reprinted with permission from Done AK: Salicylate intoxication—Significance of measurements of salicylate in blood in cases of acute ingestion. *Pediatrics,* 26:800, 1960. Copyright American Academy of Pediatrics 1960.)

Table 14–2.　Protocol Used to Estimate the Severity of Salicylate Ingestions Based Upon the Serum Salicylate Level

A. First Serum Salicylate Level (1SL)	1. If the 1SL is <30 mg/dl and the patient is objectively asymptomatic, the exposure is nontoxic and the patient may be discharged.
	2. If the 1SL is >30 mg/dl *or* the patient has objective symptoms, a second blood salicylate level should be obtained at least 2 hours after the 1SL, with reevaluation based upon the second blood level.
B. Second Serum Salicylate Level (2SL)	1. If the 2SL is <1SL, *and* <40 mg/dl, *and* at least 6 hours has elapsed since the ingestion, and the patient is asymptomatic, significant toxicity is unlikely. The patient may be discharged, with telephone follow-up 4 to 6 hours later.
	2. If the 2SL is in the "mild" category of the Done nomogram, observation should continue for at least 4 to 8 hours. Obtain baseline arterial blood gas determination and initiate IV hydration.
	3. If the 2SL is in the "moderate" category of the Done nomogram, moderate to severe toxicity is likely. The patient should be admitted (or transferred) to a major treatment facility.*
	4. If the 2SL is in the "severe" category of the Done nomogram, severe toxicity is likely. The patient should be admitted (or transferred) to a major treatment facility.
	5. If the patient's calculated elimination half-life (t½) is >15 hours, severe toxicity is present. The patient should be admitted (or transferred) to a comprehensive treatment facility.*
	6. Severe toxicity is present if the patient has any of the following manifestations: severe acidosis, marked metabolic derangement, coma, or convulsions. The patient should be admitted (or transferred) to a comprehensive treatment facility.

* Utah Bureau of Emergency Medical Services, Health Care Facility Categorization.

clinical manifestations as indicators of severity.

The greatest value of the nomogram is in the estimation of the severity of an acute ingestion early in the course of an intoxication, so that a rational judgement may be made with regard to hospitalization of the patient. It is also helpful in the identification of those individuals who are at high risk levels, so that methods of hastening the elimination of salicylate can be started before the situation becomes irreversible.

Table 14–2 summarizes the protocol used by the staff of the IRPCC in conjunction with the Done nomogram, to aid in the evaluation of the serum salicylate levels and the prediction of the severity of an acute salicylate intoxication.

CAUSES OF THE TOXIC MANIFESTATIONS

The principal pathophysiologic effects of salicylate intoxication include respiratory stimulation, uncoupling of oxidative phosphorylation, inhibition of Krebs cycle enzymes, activation of hypothalamic sympathetic centers, stimulation of lipid metabolism, inhibition of amino acid metabolism, and interference with hemostatic mechanisms. These effects result in a number of toxic manifestations, such as acid-base disturbances, fluid and electrolyte imbalance, hyperthermia, altered glucose metabolism, altered hemostatic mechanisms, CNS dysfunction, and renal abnormalities.[13–38] Death usually occurs with marked CNS depression and is related to respiratory failure and/or cardiovascular collapse.

Acid-Base Disturbance

The acid-base disturbance commonly associated with moderate to severe salicylate ingestion is the most important clinical problem in the pathogenesis of salicylate intoxication.[13,14] The defect results from an initial respiratory alkalosis, followed within a short time by compensatory mechanisms, which alter the normal renal function to permit the excretion of large quantities of bicarbonate.

Salicylates stimulate the respiratory rate and volume beyond normal homeostatic levels by both direct and indirect action.[15,16] The initial respiratory response is indirect and almost never seen clinically as a pure effect. The disturbance is characterized by an increase in the depth of respiration (hyperpnea), without an increase in rate, and is attributed to an increased production of CO_2 and an increased cellular O_2 utilization secondary to the uncoupling of oxidative phosphorylation. As salicylate gains access to the CNS, it directly stimulates the respiratory centers in the medulla.[17] This direct effect results in a marked increase in alveolar ventilation, characterized by a further increase in the depth of respiration and a marked increase in the rate of respiration (tachypnea). The resulting increase in minute volume causes the plasma CO_2 level to fall because of the greater alveolar-capillary permeability of CO_2 in relation to O_2. The hypocapnea thus produced results in a rise in the pH of the blood and is commonly referred to as respiratory alkalosis.

Homeostatic mechanisms respond to the rise in blood pH through renal mechanisms, which cause the kidneys to excrete large quantities of base in the form of bicarbonate. The result of these offsetting mechanisms is a return of the blood pH toward normal and is referred to as compensated respiratory alkalosis. This basic disturbance tends not to progress any further in adults and children older than about 4 years with mild to moderate ingestions. In the older patient, a clinical picture of mixed respiratory alkalosis and metabolic acidosis, with normal to slightly acidic pH, is an indication of moderate to severe salicylate toxicity. Infants and young children characteristically progress to a metabolic acidosis, unless the intoxication is mild.[13]

The mechanism of this age-dependent difference has not been elucidated with certainty. Some authors suggest that infants and young children may excrete a proportionally larger amount of their "buffer capacity" than adults and thus overcompensate. Although such a suggestion is plausible, it may also be that infants and young children have a decreased capacity for the plasma protein binding of salicylates, and thus a higher proportion of free drug.[7] Such a theory is supported by the fact that serum salicylate levels commonly measure both free and bound salicylate and would not reflect the increased proportion of free salicylate, which is the active component. In the case presented, the patient was judged to be severely intoxicated, as evidenced by the clinical symptoms and arterial blood gases. These findings are common in patients suffering from chronic salicylate poisoning.[18,19]

Metabolic Defects

A major effect of salicylate intoxication results from the uncoupling of oxidative phosphorylation,[20,21] inhibition of specific dehydrogenases[22] and aminotransferases,[23] and an increase in glucose demand, as outlined in Table 14–3.

Table 14–3. Factors Contributing to Metabolic Acidosis in Salicylate Intoxication

- UNCOUPLING OF OXIDATIVE PHOSPHORYLATION
  ↓
  decreased production of ATP
- ENHANCED UTILIZATION OF GLYCOLYSIS
  ↓
  accumulation of lactic and pyruvic acids
- INHIBITION OF KREBS CYCLE DEHYDROGENASES
  ↓
  accumulation of organic acids
- INHIBITION OF AMINOTRANSFERASES
  ↓
  accumulation of amino acids
- INCREASED DEMAND FOR GLUCOSE
  ↓
  stimulation of lipid metabolism
  ↓
  accumulation of ketone bodies

Within the cytochrome system of the mitochondria, the primary location of oxidative phosphorylation, O_2 is utilized to produce energy in the form of adenosine triphosphate (ATP), with CO_2 and water as byproducts. When the cytochrome system is functioning normally, 1 molecule of glucose provides 38 molecules of ATP. When uncoupling occurs, some of the energy normally stored as ATP is released as heat, and the body compensates by utilizing the less efficient glycolytic pathway as a source of energy. In addition, salicylate inhibits dehydrogenases in the Krebs cycle, resulting in the accumulation of organic acids such as oxaloacetate and α-ketoglutarate. Salicylate also inhibits specific aminotransferases, resulting in the accumulation of glutamate.

The enhanced utilization of the glycolytic pathway results in the accumulation of lactic and pyruvic acids.[23] In addition, muscle stores of glucose are rapidly depleted, and the body metabolizes fats as an energy source, which increase the production of acidic ketone bodies. The overall effect is the accumulation of organic acids, resulting in metabolic acidosis and reflected as a decrease in plasma pH.[18]

Altered Glucose Metabolism

Salicylates are capable of inducing both hyper- and hypoglycemia through mechanisms listed in Table 14–4. In large doses, salicylates rapidly deplete muscle stores of glycogen as a result of the uncoupling of oxidative phosphorylation. Salicylates also directly activate CNS sympathetic centers, resulting in a release of epinephrine from the adrenal cortex, which stimulates glucose-6-phosphatase activity.[24] Both mechanisms lead to an increase in glucose mobilization from the liver, resulting in hyperglycemia and glucosuria.

Later in the course of an intoxication, hypoglycemia may develop as a result of increased utilization of glucose in peripheral tissues and decreased carbohydrate production due to salicylate interference

Table 14–4.   Factors that Affect Glucose Metabolism

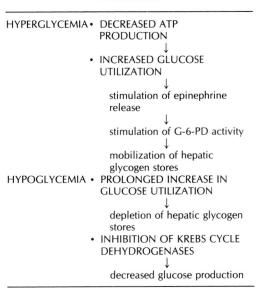

with gluconeogenesis. Hypoglycemia, therefore, may be a serious complication in chronic salicylism, or a late complication in the course of an acute ingestion. As a result, blood glucose levels should be monitored closely throughout treatment.[8–12] Blood for glucose determinations should be drawn for any patient with CNS depression and/or seizures who is suspected of ingesting salicylates.

Fluid and Electrolyte Imbalance

Fluid and electrolyte imbalances accompany the acid-base and metabolic disturbances of salicylate ingestion and contribute significantly to toxicity. Table 14–5 outlines the common factors that contribute to the water and electrolyte loss associated with salicylate intoxication. Prolonged alveolar hyperventilation is accompanied by an increase in pulmonary excretion of water. Increased metabolism and heat production result in diaphoresis (sweating), which adds to the amount of insensible water loss. Salicylates induce emesis by both a local irritant and a central effect, which may be prolonged and which

Table 14–5. Factors Contributing to Fluid and Electrolyte Loss in Salicylate Intoxication

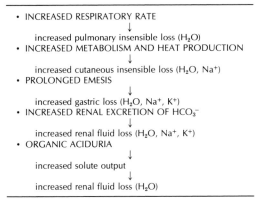

- INCREASED RESPIRATORY RATE
  ↓
  increased pulmonary insensible loss (H_2O)
- INCREASED METABOLISM AND HEAT PRODUCTION
  ↓
  increased cutaneous insensible loss (H_2O, Na^+)
- PROLONGED EMESIS
  ↓
  increased gastric loss (H_2O, Na^+, K^+)
- INCREASED RENAL EXCRETION OF HCO_3^-
  ↓
  increased renal fluid loss (H_2O, Na^+, K^+)
- ORGANIC ACIDURIA
  ↓
  increased solute output
  ↓
  increased renal fluid loss (H_2O)

accounts for considerable water and electrolyte loss.[15]

Renal compensatory mechanisms, which respond to the initial respiratory alkalosis, result in the excretion of significant amounts of bicarbonate,[14] accompanied by water, sodium, and potassium. In moderate to severe intoxication, metabolic acidosis results in an increased renal solute load, which further enhances the renal water and electrolyte loss. The additive effect of these processes results in dehydration, which is characteristic of moderate to severe salicylate intoxication. Fluid losses may be 2 to 4 liters per square meter of body surface (L/m^2) in moderate intoxication, with losses as high as 4 to 6 L/m^2 in severe intoxication.[25]

A number of factors contributes to total body depletion of potassium. The initial alkalosis favors the intracellular flux of potassium, which increases the intracellular concentration of potassium while decreasing the extracellular concentration. Therefore, serum potassium measurements obtained while the patient is alkalotic are likely to be low. As a result, those measurements would not necessarily indicate the intracellular or total body potassium. Conversely, acidosis enhances the transcellular permeability of potassium, which increases the extracellular

concentrations of potassium while decreasing the intracellular concentration. Such a shift makes potassium available for renal excretion and total body depletion.

Total body sodium is also likely to be depleted in moderate to severe salicylate ingestion. However, in most cases the relative loss of sodium is lower than the water loss, and replacement of sodium in an amount proportionate to water, as with normal saline solution for example, usually results in hypernatremia.[13]

Hematologic Manifestations

In large doses, salicylates have been reported to cause a number of hematologic defects, which are cited with varying degrees of frequency. In large measure, these effects appear to be relatively mild and of little clinical significance. However, in the overall care of the patient, they require consideration.

In therapeutic doses, acetylsalicylic acid (aspirin) increases the bleeding time by inhibiting the aggregation of platelets.[26,27] The prostaglandin thromboxane (TXA_2) appears to promote platelet aggregation and clotting. Salicylates (at least in toxic doses) inhibit TXA_2 and platelet aggregation. Cyclic endoperoxides (PGG_2 and PGH_2) are key intermediates in the synthesis of thromboxane and are inhibited by aspirin. The result is a decrease in platelet aggregation, which leads to an increase in the time required for an effective clot to form.[28,29]

This effect, although important pharmacologically, is not in our opinion a clinically significant therapeutic problem in the intoxicated patient. A commonly reported hematologic defect in salicylate intoxications is due to an apparent interference with the hepatic production of prothrombin, resulting in the prolongation of the prothrombin time. This defect is reversed or prevented by the administration of Vitamin K.[30] Another hematologic defect attributed to salicylate is a decrease in erythrocyte survival time.[31]

CNS Toxicity

CNS symptoms such as lethargy or disorientation have been associated with the early manifestations of salicylate intoxication. These may progress to hallucination, coma, and/or seizures. The degree of CNS dysfunction is apparently due to the accumulation of salicylate within the CNS.[32] Acidosis aggravates the degree of CNS dysfunction by enhancing the passage of salicylate into the CNS.[33] Many factors either produce or contribute to the CNS manifestations and include acidosis, hypernatremia, hypoglycemia, and cerebral edema.

Acute Renal Failure

A transient decrease in renal function may occur as a result of reduced renal perfusion secondary to decreased renal blood flow. Oliguria may also occur either as a manifestation of severe dehydration or secondary to a paradoxical fluid retention associated with the syndrome of inappropriate antidiuretic hormone (SIADH).[34] Both causes may result potentially in acute renal failure. However, the specific cause must be identified, since the therapies required for appropriate management are different. Dehydration is treated with fluid replacement, and SIADH is treated with fluid restriction.

Hyperthermia

When salicylate intoxication results in significant uncoupling of oxidative phosphorylation, the resulting release of energy in the form of heat is manifested clinically as hyperthermia.[19] Hyperthermia is a common finding in moderate to severe salicylate intoxications and may be life threatening. In such cases, corrective therapy must be initiated immediately, since the normal compensatory mechanism of sweating may be inhibited by dehydration.

Pulmonary Edema

Pulmonary edema has been reported to occur as a late finding in cases of severe intoxication and usually portends a poor prognosis.[35–38] The edema may be the result of fluid overload secondary to fluid retention (as seen with SIADH and acute renal failure), as a result of congestive heart failure associated with cardiac dysfunction, or from an unknown cause.

INDICATED THERAPEUTIC MEASURES

Appropriate care of the salicylate-intoxicated patient requires consideration of the basic principles of management of the toxic patient as outlined in Table 14–6.

Termination of Exposure

Decontamination of the gastrointestinal tract should be attempted as soon as possible after an acute ingestion. This is especially true in chronic salicylate intoxications, because the procedure is often overlooked, and because the prevention of absorption of even small amounts of salicylate in these cases may decrease morbidity markedly. Evacuation of the stomach is always indicated after an acute ingestion. Gastric evacuation is most ef-

Table 14–6.　Guidelines for Management of Salicylate Intoxications

TERMINATION OF EXPOSURE	• emesis/lavage
	• activated charcoal
	• catharsis
SUPPORTIVE CARE	• correction of fluid losses
	• correction of electrolyte imbalance
	• correction of acid-base disturbance
ENHANCEMENT OF ELIMINATION	• diuresis with urinary alkalinization
	• extracorporeal removal

fective within the first 4 hours. However, salicylate may remain in the stomach for prolonged periods, and gastric evacuation should be considered up to 12 hours after an ingestion.

Induction of vomiting is the preferred method of emptying the stomach in both children and adults. Forced emesis is more effective than spontaneous vomiting,[6] and the administration of an emetic is recommended even if the patient has already vomited spontaneously. Syrup of ipecac is the preferred agent for the induction of emesis, because it has no serious adverse effects when given appropriately, and because other emetics are potentially dangerous or of questionable efficacy.[39] The emetic apomorphine is a respiratory depressant in therapeutic doses and is not recommended as an emetic in patients with symptomatic salicylate intoxication, because it may exacerbate pre-existing acid-base disturbance.[40] Recommendations for the administration of syrup of ipecac are given in Table 14–7.

Induction of emesis is contraindicated in the comatose or convulsing patient because of the hazard of tracheal aspiration of the vomitus. Gastric lavage should be used instead and should be preceded by tracheal intubation with a cuffed tube and positioning of the patient on his left side, with the head slightly lower than the feet.

Table 14–7. Induction of Emesis Using Syrup of Ipecac

---

1. ADMINISTER APPROPRIATE DOSE OF SYRUP OF IPECAC.
   - Adults should receive 30 ml.
   - Children (1–12 years) should receive 15 to 20 ml.
   - Infants (<1 year) should receive 10 ml.
2. ADMINISTER CLEAR FLUID.
   - Give at least 8 fl oz of tepid water or clear liquid.
3. HAVE PATIENT WALK.
4. READMINISTER SYRUP OF IPECAC AND FLUID.
   - A maximum of one additional dose of ipecac can be administered if vomiting has not occurred within 15 to 20 minutes.
5. CONSIDER GASTRIC LAVAGE
   - if vomiting has not occurred within 15 to 20 minutes of the 2nd dose of syrup of ipecac.

The largest tolerable nasogastric or orogastric tube should be selected, and initial aspiration of the gastric contents should precede actual lavage. Lavage should be undertaken with the instillation of 200- to 300-ml aliquots of lukewarm tap water or normal saline solution. Lavage should continue until the return is clear and at least 2 to 4 L of fluid have been used. Periodically during the lavage, the position of the gastric tube should be shifted and the abdomen agitated externally, with fluid in the stomach. These procedures will ensure that a clear return is the result of an empty stomach rather than an artifact of tube placement or concretion of gastric contents.

Activated charcoal should be administered approximately 1 to 1½ hours after vomiting has stopped or immediately after lavage has been performed to adsorb any salicylate remaining in the GI tract. Ideally, the dose ratio of activated charcoal to salicylate should be 10/1. However, since the amount of salicylate remaining in the GI tract is rarely known, the commonly recommended dose of activated charcoal is 50 g in adults or 20 g in children. The powdered charcoal should be administered as a slurry in water and given orally or through a tube.

Following the administration of activated charcoal, a cathartic should be given to hasten passage of the salicylate and charcoal through the GI tract. Saline cathartics such as sodium sulfate, magnesium sulfate, or magnesium citrate are generally preferred and should be given orally in a dose of 250 mg/kg, to a maximum of 30 g /dose.[41] The dose may be repeated every 1 to 2 hours up to a total of three doses, or stopped early if a response occurs. Passage of a charcoal-laden stool is generally considered the endpoint of catharsis. It is important to note that saline cathartics produce an effect primarily by pulling water osmotically into the gut, and they are uniikely to be effective in the presence of significant dehydration.

In cases of acute salicylate intoxication in which the ingestion has occurred more than 12 hours prior to the initiation of therapy, and in cases of chronic salicylate intoxication, the need for gastric evacuation may be questionable. However, patients should still receive the benefit of intestinal decontamination. In the absence of such therapy, the patient may continue to adsorb the drug; thus exposure is prolonged and morbidity increased. Intestinal decontamination can be achieved by the administration of an appropriate dose of activated charcoal and a cathartic until a charcoal-laden stool is passed.

In the case presented, gastric evacuation was not undertaken because it was felt to be of questionable efficacy. However, decontamination of the lower intestinal tract was accomplished by the administration of activated charcoal, followed by catharsis. A charcoal-laden stool was not passed in this patient until the second day of hospitalization, presumably because of severe dehydration.

Supportive Care

Attentive supportive care is a therapeutic cornerstone in the successful management of salicylate intoxications. Patients require intensive nursing care with close monitoring of vital signs, electrolytes, and fluid balance.

Dehydration. Accompanied by an electrolyte imbalance and an acid-base disturbance, dehydration is a common finding in salicylate intoxication, and appropriate management is a requisite to successful therapy. Mild salicylate poisoning can usually be managed with oral fluids, whereas parenteral fluids are usually required to manage moderate to severe poisoning. The electrolyte imbalance and acid-base disturbance of salicylate poisoning can usually be managed safely and effectively through adequate hydration, using hypotonic solutions with potassium and bicarbonate supplementation.[13] Electrolytes should be added

to meet initial deficits and daily maintenance requirements; however, potassium should be administered only after adequate urine flow has been established.

Correction of the base deficit is managed most effectively by the gradual administration of sodium bicarbonate, whereas rapid alkali therapy is dangerous and only transiently effective.[42] On occasion, rapid alkali therapy may be indicated to obtain immediate buffering of the blood when the pH is such that the acidosis poses an immediate threat to life; however, the continued maintenance of the buffering effect can be achieved only in conjunction with correction of fluid deficit and electrolyte imbalance. Bicarbonate may also be administered in an attempt to alkalinize the urine. The following formulas can be used to calculate initial fluid, potassium, and sodium bicarbonate deficits.[43]

Fluid deficit:
 Patient's normal weight (kg)
 $\underline{-\text{ current weight (kg)}}$
 $=$ fluid loss (L)

Potassium deficit:
 Patient's normal weight (kg)
 $\times$ 0.4 L/kg
 $\times$ [ideal K^+ level $-$
  $\underline{\text{patient's } K^+ \text{ level] (mEq/L)}}$
  $=$ potassium deficit (mEq)

Sodium bicarbonate deficit:
 Patient's normal weight (kg)
 $\times$ 0.4 L/kg
 $\times$ [ideal HCO_3^- level $-$
  $\underline{\text{patient's } HCO_3^- \text{ level] (mEq/L)}}$
  $=$ sodium bicarbonate deficit (mEq/L)

In the case presented, the patient was estimated to be 10% dehydrated; this estimate was based upon the difference between recorded weight of 30 kg and a current weight of 27 kg, which was equivalent to a fluid deficit of 3 L. Calculation of the normal maintenance fluid for the next

24 hours, based upon the patient's estimated surface area, produced a figure of 1.5 L. Therefore, the patient was to receive 4.5 L of fluid during the first 24 hours of hospitalization. In order for relatively rapid rehydration to be achieved, half of the fluid (2.25 L) was infused during the first 8 hours, and the remainder over the subsequent 16 hours. Accordingly, an infusion of ½-normal saline solution was started at a rate of 300 ml/hr. No potassium was added to the initial fluid until urine output was established. The patient's potassium deficit was calculated at 15 mEq, plus a 24-hour maintenance requirement of 40 mEq.

Within the first hour of therapy, the urine output was equivalent to 7.5 ml/kg/hr, and at the end of this hour, 15 mEq/L of potassium were added to the infusion and continued for the next 23 hours at that concentration. The patient's bicarbonate deficit was calculated at 86.4 mEq. Half of the calculated deficit (44 mEq) was administered in the initial infusion, and an additional 44 mEq were administerd over the next 8 hours. A summary of the patient's fluid and electrolyte therapy is outlined in Table 14–8.

Hyperthermia. A common finding in moderate to severe salicylate intoxication, hyperthermia may be treated with tepid-water sponge baths or a cooling blanket. The aggressiveness of treatment for hyperthermia depends on the degree of fever present. Rarely will temperatures less than 40°C require treatment other than the assurance of the patient's comfort.[44,45]

Hyperpnea. Although possibly alarming and bothersome to the patient, hyperpnea is actually of benefit in that it maintains a respiratory alkalosis and thus prevents a precipitous fall in the blood pH. Hyperpnea per se does not require treatment, and respiratory depressants should be avoided in the salicylate-intoxicated patient.

Hypoglycemia. Rarely encountered in severe salicylate intoxication, hypoglycemia is most commonly encountered in infants and young children. When hypoglycemia does occur, it is a potentially life-threatening complication and requires immediate attention.[8-12] An initial dose of 2 ml/kg of 50% glucose should be given, followed by a constant infusion of 15% glucose to maintain adequate blood glucose levels.[46]

Seizures. These may occur in salicylate-intoxicated patients as either direct results of high levels of salicylate within the CNS or as indirect effects of electrolyte imbalance, prolonged acid-base disturbance, or hypoglycemia. An interesting finding has been reported by Thurston and associates that suggests that low CNS glucose levels may be present with normoglycemia.[47] Convulsions that are either severe or that continue in the presence of appropriate management of the primary cause may respond to the administration of intravenous diazepam, 0.1 to 0.3 mg/kg, to a total of 10 mg.[41] If necessary, other anticonvul-

Table 14–8. Fluid and Electrolyte Therapy during Hospitalization

TIME	SOLUTION	RATE ML/HR	Na$^+$	ADDITIONAL ELECTROLYTES K$^+$	Cl$^-$	HCO$_3^-$
0–1 hr	½ NS	300	—	15 mEq/L	—	44 mEq
2–8 hrs	D$_5$ ¼ NS	300	—	15 mEq/L	—	44 mEq/L*
9–24 hrs	D$_5$ ¼ NS	130	—	—	—	—
Day 2	Isolyte P†	70	—	—	—	—
Day 3	IV stopped, patient placed on oral fluids.					

* Bicarbonate was added to only the first liter of fluid during hours 2–8.
† Isolyte P (per liter): Na$^+$, 25 mEq; K$^+$, 20 mEq; Mg^{2+}, 3 mEq; Cl$^-$, 22 mEq; HPO$_4^{2-}$, 3 mmol; acetate, 23 mEq.

sant agents may be used if the seizures are either refractory to or recur after a therapeutic dose of diazepam. Persistent or repeated convulsive episodes are generally considered indications for the use of extracorporeal procedures to remove salicylate from the body.

Tetany. This rarely occurs as a result of frank hypocalcemia in salicylate intoxications. Tetany may appear, however, as an indication of overly aggressive bicarbonate therapy or as the result of a decrease in the proportion of ionized calcium, which occurs during the early phase of intoxication when alkalosis is present. Tetany secondary to overly aggressive bicarbonate administration requires the cessation of alkali therapy and, if needed, the intravenous administration of calcium supplements. Tetany secondary to respiratory alkalosis is difficult to treat. However, it may prove helpful to have the patient cautiously rebreathe expired air.

Hemorrhagic manifestations. These may be the result of a variety of coagulation defects. However, they are rarely of serious clinical significance. Many clinicians recommend the administration of Vitamin K_1 (phytonadione) to counteract the specific effect of salicylate inhibition of prothrombin formation.[31]

Enhancement of Elimination

Salicylate is inactivated or eliminated from the body by four parallel pathways. These are (1) conjugation with glycine to form salicyluric acid, (2) conjugation with glucuronic acid to form salicyl phenolic glucuronide or acyl glucuronide, (3) hydroxylation to gentisic acid, and (4) renal excretion of unchanged salicylate.[7,48,49]

The elimination of salicylate is unusual in that the two most quantitatively important pathways, formation of salicyluric acid and salicyl phenolic glucuronide, are saturable at therapeutic doses of salicylate. When saturation occurs, the overall elimination is measured as nonlinear, and the length of time required to eliminate the drug increases. However, since the renal excretion of unchanged salicylate is a linear process, the proportion of unchanged salicylate entering the renal tubule increases as saturation occurs. As a result, the renal elimination of salicylate becomes a quantitatively more important pathway, and methods to enhance the effectiveness of renal excretion of salicylate are indicated.

Diuresis. Simple water diuresis is of limited value since the rate of excretion of salicylate is not affected appreciably by above-normal urine volumes, and is not recommended. Osmotic diuresis with mannitol or urea has been reported to produce small increases in the renal elimination of salicylate.[50] However, such therapy may exacerbate the electrolyte imbalance and may prove to be of limited efficacy.

Forced alkaline diuresis has been shown to produce a marked increase in the elimination of salicylate.[51] The renal elimination of salicylate is exquisitely sensitive to changes in urine pH above 6, and clearance rates have been measured in humans that are increased four- to fivefold as the pH of the urine is changed from 5 to 8. These clearance rates are probably greater than would be anticipated from simple ion trapping alone. Since the pKa (the pH at which 50% is ionized) of salicylate is 3.4, approximately 97.5% of the salicylate within the renal tubule is ionized at a pH of 5.

There is no ready explanation why the clearance of salicylate should increase when the urine pH is raised from 5 to 8. It may be that methods employed to alkalinize the urine also produce a significant systemic pH gradient between the extracellular and intracellular space, thus "trapping" salicylate in the extracellular space and increasing the proportion of salicylate available for renal excretion. Although an exact explanation may be lacking, the empiric data suggest that alkaline diuresis is a valuable therapeutic tool indicated in the management of moderate and severe salicylate poisoning.

The administration of sodium bicarbonate has been widely advocated to achieve alkalinization of the urine and thus enhance elimination of salicylate from the body. However, Done and Temple report that this approach was suggested following observations undertaken in patients who were mildly to moderately intoxicated, and that urinary alkalinization is both dangerous and difficult to achieve in severely intoxicated patients.[13] This is not meant to discourage the use of urinary alkalinization as a therapeutic tool, but rather to caution against the administration of potentially dangerous quantities of bicarbonate in an attempt to alkalinize the urine and thus the production of systemic alkalosis. In addition, the restoration of any pre-existing potassium deficit is essential if urinary alkalinization is to be achieved. Other alkalinizing agents, such as tromethamine and acetazolamide, may increase intracellular pH, thus "trapping" salicylate intracellularly, and should be used cautiously.[52,53] Such agents may also produce a transient extracellular acidosis, which will complicate pre-existing pathology.

Dialysis and hemoperfusion. In certain cases, the clinical severity of the poisoning is such that extracorporeal methods employed to enhance the removal of salicylates may be lifesaving. Criteria for the institution of these procedures have been suggested,[54] and include (1) severe intoxication unresponsive to conservative measures, (2) a serum salicylate level in excess of 150 mg/dl, (3) measured elimination half-life greater than 15 hours, (4) failure to alkalinize the urine with appropriate bicarbonate therapy, and (5) renal and/or hepatic failure.

The commonly considered methods for extracorporeal removal of salicylate include exchange transfusion, peritoneal dialysis, hemodialysis, and resin hemoperfusion. Exchange transfusion has little or no place in the treatment of salicylate poisoning at the present time, because the same result can be achieved more rapidly and safely with other procedures.[55]

Peritoneal dialysis is a moderately efficient method that offers the advantages of availability in most hospitals, is relatively simple and safe, and requires less laboratory monitoring than hemodialysis. Peritoneal dialysis is less efficient than hemodialysis in achieving a rapid reduction in the salicylate level,[56,57] but can be continued without interruption for relatively long periods of time. Because salicylate is highly bound to serum proteins, peritoneal dialysis employing a 5% solution of human albumin, together with the appropriate concentrations of electrolytes, is far more efficient than the use of a protein-free dialysate.[54] Commercially available Albumisol is a 5% solution of human albumin in an isosmotic buffer, which contains the necessary quantities of essential electrolytes, with the exception of potassium and calcium.[13]

Hemodialysis is an efficient method for removal of salicylate from the body.[58,59] In facilities where this procedure can be made available and that have experienced hemodialysis teams, it should be considered in those patients who are severely intoxicated and who appear to be responding inadequately to less drastic therapy. However, the procedure suffers from numerous disadvantages, such as the need for extremely careful laboratory monitoring, technical difficulties in small children, length of time required, and the threat of dangerous blood volume fluctuations in infants.

Charcoal or resin hemoperfusion may be the most efficient and safest method for the extracorporeal removal of absorbed salicylate. Numerous animal studies have documented its efficacy in the removal of salicylate.[60,61] It also provides the advantage of relatively small blood volume shifts and a relatively short procedure. Hemoperfusion columns rarely require more than 100 to 200 ml of blood at any time, and the procedure is about two to three times more efficient than hemodialysis. Therefore, the length of the procedure is only one third to one half as long as a comparable hemodialysis procedure.

PROGNOSIS

Although accidental ingestion of salicylates is a frequent problem, over 50% of the hospitalized cases of salicylism in children have been due to chronic ingestion associated with therapeutic misuse. Salicylates also are frequently taken by adults in suicide attempts. The toxic effects of salicylates (aspirin, sodium salicylate, and methyl salicylate) are qualitatively identical when ingested in the same amounts (mg/kg of body weight). Methyl salicylate (oil of wintergreen), however, accounts for a disproportionally higher number of morbidities and mortalities. This enhanced toxicity is due to its high concentration of methyl salicylate (over 90%).

The symptoms and clinical findings exhibited by the intoxicated patient, as well as the length of hospitalization and overall outcome, will vary depending on the age and state of health of the patient, the amount of the salicylate ingested, whether the intoxication is due to an accidental ingestion or to therapeutic overdosage, and selection of appropriate therapy. Clinical findings that may contribute to the overall morbidity and mortality include severe acid-base and fluid and electrolyte disturbances, metabolic aberrations, pulmonary edema, and renal insufficiency. There do not appear to be long-term sequelae associated with the salicylates once they have been cleared from the body.

REFERENCES

1. McIntire MS, Angle CR, and Grush ML: How effective is safety packaging? *Clin Toxicol* 9:419–425, 1976.

2. Done AK, et al: Evaluations of safety packaging for the protection of children. *Pediatrics, 48*:613–627, 1971.

3. Poison Control Statistics: Annual reports. National Clearinghouse for Poison Control Centers, U.S. Government Printing Office, 1962–1975.

4. *Handbook of Nonprescription Drugs.* 6th Ed. Washington, D.C., American Pharmaceutical Society, 1979.

5. Done AK: Salicylate intoxication: Significance of measurements of salicylate in blood in cases of acute ingestion. *Pediatrics, 26*:800–807, 1960.

6. Boxer L, Anderson FP, and Rowe DS: Comparison of ipecac-induced emesis with gastric lavage in the treatment of acute salicylate ingestion. *J Pediatr, 74*:800–803, 1969.

7. Levy G: Clinical pharmacokinetics of aspirin. *Pediatrics, (Suppl), 62*:867–872, 1978.

8. Cotton EK, and Fahlberg VI: Hypoglycemia with salicylate poisoning. *Am J Dis Child, 108*:171–173, 1964.

9. Mortimer EA, and Lepow ML: Varicella with hypoglycemia possibly due to salicylates. *Am J Dis Child, 103*:583–590, 1962.

10. Hecht A, and Goldner MG: Hypoglycemic action of acetylsalicylate. *Metabolism, 8*:418–428, 1959.

11. Limbeck GA, et al: Salicylates and hypoglycemia. *Am J Dis Child, 109*:165–167, 1965.

12. David DS, et al: Aspirin induced hypoglycemia in a patient on hemodialysis. (letter) *Lancet,* 2:1092–1093, 1971.

13. Done AK, and Temple AR: Treatment of salicylate poisoning. *Mod Treatment, 8*:528–551, 1971.

14. Winters RW, et al: Disturbances of acid-base equilibrium in salicylate intoxication. *Pediatrics,* 23:269–285, 1959.

15. Tenney SM, and Miller RM: The respiratory and circulatory action of salicylate. *Am J Med,* 19:498–508, 1955.

16. Woodbury DM, and Fingl E: The salicylates. In *The Pharmacologic Basis of Therapeutics.* 5th Ed. Edited by LS Goodman and A Gilman. New York, Macmillan, 1975, pp. 328–329.

17. Brem J, et al: Salicylism, hyperventilation, and the central nervous system. *J Pediatr, 83*:264–266, 1973.

18. Done AK: Treatment of salicylate poisoning: Review of personal and published experiences. *Clin Toxicol, 1*:451, 1968.

19. Segar WE, and Holliday MA: Physiologic abnormalities of salicylate intoxication. *N Engl J Med, 259*:1191–1198, 1958.

20. Miyahara JT, and Karler R: Effect of salicylate on oxidative phosphorylation and respiration of mitochondrial fragments. *Biochem J, 97*:194–198, 1965.

21. Brady TM: The action of sodium salicylate and related compounds on tissue metabolism in vitro. *J Pharmacol Exp Ther,* 117:39–51, 1956.

22. Kaplan EH, Kennedy J, and David J: Effects of salicylate and other benzoates on oxidative enzymes of the tricarboxylic acid cycle in rat tissue homogenates. *Arch Biochem Biophys, 51*:47–61, 1954.

23. Schwartz R, et al: Organic acid excretion in

salicylate intoxication. *J Pediatr, 66*:658–666, 1965.

24. Segar WE: The critically ill child: Salicylate intoxication. *Pediatrics, 44*:440–444, 1969.

25. Temple AR: Pathophysiology of aspirin overdosage toxicity with implications for management. *Pediatrics (Suppl), 62*:873–876, 1978.

26. Al-Mondhiry H, Marcus AJ, and Spaet TH: On the mechanism of platelet function inhibition by acetylsalicylic acid. *Proc Soc Exp Biol Med, 133*:632–636, 1970.

27. Rossi EC, and Green D: Disorders of platelet function. *Med Clin North Am, 56*:35–46, 1972.

28. Marx JL: Blood clotting: The role of prostaglandins. *Science, 196*:1072-1075, 1977.

29. Smith MJH, et al: Platelets, prostaglandins and inflammation. *Agents Actions, 6*:701–704, 1977.

30. Robin ED, David RD, and Rees SB: Salicylate intoxication with special reference to the development of hypokalemia. *Am J Med, 26*:869–882, 1959.

31. Smith MJH: The metabolic basis of the major symptoms in acute salicylate intoxication. *Clin Toxicol, 1*:387, 1968.

32. Hill JB: Salicylate intoxication. *N Engl J Med, 288*:1110–1113, 1973.

33. Hill JB: Experimental salicylate poisoning: Observations on the effects of altering blood pH on tissue and plasma salicylate concentrations. *Pediatrics, 47*:658–665, 1971.

34. Temple AR, et al: Salicylate poisoning complicated by fluid retention. *Clin Toxicol, 9*:61, 1976.

35. Hrnicek G, Skelton J, and Miller WC: Pulmonary edema and salicylate intoxication. *JAMA, 230*:866–867, 1974.

36. Davis PR, and Burch PE: Pulmonary edema and salicylate intoxication. *Ann Intern Med, 80*:553–554, 1974.

37. Kahn A, and Blum D: Fatal respiratory distress syndrome and salicylate intoxication in a two-year old. *Lancet, 2*:1131–1132, 1979.

38. Sorensen SC: Adult respiratory distress syndrome in salicylate intoxication. *Lancet, 1*:1025, 1979.

39. Temple AR: Emesis and emetics. Bulletin of the Intermountain Regional Poison Control Center, Salt Lake City, Utah, 3(1), January 1976.

40. Blacow NW (ed): *Martindale's The Extra Pharmacopoeia*. 26th Edition. London, Pharmaceutical Press, 1976, p. 1720.

41. Rumack BH: *Poisindex*. Denver, Colorado, Micromedex, Inc., 1980.

42. Kreisberg RA: Diabetic ketoacidosis: new concepts and trends in pathogenesis and treatment. *Ann Intern Med, 88*:681–695, 1978.

43. Maxwell MH, and Kleeman CR (eds): *Clinical Disorders of Fluid and Electrolyte Metabolism*. 3rd Ed. New York, McGraw Hill, 1980, pp 459–478, 1563–1576.

44. Done AK: Antipyretics. *Pediatr Clin North Am, 19*:167–177, 1972.

45. Stern RC: Pathophysiologic basis for symptomatic treatment of fever. *Pediatrics, 59*:92–98, 1977.

46. Saul HS: Hypoglycemia of infants and children. In *Pediatric Therapy*. 5th Ed. Edited by HC Shirkey. St. Louis, C.V. Mosby Co., 1976, pp. 857–862.

47. Thurston JH, et al: Reduced brain glucose with normal plasma glucose in salicylate poisoning. *J Clin Invest, 49*:2139–2145, 1970.

48. Levy G, and Tsuchiya T: Salicylate accumulation kinetics in man. *N Engl J Med, 287*:430–432, 1972.

49. Levy G, Tsuchiya T, and Amsel LP: Limited capacity for salicyl phenolic glucuronide formation and its effect on the kinetics of salicylate elimination in man. *Clin Pharmacol Ther, 13*:258–268, 1972.

50. Lawson AA, et al: Forced diuresis in the treatment of acute salicylate poisoning in adults. *Q J Med, 38*:31–48, 1969.

51. Morgan AG, and Polak A: Excretion of salicylate in salicylate poisoning. *Clin Sci, 41*:475–484, 1971.

52. Strauss J, and Nahas GG: The use of amine buffer (THAM) in treatment of acute salicylate intoxication. *Proc Soc Exp Biol Med, 105*:348–351, 1960.

53. Feuerstein RC, Finberg L, and Fleishman E: The use of acetazolamide in the therapy of salicylate poisoning. *Pediatrics, 25*:215–227, 1960.

54. Schlegel RJ, et al: Peritoneal dialysis for severe salicylism: an evaluation of indications and results. *J Pediatr, 69*:553–562, 1966.

55. Spritz N, et al: The use of extracorporeal hemodialysis in the treatment of salicylate intoxication in a 2 year old child. *Pediatrics, 24*:540–543, 1959.

56. Heldorf JN, et al: Intermittent peritoneal dialysis using 5 percent albumin in the treatment of salicylate intoxication in children. *J Pediatr, 58*:226–236, 1964.

57. Etteldorf JN et al: Intermittent peritoneal dialysis in the treatment of experimental salicylate intoxication. *J Pediatr, 56*:1–10, 1960.

58. Dukes, DC, et al: The treatment of severe aspirin poisoning. *Lancet, 2*:329–331, 1963.

59. Levy RI: Overwhelming salicylate intoxication in an adult. Acid base changes during recovery with hemodialysis. *Arch Intern Med, 119*:399–402, 1967.

60. Rosebaum JL: The use of resin hemoperfusion in the treatment of acute drug intoxication. *Ind Eng Chem Prod Res Dev, 14*:99–101, 1975.

61. Chen CN, Coleman DL, Adrade JD, and Temple AR: Pharmacokinetic model for salicylate, cerebrospinal fluid, blood, organs and tissues. *J Pharm Sci, 67*:38–45, 1978.

Chapter 15

Digoxin

Brent R. Ekins

Digitalis glycosides have been used medicinally for centuries. William Withering published his now famous book on digitalis glycosides, noting his first use of the plant extract, in 1775.[1] Surprisingly, he was not aware of its cardiac effects. The knowledge of plants containing cardiac glycosides is recorded in Ebers Papyrus (ca. 15 B.C.), indicating that the ancient Egyptians were aware of the therapeutic effects of such concoctions.

Currently, digoxin and digitoxin are the most commonly available commercial products. These two preparations are similar, with the exception of their pharmacokinetic parameters (e.g., factors such as absorption and distribution characteristics, biopharmaceutic properties, and pharmacokinetic profiles). These differences are shown in Table 15–1. The use of either drug is frequently associated with toxicity, and as a result, physicians are generally acquainted with acceptable treatment measures. Acute digoxin poisoning is unique, however, in that the patients involved are often not suffering from underlying diseases, as are those using the drug chronically; the effect on electrolytes is different; and the management approach is different from that used for chronic digoxin intoxication.

Many conclusions drawn from this article for digoxin overdosage may be appropriate for digitoxin and other glycosides, as long as the previously mentioned differences are taken into account. Clinicians should become familiar with the pathophysiology of digoxin poisoning and therapeutic modalities available for the optimal management of acutely intoxicated patients.

Table 15–1.   Pharmacokinetic Parameters of Orally Administered Digoxin and Digitoxin in Patients with Normal Renal Function

PARAMETERS	DIGOXIN	DIGITOXIN
Latency	0.5 hr	1 to 2 hrs
Peak effect	3 to 6 hrs	4 to 12 days
Plasma half-life	1.5 days	4 to 6 days
Duration of action	3 to 6 days	2 to 3 weeks
Percent GI absorption	50 to 80	90 to 100
Percent bound to serum proteins	23	97
Principal excretory pathway	Renal; some GI	Hepatic and renal
Available dosage forms	Tablets: 0.125, 0.25, 0.5 mg; Elixir: 0.05 mg/ml	Tablets: 0.05, 0.01, 0.15, 0.2 mg

CASE REPORT

A 20-month-old child weighing 11.4 kg was found by his grandmother with an open bottle of her "heart medicine." There were no tablets in his mouth at the time, although several tablets were moist, and many were spread around the room. The grandmother did not think much about it at the time, assuming the child would not eat the distasteful medicine. The heart pills were identified as digoxin, 0.25 mg.

Approximately 1 hour later, the child became sick and vomited several times, including what appeared to be particles resembling pills. The grandmother at this time mentioned the events to the parents, who had not been home when the accident occurred. They phoned the Poison Control Center to determine the relationship, if any, of the apparent illness and events of the previous hour. They were unable to determine the number of tablets involved. The parents were instructed in the use of syrup of ipecac and were told to bring the child to the emergency room.

Physical examination on arrival at the ER revealed a well-developed child who was having dry vomiting and who was pale but alert. His vital signs were blood pressure, 98/54 mm Hg; pulse, 60/min and irregular, respirations, 28/min; and temperature, 37°C. Upon examination, the head, eyes, ears, mouth, nose, neck, and chest were all normal. An EKG showed first-degree AV block, intermittent secondary AV block (not of the Wenckebach type), and occasional supraventricular extrasystoles. The abdominal examination showed a soft abdomen with active bowel sounds and no organomegaly. Skin, joints, and extremities were all normal with no petechiae, ecchymoses, rashes, or swelling. The neurology evaluation showed slight decreased deep tendon reflexes. The remainder of the physical examination results were found to be within normal limits.

Laboratory values on admission included sodium, 139 mEq/L; potassium, 5.0 mEq/L; chloride, 107 mEq/L; HCO_3^- content, 19 mEq/L; BUN, 12 mg/dl; glucose, 117 mg/dl; calcium, 10 mg/dl; albumin, 4.8 g/dl; creatinine, 0.4 mg/dl. The chest x-ray examination, urinalysis, and hematologic values were all within normal limits. The initial digoxin blood level was reported as 12 ng/ml taken at $3\frac{1}{2}$ hours postingestion.

An intravenous infusion was begun, and the patient was transferred to the coronary care unit, where additional EKG findings showed runs of sinus rhythm, with first-degree AV block and second-degree 2-1 block. Heart rate decreased to 60 to 70/min, interspersed with runs of supraventricular tachycardia up to rates of 150 beats/min during the first hour of admission.

CLINICAL ASSESSMENT AND MANAGEMENT OF THE PATIENT

This case aptly presents several problems inherent in the assessment and management of this particular type of intoxication. As evidenced by the initial assessment and evaluation of the patient, few if any abnormalities were detected. Laboratory values, x-ray examination results, and most of the physical examination results were ostensibly normal.

Acute digoxin poisoning is characterized by a number of factors that need special attention. From this, an adequate therapeutic plan may be established to prevent serious complications and to preserve life. The following points should be considered: (1) manifestations and mechanisms of acute digoxin toxicity, (2) assessment of the severity of the poisoning, (3) drugs or therapeutic modalities that can decrease the toxicity of the absorbed drug, (4) how the acute poisoning situation differs from the chronic digoxin toxicity, (5) appropriate management and treatment, (6) endpoints of therapy, (7) prognosis for an acute digoxin poisoning, and (8) aspects of the acute poisoning that will need to be clarified.

MANIFESTATIONS AND MECHANISMS OF TOXICITY

Symptoms of acute digoxin poisoning appear to follow a different pattern than what standard and available pharmacology and toxicology textbooks would indicate for digoxin intoxication. Symptoms such as nausea, vomiting, diarrhea, drowsiness, fatigue, headache, blurred vision, colored vision, delirium, slow and irregular pulse, decreased blood pressure, and other cardiac arrhythmias are commonly listed as symptoms of digoxin toxicity. Few, if any, reference sources differentiate between the acute and chronic overdosage; none differentiate between pediatric and adult poisonings. A recent review documented 44 cases, of which 14 were pediatric cases.[2]

The manifestations of an acute digoxin poisoning are associated with a more limited number of symptoms and a complete lack of most of the commonly reported symptoms associated with chronic digoxin toxicity. Nausea and vomiting frequently are seen after an acute poisoning. It is thought that this effect is a result of a digoxin-mediated increase in vagal nerve activity.[3]

Various arrhythmias are expected in overdosage. Varying degrees of conduction defects, ranging from first-degree heart block to complete AV dissociation, are possible. The heart rate is generally slow and may be regular. In some patients, ventricular extrasystoles or other intraventricular abnormalities have been reported. Almost without exception, more significant abnormalities have been noted in elderly patients, some of whom have been taking the drug previously or have a history of cardiac disease. Therefore, the diseased heart, for which digitalis would be prescribed, is particularly likely to develop arrhythmias. In contrast, patients with normal hearts are not as likely to develop serious ventricular arrhythmias.[4-8]

Symptoms of acute digoxin poisoning seem to be correlated somewhat with the magnitude of the free serum digoxin level. Delayed symptoms are common with this drug, owing to a long absorption and distribution phase throughout the body. Hyperkalemia is a serious and prominent abnormality in massive overdose. The mechanism of this toxic effect is thought to be directly related to the ATPase-mediated sodium/potassium pump inhibition by digoxin.[9] Normally, this energy-dependent system maintains a high intracellular and low extracellular potassium gradient. As digoxin levels rise, this mechanism is severely damaged, and a rise in serum potassium results. The rise in extracellular potassium is accompanied by progressive intracellular potassium depletion.

As this effect becomes more pronounced, the electrical system involved in membrane stability and action potential firing is impaired. The individual cells lose their ability to respond to electrical stimuli required for muscle contraction. In the myocardium, where these cells are the pacemaker cells for the heart, this effect can be devastating, with decreased function or asystole resulting. The finding of elevated serum potassium levels is well documented, but the incidence and severity has not been uniformly studied or reported; thus, at this point no definitive statement can be made about the expected magnitude of this finding for all patients.

ASSESSMENT OF THE SEVERITY OF INTOXICATION

The symptoms and severity of this acute poisoning can be adequately assessed during the first 12 to 24 hours through monitoring of vital signs, symptoms, physiochemical indices, and serum digoxin levels. A reliable history of the ingestion may also be helpful in the prediction of the severity or outcome.

Physical examination. This drug is well absorbed, and symptoms are likely to occur during the first hours of the ingestion. Physical examination of the patient shortly after overdosage will provide a baseline for observations throughout the therapy. However, early in the time course, the physical examination cannot be relied upon in the assessment of severity, since it is likely that the patient will be asymptomatic.

Dose. The reported lethal dose for an adult is 15 mg,[10] whereas no such corresponding dose has been identified in children. Patients have survived doses as low as 70 μg/kg and 80 μg/kg, resulting in

peak serum digoxin levels of 20 ng/ml and 14 ng/ml, respectively. A dose of 440 μg/kg, resulting in peak serum digoxin level of 42 ng/ml, resulted in cardiac arrest unresponsive to treatment.[11] Precise information is limited by the lack of consistency in reports of weights, doses, and serum levels. The radioimmunoassay for digoxin was developed for widespread use in 1969,[12] yet reporting of serum digoxin levels has not gained widespread usage.

Serum potassium concentrations. There are now a number of cases documenting the high incidence of hyperkalemia associated with the acute digoxin overdosage.[4,5,8,13–16] In two cases, high serum potassium levels were reported at 9.8 mEq/L[11] and 13.5 mEq/L.[16] Both patients were unresponsive to aggressive measures, both had high serum digoxin and serum potassium levels, and both died. Bismuth and associates studied serum potassium levels in acute digitoxin overdoses.[17] They found serum potassium values useful in prognosticating the severity and outcome of acute overdoses.

The mean serum potassium concentration on admission was 6.15 ± 0.75 (2SD) mEq/L in 24 patients who succumbed, and 4.2 ± 0.52 (2SD) mEq/L in 67 patients who recovered. The difference in the mean serum values was found to be significant ($p < 0.001$). Patients with initial potassium levels below 5.0 mEq/L all survived, and no patient in whom the initial potassium level was greater than 5.5 mEq/L lived. It is presumed that the magnitude of the potassium change would be similar in acute digoxin overdoses compared to digitoxin overdosage, and that it could be used similarly to prognosticate the severity of the acute poisoning. Furthermore, almost all hospitals are able to determine quickly the serum potassium values, whereas serum digoxin levels are not done routinely at many hospitals, and others require 24 to 48 hours for such a request to be processed. The serum potassium should be monitored hourly through the course of the treatment.

Half-life. The mean half-life values found normally for infants and children are reported to be 32.5 and 38 hours respectively,[18,19] and are not considered significantly different from those found in adults with normal renal function. However, the half-life values in acute poisonings are reported to be shortened and range from 6 to greater than 35 hours in adults, and 12 hours in one pediatric patient.[8,11,13,20] This shortened half-life has not been substantiated by other authors.[5,14,21]

Some of the inherent problems in the assessment of the half-life in these patients are probably due to the fact that an adequate number of blood samples is not uniformly obtained, it is not always certain that the absorption-distribution phase of the drug has been terminated, and patients have not been monitored for a sufficient length of time to capture completely the correct elimination pattern.

The digoxin half-life can be determined by collection of three to four plasma samples drawn after the initial treatment and after the absorption and distribution phases have terminated, usually 6 to 12 hours after the ingestion. Samples drawn prior to this time will be interesting but of little direct usefulness. Early in the course of the intoxication, monitoring of plasma potassium levels is more meaningful than measurement of digoxin serum concentrations.

Plotting of the plasma digoxin levels on semilogarithmic graph paper against time of the ingestion should result in a straight line indicating that they follow first-order elimination kinetics. Significant deviation from this predicted straight line connecting the sample points may be due, in part, to continued absorption of the drug. The half-life determination is currently used to delineate drug elimination in both pediatric and adult patients. If the kinetics of a drug are altered in an overdose situation,

appropriate steps must be taken to effectively resolve the toxic state. In most cases of altered kinetics in overdosage, longer half-lives (not shorter ones) are the expected findings.

In the case presented, additional blood samples were taken at 12, 36, 60, and 96 hours postingestion, with corresponding serum digoxin values of 5.5 ng/ml, 3.5 ng/ml, 1.9 ng/ml, and 0.6 ng/ml (Fig. 15–1). The last four values were used to determine the elimination half-life in this patient. The first value obtained at 3½ hours postingestion was not included because it did not represent the elimination of the drug. It most likely had components of the absorption and distribution phases. The digoxin half-life in this child was determined through least-squares method, resulting in a half-life value of 26.05 hours. This was not felt to be significantly outside the normal range for half-life in children, as reported by Dungan and associates[18] and Hernandez and associates.[19]

PROCEDURES FOR DECREASING TOXICITY

Procedures designed to decrease the toxicity of an absorbed agent act by terminating the physiologic effect or by shortening the duration of pharmacologically active drug concentration. Techniques of active drug removal such as alkaline diuresis, peritoneal dialysis, or hemodialysis are useful in the management of severe drug overdose. These methods are effective provided the drug meets such criteria as low protein binding, high water solubility, and efficient dialyzability.

Renal elimination. Digoxin clearance is known to approximate the glomerular filtration rate, and tubular mechanisms (secretion and reabsorption) are known to have a role in digoxin elimination.[22,23] A number of papers have suggested that this be exploited by administration of potent diuretics to increase digoxin

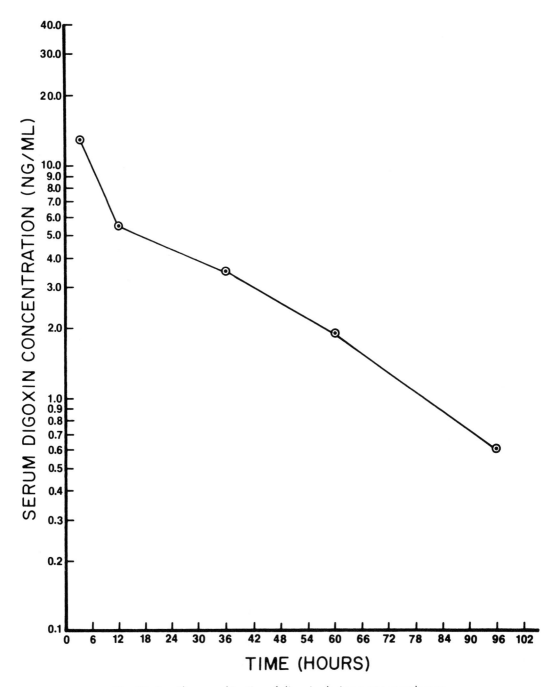

Fig. 15–1. Pharmacokinetics of digoxin during acute overdosage.

elimination.[24–28] Bloom and Nelp and Brown and associates reported no increase in digoxin elimination in normal adults given oral furosemide.[24,29] Unfortunately, in the first paper, no data were presented to support the contention that digoxin clearance was unaltered,[24] and in the second paper the furosemide was given 10 hours after the dose of digoxin.[29] This is after the normal absorption-distribution phase for digoxin and the phase in which serum-to-tissue ratios would be low, especially serum-to-myocardial tissue ratios.[30] Semple and associates[31] found that elimination rates of normal subjects given therapeutic amounts of digoxin were unaltered by a single intravenous injection of 20 mg of furosemide.

In contrast to these findings, McAllister and associates and Rotmensch and associates demonstrated that an increase in urine volume was accompanied by a proportional increase in digoxin clearance.[28,32] In both cases, when a positive effect was noted, intravenous furosemide was given shortly after the ingestion. Within the first few hours, higher serum to tissue ratios of digoxin would be expected, and more free digoxin would be presented to the glomerulus for excretion. The tissue uptake of digoxin is a slow process, which reaches its plateau 6 to 8 hours after oral doses.[33,34] It is thus conceivable that prior to the equilibration of the drug into the tissue site, significant amounts of free-circulating drug could be eliminated.

The usefulness of potent diuretics after an acute digoxin overdose seems to be somewhat correlated to the dosage form of the drug and to the time administered. Large intravenous doses of furosemide given within the first few hours of an intoxication seem to substantially increase the drug's elimination and decrease its half-life. Presently this appears to be a feasible, simple, and relatively safe method of decreasing toxicity. However, caution must be exercised in the adminis-

tration of furosemide if the time elapsed between ingestion and treatment is greater than 6 hours.

Dialysis and hemoperfusion. In most reports, the use of peritoneal dialysis and hemodialysis has not been shown to be effective in decreasing toxicity.[35,36] Digoxin fails to meet many of the required criteria for a dialyzable drug. It is highly protein bound and is present in serum in small amounts.

A recent paper described two cases in which hemoperfusion was found useful in the management of acute digoxin overdosage.[37] In one patient who inadvertently intoxicated herself, hemoperfusion with a macroreticular styrene divinylbenzene copolymer was employed. The plasma digoxin level was 4.4 ng/ml when the error was noted. Within 150 minutes of hemoperfusion, the patient said that the symptoms of her nausea had cleared. The 4-hour procedure was well tolerated, and no change occurred in the platelet count.

The second patient had deliberately taken an overdose of 17.5 mg of digoxin. She underwent hemoperfusion with cellulose-coated activated charcoal. A percutaneous femoral vein catheterization was done to obtain access to the circulation. Within 5 hours, the digoxin level had fallen from 15 ng/ml, and the platelet count remained unchanged. At the end of dialysis, the patient was fully alert and did not require continued assistance with isoproterenol or atropine, as was needed prior to hemoperfusion.

From the limited number of patients treated with charcoal hemoperfusion or resin hemoperfusion, it appears that this is a promising and potentially useful way to decrease toxicity from the already absorbed drug. However, more research is necessary before this therapy can be recommended on a routine basis. Peritoneal dialysis or hemodialysis still may be useful in the management of electrolyte abnormalities.

Digoxin-specific antibodies. There is

one case in the literature where purified Fab fragments of ovine digoxin-specific antibodies reversed severe intoxication in a patient who had taken 25 mg of digoxin in a suicidal attempt.[38] Within 5 hours, the serum potassium concentration fell from 8.7 to 4.0 mEq/L. Similarly, free digoxin concentrations fell sharply to an undetectable level. This case is unique in that it demonstrated a lack of side effects from the procedure and was effective in reversing the toxic effects.

Hess and associates further delineated this effect in animal models.[39] They found that antibody pretreatment significantly protected the animals from toxicity. They also found that the cardiac glycoside receptors of the myocardium were not blocked by the antibody-hapten complexes; these were then pharmacologically inactive.

It was suggested that the advantage of the Fab fragment antibody over the intact antibody were smaller size (permitting more rapid distribution and elimination), shorter half-life, and lower immunogenicity. At present, this active drug removal method is not widely available and should only be attempted in serious intoxications and where materials and resources are available.

DIFFERENCES BETWEEN ACUTE POISONING AND CHRONIC TOXICITY

The most important aspect of therapy involving these two situations is the recognition of the need to manage each entity

Table 15–2.   Differences in Acute Intoxication and Chronic Toxicity

	ACUTE INTOXICATION	CHRONIC TOXICITY
Types of patients most commonly involved	In many cases the patients are normal, with no history of cardiac disease.	Patients are ill, with cardiac abnormalities underlying the toxic state. The symptoms may mimic the condition for which the drug is being used.
Symptoms on admission	Nausea and vomiting are the most consistent findings. Diarrhea is occasionally observed.	Anorexia, nausea, vomiting, headache, malaise, fatigue, weakness, and drowsiness are common. Diarrhea is less common. Paresthesias and neuritic pain, along with confusion, disorientation, aphasia, delirium, hallucinations, and (rarely) convulsions are all reported. Visual changes and skin rashes are also noted.
Findings on admission	Electrocardiogram (EKG) findings indicate supraventricular arrhythmias in general, with heart block and bradycardia most commonly noted. There is a general lack of ventricular arrhythmias.	All types of arrhythmias have been attributed to digitalis glycosides. The most common arrhythmias are nonparoxysmal nodal tachycardia, atrial tachycardia with AV dissociation, and bidirectional ventricular tachycardia.
Serum potassium	Levels are normal or increased, depending on the magnitude of the overdose and the relative time course.	Levels are normal or decreased, depending on the use of potent loop diuretics, nutrition status of the patient, and the presence of other factors which are known to affect the potassium level.
Serum digoxin determinations	High levels are always expected and seem to correlate roughly with the magnitude of the rise in serum potassium and the presence of serum cardiac arrhythmias.	The levels may not identify therapeutic ranges clearly, but are generally elevated in any prominent toxic state. Borderline normal values may represent toxicity.
Serum half-life of digoxin	The half-life has been reported shortened in both adults and children, although conflicting reports have been published.	The half-life determination for both adults and children is similar.

differently. The symptoms of each are somewhat similar, but the pathophysiologic features are dissimilar. The differences between acute intoxication and chronic toxicity characteristics are presented in Table 15–2.

One of the most striking and significant findings relates to the serum potassium. The finding of hypokalemia associated with digitalis and diuretic therapy is well known.[40,42] In contrast, the acutely digoxin-poisoned individual is likely to have a mild to pronounced hyperkalemia.[4,5,11,13,15,17,38,43]

Another important finding is the lack of ventricular extrasystoles and intraventricular disturbances during acute digoxin intoxications in some patients. In these patients, including young children, young adults, and possibly older adults without prior cardiac disease, the digitalis effects on the myocardium in an acute overdose produce toxicologic symptoms that appear to be similar.[11,44] Patients with known cardiac disease are much more likely to develop ventricular arrhythmias and serious complications.

INDICATED THERAPEUTIC MEASURES

In all cases of acute intoxications, the entire situation must be assessed, other drugs must be ruled out, and the history and symptoms must be put into proper perspective. The time of ingestion, the amounts and types of drugs involved, the current clinical presentation of the patient, previous therapeutic steps that have been taken, and any other pertinent information must be collected.

The toxic dose for digoxin varies widely among all patient groups studied. It is felt that if the dose ingested is less than a normal digitalization dose (approximately 2 to 3 mg for an adult and less than 0.08 mg/kg for a child), no serious toxicity will develop. If doses can be assessed and determined to be less than these amounts, it is likely that no further therapy or treatment would be necessary other than to empty the stomach.

Measures Designed to Decrease Absorption

Although various methods are available to empty the GI tract, in studies comparing emesis and lavage, emesis has a distinct advantage over lavage in most cases.[45–47] This is particularly true in pediatric patients, owing to the size of the openings in the double lumen tube.[47] It is known that the bioavailability of digoxin is erratic and that, in massive overdoses, there may be delayed absorption due to decreased GI emptying.

Oral administration of syrup of ipecac, along with an adequate amount of fluids, is the preferred method of inducing vomiting in an alert patient. Gastric lavage using a nasogastric double lumen tube or a large-bore oral gastric hose is an alternative to the use of syrup of ipecac.

Once the stomach has been evacuated, activated charcoal and a saline cathartic are recommended. It has been shown that activated charcoal inhibits the absorption of usual or normal therapeutic doses of digoxin in normal subjects.[48] Administration of activated charcoal will absorb the glycosides remaining in the intestines, as well as any drug that is recirculated through the enterohepatic cycling of digoxin. Activated charcoal is most effective during the first hour of the intoxication prior to absorption of the drug.[9,10]

If a patient were to come into the ER for treatment after a delay, activated charcoal would still be useful, since a small portion of the absorbed drug is resecreted into the small intestine. The dose of activated charcoal is 50 to 100 g for adults and 20 to 25 g in children, given orally as a slurry. The use of other nonabsorbable, locally acting agents, such as cholestyramine, colestipol, and sodium edetate, to bind with digoxin has not been successful.[49–51]

Protective Therapy

Once digitalis toxicity has been established and various arrhythmias are present, several corrective measures are available. Atropine is perhaps the drug of choice for initial treatment. Atropine has been widely used in the treatment of digoxin poisonings and acts to reverse the increased vagal tone on the SA or AV node and to restore sinus rhythm.[10,11,15,43,52–54]

Doses of atropine should be titrated according to the needs of the patient. The initial normal adult intravenous dose is 0.4 to 0.6 mg, but much higher doses are well tolerated in management of this intoxication. The initial pediatric dose is 10 μg/kg IV over a 2- to 3-minute period. In both adult and pediatric patients, repeated doses of atropine may be given if needed. Close simultaneous monitoring with an EKG should be performed in all cases in which large doses of atropine are being used.

Phenytoin sodium (Dilantin) can convert atrial tachycardia with block to sinus rhythm and improve the impairment of the AV conduction. This drug also has the ability to reverse any ventricular arrhythmias, especially premature ventricular contractions and ventricular tachycardia.[8] As with atropine, the intravenous route is recommended for the administration of phenytoin sodium, with careful monitoring throughout the treatment. A dose of 25 to 50 mg should be given slowly IV over 5 to 10 minutes; it should be realized that following IV administration of phenytoin, a 2-hour distribution phase has been noted in healthy adult volunteers.[55] If the drug is given slowly over a period of time, excessive peak blood levels can be avoided, and more consistent and effective treatment can be maintained.

Lidocaine has also been used successfully to treat ventricular tachycardia arrhythmias, premature ventricular contractions, and bigeminy.[11,56,57] Although lidocaine would be a good drug of choice, it lacks some of the advantages noted with phenytoin sodium, particularly the ability to improve conduction through the AV node. Propranolol is reported to be useful in some types of digitalis-induced arrhythmias because of its antiadrenergic properties.[4,10,58] Generally, because of the effects of acute digoxin intoxications contrasted with those of chronic toxicity, propranolol has limited usefulness. It tends to slow the rate of depolarization, depress conduction velocity, and decrease automaticity, and it may in fact increase and intensify a pre-existing heart block.

The use of potassium salts is generally contraindicated unless a significant documented hypokalemia is detected.[42,49,59] One of the most prominent aspects of acute digoxin intoxication is a tendency to impair the energy-dependent potassium pump that maintains the high intracellular potassium concentrations. It is for this reason that patients significantly poisoned with digitalis glycosides tend to have high extracellular serum potassium levels. In addition to the effects of digitalis glycosides, which cause varying degrees of conduction defects, potassium in high doses can accentuate these abnormalities.[42,54,59]

If significant elevation of the serum potassium level occurs, immediate treatment measures to reduce this should be instituted. These may include temporary measures such as the use of glucose and insulin to drive potassium into the cells. Dialysis may be useful to correct the fluid and electrolyte imbalances. Rises in serum potassium at a gradual rate may be managed by the use of orally or rectally administered solutions of sodium polystyrene sulfonate (Kayexalate) in 70% sorbitol.

Occasionally, overdrive suppression with a temporary transvenous pacemaker is necessary to abolish ventricular tachyarrhythmias.[8,41] Despite the potential effectiveness of overdrive pacing, it should not be used unless standard measures have failed, because of the hazards of digitalis-induced decreased vulnerability threshold. Cardioversion is generally not advisable in the presence of digitalis intoxication, because malignant ventricular arrhythmias may ensue. However, when other methods have failed to control life-threatening rhythm disturbances, cardioversion can be attempted with low energy levels.

ENDPOINTS OF THERAPY

The endpoints of therapy are designed to ensure that the peak effects have passed and that the clinical picture prognosticates relative safety for the patient. Any symptomatic patient should, therefore, have a complete workup, including at least several blood level measurements taken after the distribution phase of the drug has terminated, serial chemistry determination, with special observation of the serum potassium result, and electrocardiographic monitoring. If, during the course of the intoxication, the patient develops clinical manifestations of toxicity, and the serum potassium levels begin to rise rapidly, or prominent cardiac arrhythmias develop, full-scale monitoring and protective therapy should be instituted. Measures designed to minimize and decrease absorption of the drug should be started.

The case presented is typical of a mild to moderate intoxication. The child was given three doses of atropine (0.1 mg/dose) to control episodes of bradycardia that developed. The peak effect was seen 6 to 8 hours postingestion, and all of the doses of atropine needed to control the arrhythmias were used during this time. Blood levels were continued for 60 hours from the time of ingestion, the last level being obtained after the patient's discharge. At the time of discharge, the patient was stable, the EKG was normal, and all parameters, except for the continued presence of digoxin, had returned to normal levels.

The presence of a normal EKG, the absence of noncardiac side effects, and normal physiochemical indices should be the goals of therapy. As with the patient presented, it is not necessary to achieve an absolute zero level of digoxin prior to discharge. However, a substantial decrease in the serum digoxin value should be demonstrated, and prominent pharmacologic effects should have subsided prior to discharge.

PROGNOSIS FOR ACUTE DIGOXIN OVERDOSE

The prognosis for an acute overdosage is determined largely by the prior physical health of the patient, the dose ingested, the time involved in treatment, and the presence of other simultaneously ingested drugs. Findings that may contribute to increased morbidity or mortality rates include serious cardiac manifestations, elevated serum potassium level, hypotension, renal failure, or pre-existing cardiovascular disease. Adequate care and support must be rendered in any serious overdosage to assure complete and uncompromised recovery. There do not appear to be any long-term sequelae resulting from this intoxication once it has cleared. Similarly, no late deaths are expected after an apparent recovery.

UNCLARIFIED ASPECTS OF ACUTE INTOXICATION

There remain a number of unanswered questions concerning digoxin intoxication. The unexplained lack of serious cardiac toxicity for the normal, sound heart in contrast to the heart with a history of cardiac disease needs to be explored. The basic mechanisms at the tissue level have yet to be fully clarified. Another unresolved issue is the role of substances or procedures to decrease the toxicity of absorbed drug. This includes the use of digoxin-specific antibodies and hemoperfusion devices.

The answers to these questions, and others yet to be identified, will greatly facilitate more effective approaches to the prevention and treatment of acute digoxin overdosages.

REFERENCES

1. Withering W: An account of the Foxglove and some of its medicinal uses with practical remarks on dropsy and other diseases. Birmingham, England, Swiney, 1785.
2. Ekins BR, and Watanabe AS: Acute digoxin poisonings: Review of therapy. *Am J Hosp Pharm*, 35:268–277, 1978.
3. Runge TM: Clinical implications of differences in pharmacodynamic action of polar and nonpolar cardiac glycosides. *Am Heart J*, 93:248–255, 1977.
4. Asplund J, et al: Four cases of massive digitalis poisoning. *Acta Med Scand*, 189:293–297, 1971.
5. Bertler A, Gustafson A, and Redfors A: Massive digoxin intoxication. *Acta Med Scand*, 194:245–249, 1973.
6. Fowler RS, Rathi L, and Keith JD: Accidental digitalis intoxication in children. *J Pediatr*, 64:188–200, 1964.
7. Joos HA, and Johnson JL: Digitalis intoxication in infancy and childhood. *Pediatrics*, 20:866–876, 1957.
8. Rumack BH, Wolfe RR, and Gilfrich H: Phenytoin treatment of massive digoxin overdose. *Br Heart J*, 36:405–408, 1974.
9. Smith TW, and Haber E: Digitalis. *N Engl J Med*, 289:945–951, 1973.
10. Wharton CFP: Attempted suicide by digoxin self administration and its management. *Guy's Hosp Rep*, 119:243–251, 1970.
11. Smith TW, and Willerson JT: Suicidal and accidental digoxin ingestion, report of five cases with serum digoxin level correlations. *Circulation*, 44:29–36, 1971.
12. Smith TW, Butler VP, and Haber E: Determination of therapeutic and toxic serum digoxin concentrations by radioimmunoassay. *N Engl J Med*, 281:1212–1216, 1969.
13. Citrin D, Stevenson IH, and O'Malley K: Massive digoxin overdose: Observation on hyperkalemia and plasma digoxin levels. *Scott Med J*, 17:275–277, 1972.
14. Holt DW, Traill TA, and Brown CB: The treatment of digoxin overdose. *Clin Nephrol*, 3:119–122, 1975.
15. Navab R, and Honey M: Self poisoning with digoxin: Successful treatment with atropine. *Br Med J*, 3:660–661, 1967.
16. Reza MJ, et al: Massive intravenous digoxin overdose. *N Engl J Med*, 291:771–778, 1974.
17. Bismuth C, et al: Hyperkalemia in digitalis poisoning: Prognostic significance and therapeutic implications. *Clin Toxicol*, 6:153–162, 1973.
18. Dungan WT, et al: Tritiated digoxin XVIII studies in infants and children. *Circulation*, 46:983–988, 1972.
19. Hernandez A, et al: Pharmacodynamics of 3H-digoxin in infants. *Pediatrics*, 44:418–423, 1969.
20. Hobson JD, and Zettner A: Digoxin serum half-life following suicidal digoxin poisoning. *JAMA*, 223:147–149, 1973.
21. Watanabe AS, et al: Acute digoxin poisoning: Case report and determination of elimination half-life. In *Management of the Poisoned Patient*. Edited by BH Rumack and AR Temple. Princeton, New Jersey, Science Press, 1977.
22. Doherty JE, Ferrel CB, and Towbin EJ: Localization of the renal excretion of the tritiated digoxin. *Am J Med Sci*, 258:181–189, 1969.
23. Steiness E: Renal tubular secretion of digoxin. *Circulation*, 50:103–107, 1974.
24. Bloom PM, and Nelp WB: Relationship of the excretion of tritiated digoxin to renal function. *Am J Med Sci*, 251:133–144, 1966.
25. Doherty HE, Perkins WH, and Wilson MC: Studies with tritiated digoxin in renal failure. *Am J Med*, 37:536–544, 1964.
26. Marcus FI, Kapadia GJ, and Kapadia GG: The metabolism of digoxin in normal subjects. *J Pharmacol Exp Ther*, 145:203–209, 1964.
27. Bissett JK, et al: Tritiated digoxin. XIX. Turnover studies in diabetes insipidus. *Am J Cardiol*, 31:327–335, 1973.
28. Rotmensch HH, et al: Furosemide-induced forced diuresis in digoxin intoxication. *Arch Intern Med*, 138:1495–1497, 1978.
29. Brown DD, Dormois JC, and Abraham GN: Effect of furosemide on the renal excretion of digoxin. *Clin Pharmacol Ther*, 20:395–400, 1976.
30. Doherty JE, Perkins WH, and Flanigan WJ: The distribution and concentration of tritiated digoxin in human tissues. *Ann Intern Med*, 66:116–124, 1967.
31. Semple P, Tilstone WJ, and Lawson DH: Furosemide and urinary digoxin clearance. *N Engl J Med*, 293:612–613, 1975.
32. McAllister RG, et al: Effect of intravenous furosemide on the renal excretion of digoxin. *J Clin Pharmacol*, 16:110–117, 1976.
33. Doherty JE: The clinical pharmacology of digitalis glycosides: A review. *Am J Med Sci*, 225:382–414, 1968.
34. Marks HB: Factors that affect the accumulation of digitalis glycosides by the heart. In *Basic and Clinical Pharmacology of Digitalis: Proceedings of a Symposium*. Springfield, Ill, Charles C Thomas, 1972, p. 70.
35. Ackerman GL, Doherty JE, and Flanigan WJ: Peritoneal dialysis and hemodialysis of tritiated digoxin. *Ann Intern Med*, 67:718–723, 1967.
36. Finkelstein FO, et al: Pharmacokinetics of digoxin and digitoxin in patients undergoing hemodialysis. *Am J Med*, 58:525–531, 1975.
37. Smiley JW, Warch NM, and Del Guercia ET: Hemoperfusion in the management of digoxin toxicity. *JAMA*, 240:2736–2737, 1978.
38. Smith TW, et al: Reversal of advanced digoxin intoxication with Fab fragments of digoxin-specific antibodies. *N Engl J Med*, 294:797–800, 1976.

39. Hess T, Scholtysik G, and Riesen W: The prevention and reversal of digoxin intoxication with specific antibodies. *Am Heart J, 96*:486–495, 1978.

40. Bigger JJ, and Strauss HC: Digitalis toxicity—drug interactions promoting toxicity and the management of toxicity. *Sem Drug Treat, 2*:147–177, 1972.

41. Mason DT, et al: Current concepts and treatment of digitalis toxicity. *Am J Cardiol, 27*:546–559, 1971.

42. Fisch C, and Knoebel SB: Recognition and therapy of digitalis toxicity. *Prog Cardiovasc Dis, 13*:71–96, 1970.

43. Duke M: Atrioventricular block due to accidental digoxin ingestion treated with atropine. *Am J Dis Child, 124*:754–756, 1972.

44. Inniss CN: The contrast between digitalis intoxication in children and adults. *J Natl Med Assoc, 62*:38–41, 1970.

45. Abdallah AH, and Tye A: A comparison of the efficacy of emetic drugs and stomach lavage. *Am J Dis Child, 113*:571–575, 1967.

46. Arnold FJ, et al: Evaluation of efficacy of lavage and induced emesis in the treatment of salicylate poisoning. *Pediatrics, 23*:286–301, 1959.

47. Boxer L, Anderson FP, and Rowe DS: Comparison of ipecac-induced emesis with gastric lavage in the treatment of acute salicylate ingestion. *J Pediatr, 74*:800–803, 1969.

48. Härtel G, Manninen F, and Reissell P: Treatment of digoxin intoxication. *Lancet, 2*:158–159, 1973.

49. Bernstein MS, Neschis M, and Collini F: Treatment of acute massive digitalis poisoning by administration of chelating agent. *N Engl J Med, 261*:961–963, 1959.

50. Caldwell JH, and Greenberger NJ: Cholestyramine enhances digitalis excretion and protects against lethal intoxication. *J Clin Invest, 49*:16a, 1970.

51. Bazzano G, and Sansone-Bazzano G: Digitalis intoxication: Treatment with a new steroid binding resin. *JAMA, 220*:828–830, 1972.

52. Miller PH: Efficacy of atropine in the treatment of digitalis induced AV block. *Dis Chest, 56*:229–230, 1969.

53. Petch CP: Sinoatrial heart-block. *Lancet, 2*:1313–1314, 1970.

54. Rios JC, Dziok CA, and Ali NA: Digitalis-induced arrhythmias: Recognition and management. *Cardiovasc Clin, 2*:261–279, 1970.

55. Gugler R, Manion CV, and Azarnoff DL: Phenytoin: Pharmacokinetics and bioavailability. *Clin Pharmacol Ther, 19*:135–142, 1976.

56. Collinsworth KA, Kalman SM, and Harrison DC: The clinical pharmacology of lidocaine as an antiarrhythmic drug. *Circulation, 50*:1217–1230, 1974.

57. Rosen MR, Hoffman BF, and Wit AL: Electrophysiology and pharmacology or cardiac arrhythmias v. cardiac antiarrhythmic effects of lidocaine. *Am Heart J, 89*:526–536, 1975.

58. Buchanan J: Self poisoning with digitalis glycosides. *Br Med J, 3*:661–663, 1967.

59. McNamara DG, Brewer EJ, and Ferry GD Jr: Accidental poisoning of children with digitalis. *N Engl J Med, 271*:1106–1108, 1964.

Chapter 16

Acetaminophen

Peter A. Czajka

Acetaminophen (paracetamol) has been used as a mild analgesic and antipyretic since the early 1950s.[1] The first case of acute acetaminophen overdosage was recorded in the medical literature in 1967.[2] Subsequently, clinicians began to recognize the problem as reflected in the progressive number of indexed entries in four major medical journals (Fig. 16–1).

Currently, acetaminophen is contained in over 100 medicinal formulations and accounts for approximately 29% of dosage units on the market (cf aspirin, with 71%).[3] In the United Kingdom, where acetaminophen is used more widely, increased availability of acetaminophen is directly correlated with a rise in deaths associated with acetaminophen overdosage.[4] Because of the widespread availability of acetaminophen, clinicians should be readily familiar with the potentially toxic and lethal consequence of acetaminophen overdosage.

CASE REPORT

A 16-year-old white female weighing 43 kg had ingested approximately 25 500-mg acetaminophen tablets during an argument with her husband. After realizing she did not truly intend suicide, she went to an emergency room 4 hours after the ingestion. She claimed to have taken only her oral contraceptive pill that morning and denied recent exposure to other drugs, including ethanol. This anxious patient denied any discomfort, nausea, vomiting, or right upper quadrant abdominal pain.

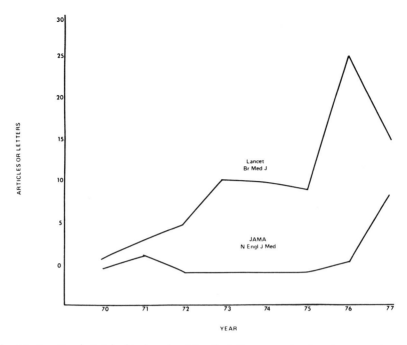

Fig. 16–1. Yearly total of indexed entries that discuss acetaminophen overdosage.

Physical examination revealed a well-developed, well-nourished female in no apparent distress. Her vital signs were blood pressure, 124/60 mm Hg; pulse, 112/min and regular; respirations, 16/min; and temperature, 37°C. Results of examination of the head, eyes, ears, nose and throat were normal, and no scleral icterus was present. The lungs were clear and the heart was not enlarged. No murmur or gallops were detected upon auscultation, but the patient appeared to have sinus tachycardia.

Normal bowel sounds were heard in the abdominal examination. The liver spanned approximately 8 cm and was mildly tender to palpation. Urogenital and rectal examination results were normal. Extremities were normal in appearance, without petechiae or purpura. This patient also had normal cerebral and cerebellar function. Cranial nerves were grossly intact, and no abnormal reflexes were elicited. On admission to the emergency room, her EKG, chest x-ray examination, electrolytes, urinalysis and complete blood count were within normal limits.

CLINICAL ASSESSMENT AND MANAGEMENT OF THE PATIENT

The presence of significant pathology is not ostensibly evident from a review of this patient's physical examination and preliminary laboratory tests. However, the appropriate assessment and management of a suspected acetaminophen overdosage demands consideration of the following: (1) manifestations and mechanisms of acetaminophen toxicity, (2) assessment of the potential severity, (3) drugs that alter the toxicity, (4) appropriate management, (5) the endpoints of therapy, (6) general prognosis, (7) unclarified aspects of acetaminophen toxicity.

MANIFESTATIONS AND MECHANISMS OF ACETAMINOPHEN TOXICITY

The symptoms of acute acetaminophen poisoning have been characterized in three phases.[5] In the first phase, which occurs within the first day of the ingestion, the patient is usually in no acute distress, but may complain of nausea, vomiting, and diaphoresis. During the second phase, 24 to 72 hours after the ingestion, the patient apparently improves, but serum concentrations of hepatic enzymes begin to rise, and the right-upper-quadrant abdominal area may be tender to palpation. The third phase, which typically occurs 3 to 5 days after the ingestion, is characterized by signs of hepatic necrosis (jaundice, increased prothrombin time, and hypoglycemia), hepatic encephalopathy, possibly renal failure, and (rarely) cardiac abnormalities.

The patient presented was temporally in the first phase, but mild right-upper-quadrant tenderness was elicited within 6 hours of ingestion. Clearly, this patient was in no acute distress and had no physical complaints or pathologic findings.

However, when acetaminophen toxicity becomes manifest 3 to 5 days after the ingestion, patients may experience hepatic, renal, and myocardial dysfunction.

Hepatotoxicity

The proposed mechanism of the hepatotoxicity of an acetaminophen overdosage implicates a metabolite (Fig. 16–2). In therapeutic amounts, acetaminophen is eliminated by formation of sulfate (20% to

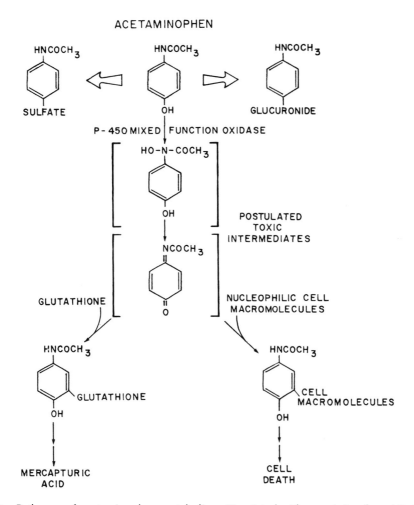

Fig. 16–2. Pathways of acetaminophen metabolism. (Reprinted with permission from Mitchell JR, et al: Acetaminophen-induced hepatic injury: Protective role of glutathione in man and rationale for therapy. *Clin Pharmacol Ther,* 16:676, 1974.)

30%) or glucuronide (45% to 55%) conjugates, which are excreted in the urine with small amounts (0% to 2%) of unchanged drug.[6] In addition, some of the drug (15% to 25%) is metabolized by the cytochrome P-450 mixed-function oxidase system in the liver. (A recent paper has cited numerous studies that differ on the relative extent of metabolism by the three proposed pathways.[7]) This pathway produces an intermediary metabolite (Fig. 16–2), which possesses a highly reactive arylating moiety.[8] With therapeutic doses, this intermediate reacts with the hepatic stores of glutathione to ultimately form mercapturic acid, a nontoxic metabolite excreted in the urine.

With an acute overdosage of acetaminophen, metabolism proceeds in generally the same fashion. However, the available hepatic stores of sulfate and glutathione apparently become depleted.[6,8] Consequently, with less sulfate available, more acetaminophen remains to be metabolized by the alternative mechanisms, namely conjugation with glucuronic acid or glutathione.

It is theorized that more of the drug is metabolized by the cytochrome P-450 system, either coinciding with or resulting from sulfate depletion, and this eventually depletes the hepatic stores of glutathione. With inadequate concentrations of glutathione, the intermediary metabolite covalently bonds to the cellular protein macromolecules to cause hepatocellular death.[8] The role of the cytochrome P-450 system in the production of hepatonecrosis has been demonstrated in rats pretreated with piperonyl butoxide, an inhibitor of this metabolic pathway. When hepatotoxic amounts of acetaminophen were administered, no apparent toxicity developed.[9]

Hepatic glutathione concentrations have been measured in animals before and after exposure to hepatotoxic amounts of acetaminophen. The findings indicate that glutathione stores must be depleted by 70% of their normal concentration for hepatonecrosis to occur.[8] Indirect evidence of these findings has been demonstrated in humans and will be discussed in a later section on drugs that alter the hepatotoxicity of acetaminophen.

Renal Toxicity

Renal failure resulting from acute tubular necrosis has been associated with acute acetaminophen overdosage. In patients who develop severe hepatonecrosis, 10% to 40% have been estimated to develop renal tubular necrosis.[10] The cause of this renal damage is still the subject of controversy. An animal study suggests that the renal lesion is produced by glutathione depletion in the kidney,[11] analogous to the mechanism of hepatotoxicity. However an analysis of 160 patients with fulminant hepatic failure revealed that the frequency of renal failure in acetaminophen-poisoned patients (53%) was not significantly higher (p>0.05) than in those patients with hepatic failure due to other causes (38%).[12] Whether acute tubular necrosis is a direct effect of an acetaminophen metabolite or a secondary complication of hepatic failure, patients who potentially may develop hepatotoxicity should have their renal function closely monitored.

Cardiac Abnormalities

In association with hepatonecrosis, a few patients have developed ST-segment abnormalities and T-wave flattening,[13] pericarditis,[14] or myocardial necrosis.[15] The cause and incidence of these cardiac abnormalities within the framework of acute acetaminophen poisoning are presently unknown.

ASSESSMENT OF POTENTIAL SEVERITY OF INTOXICATION

The severity of many acute intoxications, except those with acetaminophen, can be adequately assessed within the first

12 to 24 hours after the exposure through monitoring of symptoms, biochemical indices, and vital signs. However, the delayed onset of significant findings until 3 to 5 days after an acute acetaminophen overdosage obviates the utility of many traditional methods of assessment.

Physical examination. Shortly after an acute overdosage of acetaminophen, physical examination of the patient provides a baseline for future observation, since most patients are initially asymptomatic. In addition, the presence of abnormal findings within the first few hours after a suspected acetaminophen overdosage should suggest concomitant exposure to other drugs or the presence of an underlying disease. Therefore, physical examination alone cannot be relied upon to adequately assess the severity of acute acetaminophen toxicity.

Dose. The smallest dose reported to have produced hepatotoxicity in an adult is 5.4 g, whereas 10 g has produced hepatic coma and death.[16] However, the amount of acetaminophen ingested does not accurately estimate the potential severity. This concept was demonstrated in five patients who claimed they had each ingested from 10 to 50 g of acetaminophen, but only one developed slight SGOT (serum glutamic-oxaloacetic transaminase) elevations. All patients had nontoxic plasma concentrations of acetaminophen, and two patients had nontoxic plasma half-lives of acetaminophen.[17]

Hepatic enzyme concentrations. Experience with acetaminophen-intoxicated patients demonstrates that hepatic enzyme concentrations do not rise significantly shortly after the ingestion.[18,19] Since acetaminophen hepatotoxicity becomes manifest 2 to 3 days after the ingestion, hepatic enzyme concentrations should not be expected to rise before that time. However, peak concentrations may prognosticate the subsequent clinical course. Peak SGOT concentrations in excess of 400 units/L have been correlated with liver

biopsies that demonstrated severe centrizonal necrosis in acetaminophen-poisoned patients.[19]

Similarly, peak concentrations of bilirubin in excess of 4 mg/dl and prothrombin time ratios in excess of 2.2 on the third and fifth days after ingestion were associated with death or encephalopathy. At lower values, death did not occur.[18] These observations substantiate the nonpredictive value of hepatic enzyme concentrations as initial methods of assessing the severity of an acetaminophen overdosage. However, these biochemical indices can be useful as baseline measurements, indicators of underlying disease, prognosticators of the later clinical course, and measures of the efficacy of treatment.

Nomogram. Because of the limited value of conventional methods of assessment, a nomogram was developed for acetaminophen poisoning.[5] This nomogram (Fig. 16–3) was based on observations of over 30 patients.[20] Its utility in differentiating patients who are unlikely to develop toxicity has been confirmed by

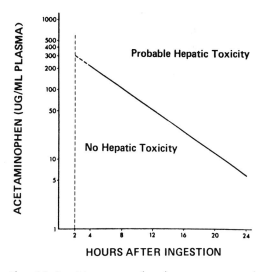

Fig. 16–3. Nomogram for the assessment of acute acetaminophen overdosage. (Reprinted with permission from Rumack BH, and Matthew H: Acetaminophen poisoning and toxicity. *Pediatrics,* 55:871, 1975. Copyright American Academy of Pediatrics 1975.)

a contemporary multiclinic study.[21] When this nomogram is used, a single determination of the plasma acetaminophen concentration is usually sufficient, but the plasma should be collected at least 4 to 6 hours after the ingestion. This interval allows for full absorption from the gastrointestinal tract. Obviously, the approximate time of ingestion must also be reasonably certain within a 2-hour variance.

Since plasma concentrations of acetaminophen can assume a crucial role in patient assessment, the analytic method must be accurate. Recently, the accuracy of colorimetric and gas chromatographic assays has been questioned.[22,23] A high-pressure liquid chromatographic method has been described that appears to be reasonably accurate throughout the plasma concentrations usually observed.[24]

Half-life. Determination of the plasma half-life of acetaminophen can aid the initial assessment of acetaminophen toxicity. In healthy adults who consumed 1.5 to 1.8 g of acetaminophen, the half-life of acetaminophen averaged 2 hours. For patients who experienced acetaminophen-induced hepatotoxicity, the mean half-life was 7.6 hours. These findings led to the generalization that hepatotoxicity was likely when the half-life exceeded 4 hours, and that hepatic coma was possible when the half-life exceeded 12 hours.[20] However, intersubject variation in elimination rates undoubtedly exists. As evidence for this variation, mean half-lives of 1.95 hours,[25] 1.9 hours,[26] approximately 4 hours,[27] and 1.5 to 3.0 hours[7] were reported for healthy adults who received nontoxic doses of acetaminophen.

Acetaminophen half-life determination begins with the collection of three to four plasma samples that are drawn 2 to 3 hours apart. They should be collected after most of the drug has been absorbed, usually 4 to 6 hours after the ingestion.[26] A plot of these concentrations on a semilogarithmic graph should produce a reasonably straight line and an estimate of half-life.

Although the relative predictive value of a half-life determination and comparison to the nomogram has yet to be evaluated, the half-life can be determined irrespective of the time of ingestion, an obvious advantage in the uncooperative patient. However, the time required to collect sufficient samples to determine a half-life may delay recognition of severely poisoned patients and should not delay treatment. Until studies have demonstrated the superiority of one method, the first plasma concentration of acetaminophen should be compared to the nomogram and the assessment confirmed by half-life estimation, when the initial concentration falls near the discriminating line of the nomogram.

In the case presented, the patient had no abnormal physical findings or complaints. By her account, she had ingested 12.5 g of acetaminophen. Approximately 6 hours after the ingestion, her biochemical indices of liver function were reported as SGOT, 29 units/L; SGPT, 24 units/L; total bilirubin, 0.7 mg/dl; and prothrombin time, 12.0 seconds, with the control, measured at 11.3 seconds. The peak SGOT concentration of 76 units/L was recorded 48 hours after the ingestion and gradually declined to the baseline concentration within 5 days. Similarly, her SGPT peaked at 48 units/L, and total bilirubin peaked at 1.5 mg/dl, both 12 hours after ingestion.

All other laboratory test results were within normal limits. The patient's initial right-upper-quadrant abdominal pain subsided within 12 hours of the ingestion, and she remained asymptomatic. The plasma concentration of acetaminophen at 6 hours after the ingestion was 15 μg/ml, but a half-life was not determined. Results of all methods of assessment, except the history of the amount ingested, suggested that this patient should not develop hepatotoxicity.

DRUGS THAT ALTER TOXICITY

Since acetaminophen toxicity is related to the production of a toxic intermediary metabolite, a substance that alters the metabolism of acetaminophen could alter the degree of toxicity.

Increased toxicity. Agents that can induce the activity of the microsomal P-450 mixed-function oxidase enzymes (Fig. 16–2) can increase the utilization of this metabolic pathway. It can be seen intuitively that with these induced enzymes, more of the toxic intermediary metabolite will be formed; hence, greater toxicity will result. The deleterious effect of enzyme induction was demonstrated in rats and mice treated with phenobarbital prior to the administration of acetaminophen.[5] When compared to procedures in which animals received acetaminophen alone, phenobarbital pretreatment markedly potentiated the hepatic necrosis.

These findings were corroborated in acetaminophen-poisoned patients who had chronically taken known enzyme-inducing drugs (barbiturates, ethanol). These patients developed significantly more hepatic necrosis, ($p < 0.05$) with a higher incidence of death and acute renal failure, as compared to patients not regularly exposed to enzyme-inducing drugs.[28] Therefore, the risk of acetaminophen toxicity may be exacerbated in patients regularly exposed to an enzyme-inducing substance.

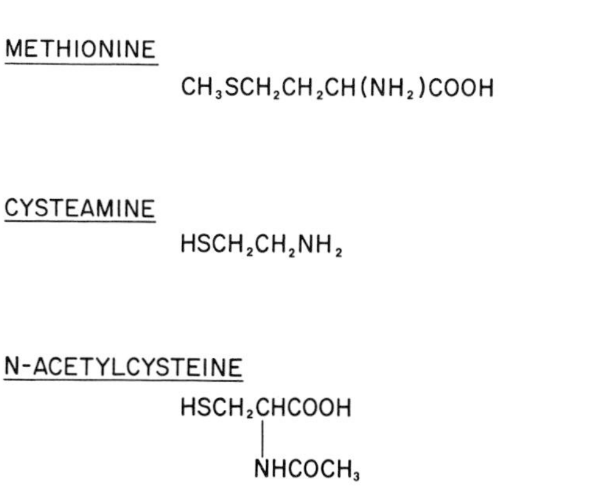

Decreased toxicity. Possible ways to decrease acetaminophen toxicity include the inhibition of the P-450 enzyme system or substitution of a sulfhydryl-containing compound in the hepatocyte. These mechanisms were demonstrated in mice pretreated with piperonyl butoxide, an inhibitor of the P-450 enzyme system. The mice did not develop hepatotoxicity when toxic amounts of acetaminophen were administered. Unfortunately the toxicity of piperonyl butoxide precludes its use in humans.

In the same report, other mice were pretreated with cysteine, a precursor of glutathione. These animals did not develop hepatic damage when they received toxic doses of acetaminophen.[29] This finding led to the investigation of similar protective compounds. Glutathione was administered, but could not adequately penetrate the hepatocyte to offer much protection. Subsequently, precursors to glutathione (cysteine, methionine) or agents that possess a sulfhydryl moiety (cysteamine, N-acetylcysteine), as shown in Figure 16–4, prevented hepatotoxicity in animals.[30]

Presently, methionine, cysteamine, and N-acetylcysteine are used to treat acute acetaminophen overdosage in humans.[31] N-acetylcysteine (Mucomyst) is readily available in this country, but only as a new investigational drug for this indication. A comparison of these agents in reports of acetaminophen-poisoned patients.[21,32–36] is presented in Table 16–1.

GLUTATHIONE

$$H_2NCHCH_2CH_2CONHCHCONHCH_2COOH$$

COOH   CH_2SH

CYSTEINE

$$HSCH_2CH(NH_2)COOH$$

METHIONINE

$$CH_3SCH_2CH_2CH(NH_2)COOH$$

CYSTEAMINE

$$HSCH_2CH_2NH_2$$

N-ACETYLCYSTEINE

$$HSCH_2CHCOOH$$

NHCOCH_3

Fig. 16–4. Glutathione and similar agents.

Table 16–1.   Comparison of Supportive and Protective Treatment

TREATMENT	TIME GIVEN (HR)	N	PERCENT WITH HEPATOTOXICITY*	PERCENT WITH RENAL FAILURE	PERCENT DEATHS	REFERENCE
Supportive only						
	—	52	60	12	6	32
	—	20	55	10	5	34
	—	54	51	7	6	36
	—	12	67	—	0	21
Methionine						
PO	<10	30	10	0	0	35
PO	<12	15	20	0	0	36
Cysteamine						
IV	<10	23	13	0	0	33
IV	<10	20	0	0	0	36
IV	>10	12	66	8	8	36
IV	>10	13	62	8	8	32
IV	>10	16	50	19	6	33
N-acetylcysteine						
IV	<10	29	3	0	0	32
PO	<10	49	17	—	0	21
IV	>10	20	70	15	5	32
PO	>10	51	45	—	0	21

*Hepatotoxicity indicated by SGOT > 1000 units/L.

All three agents, when appropriately administered, were obviously more effective than supportive measures alone. The data also indicate that for these agents to be optimally effective, they should be administered within 10 hours of the ingestion. This temporal relationship seems logical, considering that, in order to have a protective effect, the agent should be present in the hepatocyte, while the toxic intermediary metabolite depletes the hepatic stores of glutathione.

Even though the adverse effects of these therapies have been reported to be primarily nausea and vomiting, at times severe,[30] methionine and cysteamine may induce hepatic coma in some patients with severe hepatotoxicity or cirrhosis.[31,37] Until a comparative controlled trial of these agents is adequately performed and the results of the multicenter trial of N-acetylcysteine are available,[21] all three agents appear to be effective when given within 10 hours of the ingestion.

Unaltered toxicity. The effectiveness of conventional supportive therapy is unsatisfactory (Table 16–1). Similarly, unsatisfactory results have been reported when the following modalities were used: corticosteroids and antihistamines, vitamin E, heparin, hemodialysis, charcoal hemoperfusion, dimercaprol, cholestyramine, penicillamine, and forced diuresis.[30,31,36]

The patient presented denied recent exposure to any known enzyme-inducing substance. Based on the history of the amount ingested, and pending the determination of her plasma acetaminophen concentration, protective therapy appeared to be indicated. She received therapy with N-acetylcysteine administered orally.

APPROPRIATE THERAPY

As with any intoxication, the establishment of adequate vital signs is of paramount importance. If an acetamino-phen-intoxicated patient has life-threatening symptoms shortly after the ingestion, other drugs or underlying diseases should be suspected. After acceptable vital signs have been assured, determination of the time and amount of the overdose by history is mandatory. If definitely less than 3 g of acetaminophen was ingested in an adult, toxicity would be unlikely, and only gastric evacuation would be indicated. However, if the amount is unknown or exceeds 3 to 5 g of acetaminophen (140 mg/kg in children), further treatment should be performed and acetaminophen plasma concentration determined.

Nonspecific Treatment

Generally, patients should receive syrup of ipecac, with copious amounts of fluid, to evacuate the stomach. If contraindications to emesis are present (coma, seizures, or no gag reflex), gastric lavage with the largest tolerable nasogastric tube should be performed. Following gastric evacuation, activated charcoal and a saline cathartic can be useful if administered within an hour of the ingestion[35] or when additional drugs are suspected.

Most of the acetaminophen is probably absorbed within 3 to 4 hours after ingestion.[26] The residual activated charcoal may absorb orally administered protective therapy (N-acetylcysteine).[21] If activated charcoal is administered within 1 hour of ingestion, gastric lavage should be repeated until the gastric aspirate is essentially clear of charcoal before the administration of N-acetylcysteine. In cases with questionable time of ingestion, it would be prudent to avoid administering activated charcoal.

During the initial treatment and subsequent clinical course, laboratory indices of liver function (SGOT, SGPT, bilirubin, PT) and renal function tests (BUN,

creatinine, urinalysis) should be monitored periodically.

Protective Therapy

Of the three protective agents, N-acetylcysteine is readily available in this country as Mucomyst, in 10% and 20% solutions. It is administered orally in an initial dose of 140 mg/kg. Beginning 4 hours later, 70 mg/kg is administered every 4 hours for 17 doses. Mucomyst should be diluted with carbonated beverage (Pepsi-Cola, Coca-Cola, Fresca) or grapefruit juice to make a 5% solution. If the patient vomits a dose within 1 hour of administration, it should be repeated.[21] The Rocky Mountain Poison Center may be called at (800) 525–6115 to allow the use of N-acetylcysteine under its investigational FDA license. In time, N-acetylcysteine may be approved by the FDA for this indication and route of administration, or other dosage schedules, therapies and routes of administration may be proven more efficacious.

In the emergency room, the patient presented promptly received syrup of ipecac, which produced 1.5 L of nonbloody vomitus without tablet fragments. Activated charcoal was not administered. She was admitted for treatment with N-acetylcysteine and received a loading dose of 6 g (140 mg/kg), which was not kept down even after repeated administration. However, maintenance doses of 3 g (70 mg/kg) every 4 hours were retained without complaints.

ENDPOINTS OF THERAPY

Frequently, preventive therapy with agents like N-acetylcysteine must be initiated prior to determination of the patient's acetaminophen plasma concentration. Since the overall effectiveness of protective therapy greatly diminishes when started 10 hours after the ingestion (Table 16–1), the initiation of therapy in many cases must be based upon the amount ingested as determined from the history. This delay in laboratory assessment can be minimized by the ready availability of acetaminophen analysis. Therefore, protective therapy should continue until the results are reported and evaluated.[39]

If the plasma acetaminophen concentration indicates that the risk of hepatotoxicity is minimal, the continuation of protective therapy is not indicated. However, if hepatotoxicity is suggested by the plasma acetaminophen concentration, the full course of protective therapy should be administered. In either situation, after the cessation of therapy, liver and renal functions should be monitored to assess the adequacy of treatment and to identify possible complications. Repeated full courses of protective therapy appear unjustifiable[40] based upon consideration of the mechanism of toxicity of acetaminophen.

In the case presented, when the plasma concentration of acetaminophen, which was drawn 6 hours after ingestion, was reported as 15 μg/ml, the N-acetylcysteine therapy was stopped. The patient received a total of three maintenance doses. Ultimately, the patient was discharged following a psychiatric evaluation and was observed as an outpatient for 1 week after discharge.

GENERAL PROGNOSIS

The outcome of an acute acetaminophen overdosage is generally determined by the amount ingested, the time interval between ingestion and treatment, the plasma concentration of acetaminophen, the selection of appropriate therapy, and the additional toxicity of other drugs concomitantly ingested. In patients who receive only supportive therapy, the mortality rate is 5% to 6%. Similar mortality rates are reported in patients who started protective therapy more than 10 hours after the ingestion. When appropriately administered, protective therapy apparently minimizes the risk of death (Table 16–1).

Histologically, severe acetaminophen-induced hepatotoxicity is characterized by diffuse centrilobular necrosis. Liver biopsies of 22 out of 100 patients who had been intoxicated with acetaminophen revealed centrizonal necrosis of hepatocytes. Lesser damage was found in the remaining 78 patients and was expressed by an abundance of lipofuscin pigment granules, sparse focal hepatonecrosis, and some phagocytosis of lipofuscin. Biopsies were repeated for 39 patients representing both groups 3 months later and demonstrated that the central necrotic zones were completely reconstituted except for one patient.[41] In another series, increased fibrous tissue without evidence of cirrhosis was detected in biopsy specimens 3 months after the initial biopsy.[18]

UNCLARIFIED ASPECTS OF ACETAMINOPHEN TOXICITY

Several questions concerning acetaminophen toxicity currently do not have satisfactory answers. A puzzling phenomenon surrounds the rare reports of acute toxicity in children under 12 years of age.[42,45] A small series of acetaminophen-intoxicated children under 6 years of age, who were assessed as toxic by the plasma concentration-versus-time nomogram, did not develop clinically significant toxicity.[21] Clearly, acetaminophen toxicity is different in young children. Another unresolved issue is the potential for development of hepatotoxicity with chronic use of acetaminophen.[46,47] Similarly, the effects of acetaminophen in patients with underlying hepatic disease are still unknown.[48-50] Futher investigation should provide some answers to these questions and perhaps suggest a method of prevention.

REFERENCES

1. Spooner JB, and Harvey JG: The history and usage of paracetamol. *J Int Med Res (Suppl 4)*, 4:1–6, 1976.
2. Davison DGD, and Eastham WN: Acute liver necrosis following overdose of paracetamol. *Br Med J*, 2:497–499, 1967.
3. Rumack BH: Aspirin versus acetaminophen: A comparative view. *Pediatrics*, 62(*Suppl*),943–946, 1978.
4. Volans GN: Self-poisoning and suicide due to paracetamol. *J Int Med Res (Suppl 4)*, 4:7–13, 1976.
5. Rumack BH, and Matthew H: Acetaminophen poisoning and toxicity. *Pediatrics*, 55:871–876, 1975.
6. Davis M, et al: Paracetamol overdose in man: Relationship between pattern of urinary metabolites and severity of liver damage. *Q J Med*, 45:181–191, 1976.
7. Peterson RG, and Rumack BH: Pharmacokinetics of acetaminophen in children. *Pediatrics*, 62(*Suppl*), 877–879, 1978.
8. Mitchell JR, et al: Acetaminophen-induced hepatic injury: Protective role of glutathione in man and rationale for therapy. *Clin Pharmacol Ther*, 16: 676-684, 1974.
9. Mitchell JR, et al: Acetaminophen-induced hepatic necrosis: 1. Role of drug metabolism. *J Pharmacol Exp Ther*, 187:185–194, 1973.
10. McJunkin B, et al: Fatal massive hepatic necrosis following acetaminophen overdose. *JAMA*, 236:1874–1875, 1976.
11. Mitchell JR, et al: Molecular basis for several drug-induced nephropathies. *Am J Med*, 62:518–526, 1976.
12. Wildinson SP, et al: Frequency of renal impairment in paracetamol over-dosage compared with other causes of acute liver damage. *J Clin Pathol*, 30:141–143, 1977.
13. Will EJ, and Tomkins AM: Acute myocardial necrosis in paracetamol poisoning. *Br Med J*, 2:430–431, 1971.
14. Pimstone BL, and Uys CJ: Liver necrosis and myocardiopathy following paracetamol overdosage. *S Afr Med J*, 42:259–262, 1968.
15. Sanerkin NG: Acute myocardial necrosis in paracetamol poisoning. *Br Med J*, 2:478, 1971.
16. Prescott LF: Hepatotoxic dose of paracetamol. *Lancet*, 3:142, 1977.
17. Ambre J, and Alexander M: Liver toxicity after acetaminophen ingestion. *JAMA*, 238:500–501, 1977.
18. Clark R, et al: Hepatic damage and death from overdose of paracetamol. *Lancet*, 1:66–70, 1973.
19. James O, et al: Liver damage after paracetamol overdose. *Lancet*, 1:579–581, 1975.
20. Prescott LF, et al: Plasma-paracetamol half-life and hepatic necrosis in patients with paracetamol overdosage. *Lancet*, 1:519–522, 1971.
21. Rumack BH, and Peterson RG: Acetaminophen overdose: Incidence, diagnosis, and management in 416 patients. *Pediatrics*, 62(*Suppl*):898–903, 1978.
22. Mace PKF, and Walter G: Salicylate interference with plasma paracetamol method. *Lancet*, 4:1362, 1976.
23. Gilbertson AA, et al: Cysteamine or N-acetylcysteine for paracetamol poisoning? (reply). *Br Med J*, 1:856–857, 1978.
24. Blair D, and Rumack BH: Acetaminophen in serum and plasma estimated by high-pressure liquid chromatography: A micro-scale method. *Clin Chem*, 23:743–745, 1977.
25. Nelson E, and Morioka T: Kinetics of the metabolism of acetaminophen by humans. *J Pharm Sci*, 52:864–868, 1963.
26. Albert KS, Sedman AJ, and Wagner JG: Pharmacokinetics of orally administered acetaminophen in man. *J Pharmacokinet Biopharm*, 2:381–393, 1974.
27. Miller RP, Roberts RJ, and Fischer LJ: Acetaminophen elimination kinetics in neonates, children and adults. *Clin Pharmacol Ther*, 19:284–294, 1976.
28. Wright N, and Prescott LF: Potentiation by previous drug therapy of hepatotoxicity following paracetamol overdosage. *Scott Med J*, 18:56–58, 1973.
29. Mitchell Jr, et al: Acetaminophen-induced hepatic necrosis. IV. Protective role of glutathione. *J Pharmacol Exp Ther*, 187:211–217, 1973.
30. Anon: Paracetamol (acetaminophen) and the liver. *Br Med J*, 1:537–538, 1975.
31. Anon: Treatment of paracetamol poisoning. *Br Med J*, 2:481–482, 1977.
32. Prescott LF, Stewart MJ, and Proudfoot AT: Cysteamine or N-acetylcysteine for paracetamol poisoning? *Br Med J*, 1:856, 1978.
33. Smith JM, et al: Late treatment of paracetamol poisoning with mercaptamine. *Br Med J*, 1:331–333, 1978.
34. Douglas AP, Hamlyn A, and James O: Controlled trial of cysteamine in treatment of acute paracetamol (acetaminophen) poisoning. *Lancet*, 1:111–115, 1976.
35. Crome P. et al: Oral methionine in the treatment of severe paracetamol (acetaminophen) overdose. *Lancet*, 4:829–830, 1976.
36. Prescott LF, et al: Cysteamine, methionine and pencillamine in the treatment of paracetamol poisoning. *Lancet*, 3:109–113, 1976.
37. Phear EA, et al: Methionine toxicity in liver disease and its prevention by chloretracycline. *Clin Sci*, 15:94–117, 1956.
38. Levy G, and Houston JG: Effect of activated charcoal on acetaminophen absorption. *Pediatrics*, 58:432–435, 1976.
39. Peterson RG, and Rumack BH: Toxicity of acetaminophen overdose. *JACEP*, 7:202–205, 1978.
40. Peterson RG, and Rumack BH: N-acetylcysteine for acetaminophen overdosage. *N Engl J Med*, 296:515, 1977.
41. Lesna M, et al: Evaluation of paracetamol-induced damage in liver biopsies. *Virchows Arch (Path Anat)*, 370:333–344, 1976.
42. Glasco SP: Toxicity of paracetamol in children. *Br Med J*, 2:235, 1976.

43. Crome P, et al: Toxicity of paracetamol in children. *Br Med J*, 2:475, 1976.
44. Robertson WO: Changing perspectives on acetaminophen. *Am J Dis Child, 132*:459–460, 1978.
45. Nogen AG, and Bremner JE: Fatal acetaminophen overdosage in a young child. *J Pediatr, 92*:832–833, 1978.
46. Barker JD, deCarle DJ, and Anuras S: Chronic excessive acetaminophen use and liver damage. *Ann Intern Med, 87*:299–301, 1977.
47. Ware AJ, et al: Acetaminophen and the liver. *Ann Intern Med, 88*:267–268, 1978.
48. Rosenberg DM, et al: Acetaminophen and hepatic dysfunction in infectious mononucleosis. *South Med J, 70*:660–661, 1977.
49. Johnson GK, and Tolman KG: Chronic liver disease and acetaminophen. *Ann Intern Med, 87*:302–304, 1977.
50. Bonkowsky HL, Mudge GH, and McMurtry RJ: Chronic hepatic inflammation and fibrosis due to low doses of paracetamol. *Lancet, 1*:1016–1018, 1978.

Chapter 17

Iron

Anthony S. Manoguerra

The potentially lethal effects of the ingestion of large amounts of iron have been known for well over 100 years. However, it is only since the 1940s that attention has been focused on this frequent problem. Forbes is credited for having brought the issue of acute iron poisoning to the attention of the medical profession in 1947.[1] Since then, numerous papers have been published, attempting to increase the medical profession's awareness of the toxicity of iron and the seriousness of the problem. In spite of these reports, there appears to be a general lack of appreciation among health professionals and the general public of the hazard of iron-containing preparations.

Data from the National Center for Health Statistics, Mortality Statistics Branch, show that from 1969 through 1973, 48 children under 5 years of age died from accidental iron poisoning. For the same period, the National Clearinghouse for poison control centers received 2001 voluntary reports of iron ingestions in children under 5 years of age, of which 543 were hospitalized for 1 to 9 days.[2] Local statistics from the Regional Poison Center, University of California, San Diego, show that prior to 1977, iron poisonings accounted for approximately 3.5% of all accidental poisonings reported to the Center. However, in 1977 this incidence dropped dramatically to 1.3% and stayed consistently at about 1.5% through 1979.[3] On June 2, 1977, the Poison Prevention Packaging Act was expanded to include all iron-marketed products containing 500 mg or more of elemental iron per container. This abrupt decline in the incidence of iron ingestions can be attributed in part to the child-resistant packaging.

CASE REPORT

A 13-month-old white male child was in good health until the day of admission, when he ingested approximately 30 ferrous sulfate tablets. About 4 weeks previously, the child had begun to walk, and the mother had placed the iron tablets in a drawer about 3 feet above floor level. The child apparently opened the drawer and consumed the tablets.

The mother found him sitting on the floor with the empty container in his mouth. Since the child did not appear ill, he was taken to a babysitter. The sitter, who was a nurse, knew about the toxicity of iron and administered syrup of ipecac, and the child was taken to the hospital. On the way, he vomited greenish, chalky material. On arrival at the emergency room, the child was pale and obtunded and vomited greenish material. A nasogastric tube was inserted, and 150 ml of sodium bicarbonate administered. Vital signs were temperature, 96.4°F; blood pressure, 88 mm Hg and palpable; pulse, 130/min; and respiration, 40/min.

Physical examination was unremarkable except for a fluctuating state of consciousness, varying from an almost-awake state with spontaneous crying to an obtunded state responsive only to deep pain. Pertinent laboratory studies showed a serum pH of 7.21, Po_2 of 147 (on oxygen), Pco_2 of 30, base excess of -15, bicarbonate level of 15 mEq/L, potassium level of 3.7 mEq/L, and WBC of 20,300 (no/mm^3). A flat plate x-ray examination of the abdomen showed no iron tablets present. Serum iron level was 942 μg/ml. Total iron binding capacity (TIBC) was unavailable.

The patient was admitted to the intensive care unit. Deferoxamine, 1 g, was given intramuscularly. Intravenous lines were placed, and fluids were administered to combat hypotension. A deferoxamine infusion was begun at 15 mg/kg/hr. Diuresis was induced with furosemide, and the urine was orange-red in color.

Stools were positive for blood. The serum iron level 6 hours after admission was 315 μg/100 ml and at 24 hours was 130 μg/100 ml. The urine was clear yellow in color. At 48 hours postingestion, the patient was alert and active, all laboratory values were within normal limits, and the patient was tolerating oral feedings. The child was discharged on the third day after admission. Follow-up examinations at 10 days and 2 months after ingestion were normal.

CLINICAL ASSESSMENT AND MANAGEMENT OF THE PATIENT

In the assessment of this patient, the following points should be considered: (1) toxic manifestations of iron poisoning, (2) cause of the toxic effects, (3) quantity of iron necessary to produce these effects, (4) laboratory tests that can confirm the diagnosis and help to assess the severity of the poisoning, (5) appropriate therapeutic measures, (6) endpoints of therapy, and (7) prognosis.

TOXIC MANIFESTATIONS OF IRON INTOXICATION

The clinical features of iron intoxication can be divided into four stages and are summarized in Table 17–1.[4]

Stage 1 occurs usually between 1 to 6 hours after ingestion and includes nausea, vomiting, and diarrhea, which may be occasionally bloody in nature. Shock may

Table 17–1. Stages of Iron Poisoning

STAGE	ONSET	SYMPTOMS
1	1 to 6 hrs	Gastrointestinal bleeding, vomiting, diarrhea, shock, lethargy, coma
2	6 to 24 hrs	Apparent improvement
3	12 to 24 hrs	Metabolic acidosis, fever, leukocytosis, liver and renal failure with related findings
4	Weeks	Intestinal scarring with possible obstruction

follow as a result of fluid and blood loss into the GI tract, and also as a result of a direct vasodilatory effect of ferritin,[5] released from the damaged GI mucosa. Lethargy and coma may also be present.

Stage 2 occurs 6 to 24 hours after ingestion and is a period of improvement in clinical condition. Patients given adequate treatment may progress from this stage to complete revovery. Untreated or severely poisoned patients will progress to Stage 3.

Stage 3 usually occurs in the first 24 hours after ingestion and is characterized by severe metabolic acidosis and liver and kidney failure, with resultant derangements in biochemical, hematologic, and electrolyte indices. Death usually occurs as a result of a multiplicity of factors.

Stage 4 follows if the patient survives stage 3 and involves intestinal obstruction, which may occur several weeks after the acute poisoning episode.

The symptoms expressed by the patient in the case presented are classic for acute iron poisoning.

CAUSE OF THE TOXIC EFFECTS

Iron has a corrosive effect on the GI mucosa, leading to excessive bleeding, fluid loss, and the resultant hypotension,[6] which is further exacerbated by the ferritin release.[5] The depression of the CNS appears to be a direct effect of iron.[5]

The mucosal damage in the GI tract allows for rapid absorption of the iron into the systemic circulation, where it is taken up by serum proteins. As the iron-binding capacity of the blood becomes saturated, free iron is produced, which can then be deposited in soft tissue, particularly in the liver, leading to hepatic necrosis. The cause of the acidosis is speculative. Proposed theories are that iron interferes with Krebs cycle metabolism, causing the accumulation of organic acids, and that hydrogen ions are released in the conversion of ferrous iron to ferric iron in the blood.[7] Because the

acidosis can be seen early in the course of the intoxication, the second theory may be most plausible.

Fever and leukocytosis result from bacterial invasion of the damaged intestinal mucosa, which may lead to sepsis. Acute hepatic necrosis leads to clotting abnormalities, and hypoglycemia, and if damage is severe, hepatic coma may result.

Autopsy findings in reported cases have shown hemorrhagic necrosis,[1,8,9,10,11] subendocardial hemorrhage,[9] GI ulcerations,[1,8,9,10,11] and renal tubular degeneration.[11]

QUANTITY OF IRON NECESSARY TO PRODUCE TOXIC EFFECTS

An accurate determination of the minimum toxic dose in humans has yet to be made. Many estimates of the toxic dose have been proposed in the literature, based on either case report data or extrapolations from animal data. Fatal poisonings in children have occurred with as little as 300 to 600 mg of elemental iron.[11]

As a general rule, if there is a serious question as to the severity of iron toxicity, it is better to institute diagnostic and therapeutic measures early than to wait for the late (and sometimes irreversible) consequences of iron poisoning. Any child who has ingested 30 mg of elemental iron per kg of body weight, whether or not symptoms are present, should be admitted to the hospital. For a 2-year-old child, this would mean an ingestion of seven adult ferrous sulfate tablets. In such patients, vigorous treatment and close monitoring of biochemical and hematologic indices are essential.

Since the elemental iron content of a product varies according to the iron salt present, and because presently the *Physician's Desk Reference* lists more than 100 commercial preparations of iron, it is important for the clinician to be familiar with

Table 17–2. Commonly Used Iron Preparations. (Adapted, with permission from the NEW YORK STATE JOURNAL OF MEDICINE, copyright by the Medical Society of the State of New York. Snyder R, Mofenson JC, and Geensher J: Acute iron poisoning in infancy. *NY State J Med*, 74:2215–2217, 1974.)

PRODUCT	EQUIVALENT OF ELEMENTAL IRON (mg)
Ferrous sulfate	
Form described in text	
Tablets—0.3 g	60
Elixir—0.150 g/5 ml	30
Spansules—225 mg	45
Fer-In-Sol	
Pediatric drops—125 mg/ml	25
Mol-Iron	
Tablet—195 mg	39
Liquid—195 mg/4 ml	39
Drops—125 mg/ml	25
Ferrous sulfate, U.S.P.	
Tablet—300 mg	60
Elixir—200 mg/5 ml	40
Solution—125 mg/ml	25
Ferrous gluconate	
Fergon	
Tablets—320 mg	36
Elixir—300 mg/5 ml	34
Ferrous gluconate, U.S.P.	
Tablets—160 mg, 320 mg	18, 36
Elixir—300 mg/5 ml	34
Ferrous choline citrate	
Chel Iron	
Tablet—0.33 g	40
Liquid—per 5 ml	50
Drops—per 1 ml	25
Ferrolip	
Syrup—5 ml	50
Syrup—5 ml	20
Tablet—0.33 g	40
Drops—1 ml	25
Ferrous fumarate	
Ircon	
Tablets—200 mg	66.6
Feostat	
Tablets—200 mg	66.6
Suspension—60 mg/5 ml	20
Chewable tablet—60 mg	20

the iron content of various products. In general, ferrous sulfate is 20% elemental iron, ferrous fumarate is 33% elemental iron, and ferrous gluconate is 12% elemental iron. Most iron-containing products list the elemental iron content on the label. If the label states the amount of iron, and then in parentheses lists the iron salts, the amount listed is the elemental iron content of the product. For instance, if the label says "Iron (as ferrous fumarate) 12 mg," the 12-mg amount is elemental iron. If, on the other hand, the iron salt is listed (e.g. "Ferrous fumarate, 36 mg"), the clinician must calculate the elemental iron content (in this case, 12 mg), using the fact that ferrous fumarate is 33% elemental iron. Table 17–2 summarizes the elemental iron content of some of the commonly used iron preparations.

LABORATORY TESTS

To confirm the diagnosis of iron ingestion, McGuigan has proposed the use of the qualitative deferoxamine color test.[13] This involves the addition of deferoxamine to gastric fluid, which has been prepared by the addition of 30% hydrogen peroxide and distilled water. Iron, present in the gastric fluid, will produce a color ranging from light orange (small amounts of iron) to dark red (large amounts of iron). When applied to gastric samples from 11 suspected iron ingestions, the test appeared reliable. No color changes are seen in control gastric samples.

A method that is more routinely used is the abdominal roentgenogram. Iron tablets are radiopaque and will be visible on the film.[14] If tablets can be seen, then the diagnosis can be confirmed. The absence of tablets on the roentgenogram, however, does not rule out iron ingestion, since dissolution of the tablets may have occurred.

For an assessment of the severity of an iron ingestion, the serum iron determination coupled with the iron-binding capacity determination is the best method currently available. In general, if the serum iron level exceeds the iron-binding capacity, the potential for systemic toxicity is present. In the utilization of serum iron level, it is important to be sure that absorption of the iron from the GI tract has been stopped. If the blood sample was drawn prior to removal of unabsorbed iron from the GI tract by emesis, lavage, and catharsis, a second level should be taken to be sure that the serum iron has reached the plateau level. From case report data, it appears that the serum iron level will usually reach a maximum 6 hours after ingestion.

In some institutions, serum iron determinations are available on a rapid response basis, but iron-binding capacity determinations are not. To compensate for this, Fischer has proposed a rapid test to determine if the iron-binding capacity has been exceeded.[15] This test, however, has not undergone extensive evaluation, and its accuracy is unknown.

I suggest the following procedures when a serum iron determination is available without an iron-binding capacity determination. If the serum iron level exceeds the normal value of 110 μg/100 ml but is less than 350 μg/100 ml, it is unlikely that any free iron exists, and the patient need not be admitted to the hospital unless symptoms are present.

If the serum iron level is greater than 350 μg/100 ml, or if symptoms are present, the patient should be admitted to the hospital. The provocative chelation test should then be performed to determine if any free iron exists in the patient's blood. In this test, 25 to 50 mg/kg (1 g maximum) of deferoxamine is administered intramuscularly. If the iron level exceeds the iron-binding capacity, the free iron will be chelated by the deferoxamine and eliminated in the urine, producing a "vin rose" color.

Unfortunately, this test is not completely accurate, as evidenced by an unpublished case seen in our institution. The child had a serum level of 1980 μg/100 ml. When deferoxamine was given, however, the urine retained its yellow color. Laboratory analysis of the urine showed large amounts of iron present. Subsequent deferoxamine injections reduced the serum iron level, but the urine never achieved the characteristic "vin rose" color. Patients with serum iron levels greater than 500 μg/100 ml will undoubtedly have free iron present in their blood and should be started on deferoxamine therapy.

Other laboratory tests that should be performed include complete blood count, liver and renal function tests, electrolyte, blood sugar, and blood gas determinations, clotting studies, and tests of stool and gastric contents for the presence of blood.

APPROPRIATE THERAPEUTIC MEASURES

The serious consequences of an acute iron poisoning can be avoided if vigorous treatment is begun early to remove the iron from the intestinal tract. If the patient is awake and alert, emesis can be induced with syrup of ipecac. If the patient is unconscious, gastric lavage can be performed. The administration of 50 to 100 ml of either a 5% sodium bicarbonate or sodium dihydrogen phosphate solution has been advocated to convert the iron to ferrous carbonate or ferrous phosphate, which are poorly absorbed and less irritating.[16,17] This conversion to the phosphate and bicarbonate salt has been shown to have a protective role in animals, but this has not been proven in humans. A convenient method of preparing a sodium dihydrogen phosphate solution is to dilute one part of Fleet's Enema with four of water.

When the phosphate solution is administered, the 100-ml dosage should not be exceeded; if the solution is to be used for lavage, it should be further diluted to half strength with water and then only used for two or three lavage exchanges. Administration of large amounts of the phosphate solution can lead to hyperphosphatemia and hypocalcemia, as in a case reported by Bachrach.[18] In this case, gastric lavage was administered, with half-strength Fleet's Enema solution, to a total of 1380 ml, resulting in severe hypocalcemia, hyperphosphatemia, hypernatremia, and acidosis. This can be avoided by observation of the above dosage recommendations.

Since the first reported use of deferoxamine in 1963,[19] it was standard practice to administer deferoxamine orally, the intent being to chelate the iron in the GI tract and retard absorption. This procedure is no longer recommended, as it has not been proven effective and may enhance rather than retard the absorption. Whitten and associates demonstrated the ability to produce iron poisoning in dogs by the oral administration of the iron-deferoxamine complex.[20] These investigators also studied three "mentally defective" children and found that oral deferoxamine did not retard the absorption of administered doses of iron.

Following the induction of emesis or completion of lavage, an abdominal x-ray examination should be performed to look for undissolved tablets in the GI tract, since iron is radiopaque and can be seen on x-ray film. If tablets are visible in the stomach, emesis or lavage should be repeated. If the tablets are in the bowel, a cathartic should be administered to hasten movement of the tablets through the intestine. Activated charcoal will not absorb iron and should not be used.[21] Intravenous fluids should be administered to combat shock, and sodium bicarbonate and electrolytes should be administered to reverse acidosis and replace losses.

Deferoxamine chelation therapy should be instituted in any patient who has one of the following: a serum iron level greater than 350 μg/100 ml and evidence of free iron, a serum iron level greater than 500 μg/100 ml, severe clinical symptoms when a serum iron determination is unavailable, or a positive provocative deferoxamine test.

Deferoxamine binds free iron, ferritin, hemosiderin, and iron taken up by the reticuloendothelial system, but does not affect cytochrome iron or hemoglobin. Deferoxamine forms the soluble complex ferrioxamine, which is readily eliminated by the kidneys. The dosage in a normotensive patient should be 1 g intramuscularly, regardless of the age of the patient, followed by 1 g every 4 to 12 hours, depending on the clinical and laboratory response, to a maximum of 6 g per day. If the patient is hypotensive, the intravenous route must be used, in which case the infusion rate should not exceed 15 mg/kg/hr. The 6-g/day maximum is stated in the package insert for this product, but the reason for this maximum dose is unclear. A 1-g dose of deferoxamine will chelate 85 mg of iron. Therefore, in massive iron poisonings, maximum doses of deferoxamine may not halt the progression of the toxic effects.[8]

Adverse effects of deferoxamine include pain and induration at the site of intramuscular injection, generalized erythema and urticaria, indicative of allergic reactions, and hypotension when the drug is administered too rapidly by the intravenous route.

When the clinical condition of a severely poisoned patient is not significantly improved following the use of deferoxamine, the clinician must turn to other forms of therapy to decrease the iron load. Three modalities have potential use: peritoneal dialysis, hemodialysis, and exchange transfusion. Although free iron is not dialyzable,[22] the chelated deferoxamine complex can be removed by either peritoneal dialysis or hemodialysis. Perhaps the best clinical results, however, have been obtained with exchange transfusion. There is excellent experimental evidence from studies using animals that exchange transfusion is many times more effective than deferoxamine administration in removing iron from the body.[23] These methods are of particular importance in a patient with renal shutdown.

ENDPOINTS OF THERAPY

The endpoints of therapy in the acutely intoxicated patient are directed toward the stabilization of the pathophysiologic changes produced by the ingestion of iron (e.g., shock, metabolic acidosis, and biochemical and hematologic abnormalities), and in the removal of iron from the patient's body. Deferoxamine treatment should be continued until the serum level is below 350 μg/100 ml. In addition, when all of the free iron has been chelated, the "vin rose" color of the urine will no longer be seen.

PROGNOSIS

Throughout the 1950s, the mortality rate for acute iron poisoning was said to approach 50%.[24] Since that time, with improvements in supportive techniques and the use of deferoxamine, the mortality rate has declined and is probably close to 5%.[6] The best guides to prognosis are the presence or absence of vasomotor instability, shock, or coma, and the serum iron level relative to TIBC within the first 4 to 5 hours after iron ingestion. The presence of hypotension, frank shock, or coma is a clear indication for immediate institution of parenteral therapy with deferoxamine, along with measures for correction of shock and electrolyte abnormalities. In the absence of coma or shock, a serum iron level greatly in excess of the TIBC is a poor prognostic sign, and parenteral therapy with deferoxamine should be instituted. Serum iron levels that remain below the total iron binding capacity in the first 4 to 5 hours after iron ingestion indicate that the patient probably will do well without deferoxamine therapy.

The sequelae of the corrosive effects of iron on the GI tract are predominately gastric and pyloric stenosis or stricture. The incidence of these complications is unknown, but numerous cases have been reported.[24,25] This should be considered in any patient who developed severe GI symptoms owing to acute ingestion of iron.

REFERENCES

1. Forbes G: Poisoning with a preparation of iron, copper and manganese. *Br Med J*, 1:367–370, 1947.
2. Federal Register, 41:22261, June 2, 1976.

3. Unpublished data, Regional Poison Center, University of California, San Diego, 1975–79.

4. Jacobs J, Greene H, and Gendel BR: Acute iron intoxication. *New Engl J Med, 273*:1124–1127, 1965.

5. Brown RK, and Gray JD: Mechanism of acute ferrous sulfate poisoning. *Can Med Assoc J, 73*:192–197, 1955.

6. Greengard J: Iron poisoning in children. *Clin Toxicol, 8(6)*: 575–597, 1975.

7. Reissman KR, and Coleman TJ: Acute intestinal iron intoxication II. Metabolic, respiratory and circulatory effects of absorbed iron salts. *Blood, 10*:46–51, 1955.

8. Gleason WA, de Mello DE, de Castro FJ, and Connors JJ: Acute hepatic failure in severe iron poisoning. *J Pediatr, 95*:138–140, 1979.

9. Manoguerra AS: Iron poisoning: Report of a fatal case in an adult. *Am J Hosp Pharm, 33*:1088–1090, 1976.

10. Coney TJ: Ferrous sulfate poisoning. *J Pediatr, 64*:218–226, 1964.

11. Greenblatt DJ, Allen MD, and Koch-Weser J: Accidental iron poisoning in children. *Clin Pediatr, 15*:835–838, 1976.

12. Rumack BH (ed): *Poisindex.* Denver, Colorado, Micromedex, Inc., 1979.

13. McGuigan MA, et al: Qualitative deferoxamine color test for iron ingestion. *J Pediatr, 94*:940–942, 1979.

14. Staple TW, and McAlister WH: Roentgenographic visualization of iron preparation in the gastro-intestinal tract. *Radiology, 83*:1051–1056, 1964.

15. Fischer DS: A method for rapid detection of acute iron toxicity. *Clin Chem, 13*:6–11, 1967.

16. Sesson TRC, and Bronson WR: Studies in the treatment of acute iron poisoning. *Am J Dis Child, 96*:463–465, 1958.

17. Bronson WR, and Sisson TRC: Studies on acute iron poisoning. *Am J Dis Child, 99*:18–26, 1960.

18. Bachrach L, Correa A, Levin R, and Grossman M: Iron poisoning: Complications of hypertonic phosphate lavage therapy. *J Pediatr, 94*:147–149, 1979.

19. Henderson F, Vietti TJ, and Brown EB: Desferrioxamine in treatment of acute toxic reaction to ferrous gluconate. *JAMA, 186*:1139–1142, 1963.

20. Whitten CF, et al: Studies in acute iron poisoning. I: Desferrioxamine in the treatment of acute iron poisoning: Clinical observations, experimental studies and theoretical considerations. *Pediatrics, 36*:322–334, 1965.

21. Hayden JW, and Comstock EG: Use of activated charcoal in acute poisoning. *Clin Toxicol, 8(5)*:515–533, 1975.

22. Winchester JF, Gelfand MS, Knepshield JH, and Schreiner GE: Dialysis and hemoperfusion of poisons and drugs—update. *Trans Am Soc Artif Intern Organs, 23*:762–842, 1972.

23. Mavassaghi N, Purugganan GG, and Leiken S: Comparison of exchange transfusion and deferoxamine in the treatment of acute iron poisoning. *J Pediatr, 75*:604–608, 1969.

24. Aldrich R: Acute iron toxicity. In *Iron in Clinical Medicine.* Edited by RO Wallerstein and SR Mettier. Berkeley, University of California Press, 1958.

25. Ghandi R, and Robarts F: Hourglass stricture of the stomach and pyloric stenosis due to ferrous sulfate poisoning. *Br J Surg, 49*:613–617, 1962.

Chapter 18

Isoniazid (INH)

Richard L. Kingston
Kusum Saxena

Since its introduction into clinical medicine 20 years ago, isoniazid (INH, Fig. 18–1) has become the cornerstone of treatment for active tuberculosis (TB) and prophylaxis of positive TB skin reactors. Such widespread use, however, provides a ready availability of the drug, with the potential for accidental, or suicidal overdosages. Various authors have reported a high incidence of INH overdosages in the American Indian population, where TB is prevalent and suicide common.[1-6] Throughout the United States, however, the overall incidence of INH overdosage is relatively low when compared to the more common drugs of misuse and abuse (e.g., opiates, sedative-hypnotics, CNS stimulants), but it is considered one of the most severe types of drug overdoses. The mortality following INH-induced convulsions has been reported to be as high as 19%, and there are reports of survival with permanent brain damage.[7]

Due to the seriousness of INH overdosage and its widespread therapeutic use, clinicians should become familiar with the clinical diagnostic considerations, the mechanism(s) of INH-induced toxic effects, the laboratory tests indicated, and the therapeutic measures available for the optimal management of patients that have been intoxicated with INH.

CASE REPORT

A 60-year-old white female in a comatose state was brought to the emergency room by paramedics and a drug overdose was suspected. According to the paramedics, they were summoned to the patient's

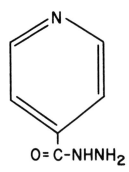

Fig. 18–1. Structure of isoniazid (isonicotinic acid hydrazide.).

examinations were found to be grossly within normal limits.

Laboratory analysis of blood gases revealed: pH, 6.77; P_{O_2}, 60 mm Hg; P_{CO_2}, 25 mm Hg; and HCO_3^-, 10 mEq/L. Blood glucose was 32 mg/dl. Serum electrolytes were sodium, 144 mEq/L; potassium, 4.0 mEq/L; chloride, 95 mEq/L; blood urea nitrogen, 18 mg/dl; and serum creatinine, 1.2 mg/dl. A serum lactate level of 270 mEq/L (normal: 9 to 16 mEq/L) was also reported. The remainder of the biochemical and hematologic indices were within normal limits.

apartment by neighbors when the patient failed to respond to telephone calls and knocking at her apartment door. At the scene, the patient was lethargic but oriented to time and place, and was able to give a sketchy history of heavy alcohol drinking during the previous week. Although an empty bottle of INH 300-mg tablets (No. 100) was found nearby, the patient denied ingesting anything other than alcohol. En route to the ER, the patient became comatose and suffered two generalized seizures.

On admission to the ER, physical examination revealed a normally developed, slightly undernourished white female, deeply comatose, hypotensive, with moderate respiratory depression, and obvious ethanol on her breath. Vital signs at this time were blood pressure, 115/50 mm Hg; pulse, 140 beats/min and regular; respirations, 12/min; and temperature, 35.0°C. The head was normocephalic; the pupils were equal, round, and reactive to light, and fundi were not seen. The chest was clear to auscultation and percussion. The neck was supple, with the thyroid palpable, and the heart showed no abnormal rhythms and no S_3 or S_4. No murmurs were heard. The abdomen was distended with no bowel sounds, and the liver was not palpable. There were no masses felt. The extremities were cold. Results of the neurological

CLINICAL ASSESSMENT AND MANAGEMENT OF THE PATIENT

In evaluating a patient such as the one presented in this report, the clinician faces a number of problems all of which demand immediate attention. A systematic approach must be organized, including basic medical considerations as well as a toxicologic evaluation.

Since the only drug found at the scene was INH, its toxicity must be considered in the overall assessment of clinical status. In reviewing the patient's clinical course thus far, the following should be considered: (1) clinical diagnostic considerations, (2) substances or syndromes that are capable of producing these signs and symptoms, (3) manifestations and mechanisms of INH toxicity, (4) indicated laboratory tests, (5) indicated therapeutic measures, and (6) general prognosis.

DIAGNOSTIC CONSIDERATIONS

The history presented by the patient was at best questionable. Initially, the patient indicated that she had been drinking during the previous week, but denied ingesting any INH tablets or other drugs. We were presented with a 60-year-old comatose female patient who had suffered two episodes of convulsions en route to the ER and was in profound acidosis. Additionally, she was hypotensive, hypoglycemic, in moderate respiratory distress, and appeared to be intoxicated.

As mentioned earlier, the patient's symptoms required immediate attention. To maintain oxygenation, a cuffed endotracheal tube was inserted and respiratory assistance was provided. Additionally, an intravenous line was started, bladder catheterization was performed, and blood and urine samples, 10 and 100 ml respectively, were collected and sent to the toxicology laboratory for serum drug analysis and urine drug screening. At the same time, two doses of naloxone hydrochloride (Narcan), 0.4 mg each, were administered intravenously, as were 50 ml of 50% dextrose in water. However, no demonstrable clinical effects were observed in the patient after the administration of either agent. Thereafter, two ampules of sodium bicarbonate (50 mEq each) also were administered, with a minimal increase in the patient's arterial blood pH.

Initial toxicologic analysis of serum and urine samples revealed no detectable amount of salicylates, barbiturates, and opiates. Serum ethanol level was 0.06 g/dl. At this point, the patient developed status epilepticus, which ultimately responded to the administration of diazepam, 10 mg IV.

The clinical diagnostic considerations thus far indicated that the patient was unresponsive to the administration of naloxone and glucose, and that she probably had not been intoxicated with salicylates, barbiturates, or opiates. Additionally, the patient had resumed seizing and appeared to be in severe refractory acidosis.

POSSIBLE CAUSES OF THE TOXIC EFFECTS

In a patient with coma and seizures, for whom results of the neurologic examination are grossly within normal limits, a large number of possibilities exists for the causes of the symptoms. Many of the toxicologic causes for coma and seizures were ruled out in our patient by lack of confirming symptoms. Most characteristic in this case was the presentation of coma and seizures with severe refractory acidosis.

Metabolic acidosis can be caused by a number of substances and/or drugs. In physiologic terms, it is a condition resulting from accumulation of an acid (other than carbonic) in the extracellular fluid, or loss of bicarbonate from the extracellular fluid. Metabolic acidosis, secondary to various poisonings or drug overdosages, can be screened by using the concept of "anion gap" [e.g., anion gap = extracellular concentration of $(Na + K) - (Cl + P_{CO_2})$]. The normal range of anion gap is 8 to 16 mM/L, with the mean about 12 mM/L.

Metabolic acidosis without an increase in the anion gap usually represents a bicarbonate loss with an increase in serum chloride. The most common examples of this type of metabolic acidosis are listed in Table 18–1, Part A. Metabolic acidosis with an increased anion gap usually represents an accumulation of acid other than carbonic acid. Most cases of acidosis with a pharmacologic or toxicologic cause are of this type (Table 18–1, Part B).

In the assessment of our patient's metabolic acidosis, a significant anion gap of greater than 43 was noted. Additionally, a serum lactate level of 270 mEq/L (normal: 9 to 16 mEq/L) was reported. These signs and symptoms were indicative of severe lactic acidosis. There are many physiologic causes that can induce lactic acidosis (Table 18–1, Part C). Further differentiation of these causes yields three possible toxicologic causes: (1) ethanol, (2) phenformin, or (3) INH intoxication.

The patient in this case had no known history of diabetes or past use of phenformin. Although ethanol ingestion can produce lactic acidosis, the patient's serum level of ethanol and the degree of

Table 18–1.   Disease States and/or Drugs Capable of Producing Metabolic
or Lactic Acidosis

	CLASSIFICATION	CAUSES

Part A	Metabolic acidosis *without* an increase in anion gap	Diarrhea
		Ureteral enterostomy (especially sigmoid)
		Acidifying agents
		    Carbonic anhydrase inhibitors (diamox, sulfamylon)
		    Ammonium chloride
		Hyperalimentation
		Dilution by rapid saline infusion (questionable)
		Cholestyramine

Part B	Metabolic acidosis *with* an increase in anion gap	Uremic acidosis Diabetic ketoacidosis Lactic acidosis Salicylate intoxication Methanol acidosis Ethylene glycol intoxication Paraldehyde

Part C	Lactic acidosis	Epinephrine
		Cardiovascular insufficiency
		    (a) Shock
		    (b) Cardiopulmonary bypass
		Acute hypoxemia
		Leukemia
		Diabetes mellitus
		Phenformin therapy
		INH intoxication
		Ethanol intoxication
		Spontaneous (idiopathic)

acidosis did not strongly support this as the primary cause. INH has been reported to cause metabolic acidosis with high serum lactate levels.[8–10] Although our patient had a questionable history, the empty bottle of INH tablets found nearby indicated that INH should be strongly considered as a possible explanation of the clinical and toxicologic manifestations present in our patient.

MANIFESTATIONS AND MECHANISMS OF INH TOXICITY

Acute ingestion by adults of 6 to 10 g of INH (20 to 30 INH tablets, 300 mg each) is uniformly associated with severe toxicity and a significant mortality rate. Furthermore, as little as 1.5 g of INH may induce minor toxicity, and 15 g or more is often fatal without appropriate therapy.[3,11,12] Symptoms of INH overdosage may begin as early as 30 minutes and as late as 4 hours after ingestion. The first signs and symptoms include nausea, vomiting, ataxia, blurred vision, and tachycardia. The patient may then lapse into coma, and grand mal or localized seizures may begin. There may be a rapid progression to intractable coma, marked hyperreflexia or complete areflexia, cyanosis, and even death.

Physical examination and laboratory studies may reveal metabolic acidosis with high serum lactate level, hyperpyrexia, severe hypotension, increased pulse rate, leukocytosis, mild hypokalemia, increased urinary excretion of pyridoxine, oliguria, and anuria. Hyperglycemia, glycosuria, and ketonuria may be present, suggesting the possibility of diabetic ketoacidosis and coma.[1–5,8,10–15] In addition, hepatic toxicity evidenced by transient increase in serum transaminase has been reported after acute ingestions but is not a consistent finding.[2,10,16]

The patient presented in this case report was lethargic and disoriented when initially evaluated by the paramedics and lapsed into coma en route to the ER. Seizures began soon after the CNS status deteriorated. This sequence of events happened in a period of approximately 1½ hours. On physical examination in the ER, the patient was hypotensive, hypothermic, tachycardic, acidotic, and in severe intractable coma. The laboratory findings were all within normal limits, with the exception of hypoglycemia, severe lactic acidosis, and an ethanol level of 0.06 g/dl.

The toxicologic effects exhibited by our patient were consistent with an INH intoxication, with the exception of hypoglycemia and hypothermia. Hyperglycemia and hyperpyrexia are the commonly seen features in INH intoxication. The hypoglycemia present in our patient probably was due to excessive alcohol intake or poor dietary intake during the week prior to admission. The hypothermia, which was also present, is a common feature in hypoglycemic individuals and subjects given the inhibitor of glucose utilization, 2-deoxy-D-glucose.[17]

The manifestations of INH intoxication, therefore, may rapidly progress in severity after the initial symptoms are noted. The most striking systemic effects are the CNS toxicity (convulsions) and metabolic (lactic) acidosis.

Central Nervous System Effects

The most consistent CNS toxicity associated with INH intoxication is that of convulsions. Published case reports indicate that human ingestions of 80 to 150 mg/kg usually result in severe seizures, with a high likelihood of mortality.[2,3] The mechanism by which toxicity is produced is not completely understood. It has been postulated that the CNS-convulsive effects are directly associated with disruption of the glutamic acid-gamma-aminobutyric acid system.[18–20]

In the CNS, synaptic transmission is inhibited by gamma-aminobutyric acid (GABA). Synthesis of GABA requires the enzyme L-glutamic acid decarboxylase (GAD), and the coenzyme pyridoxal 5-phosphate (the active form of Vitamin B_6). By depleting the stores of Vitamin B_6 (pyridoxine), which is required for the decarboxylation of glutamic acid to GABA, INH effectively decreases the activity of GABA.

The CNS changes in GABA content and GAD activity, therefore, may be the inciting mechanism in INH-induced seizures.[19] Reilly and associates have reported the only systematic attempt to document the dosage of INH required to induce seizures in humans.[21] Their research was carried out in order to evaluate the role of INH as an adjunct to "shock therapy" in patients in mental institutions. INH in oral doses of 15 mg/kg lowered the seizure threshold for photic stimulation. However, doses as large as 30 to 40 mg/kg were not reliable convulsants.

Metabolic (Lactic) Acidosis

Although the underlying cause is not entirely clear, metabolic acidosis in INH intoxication has been postulated to be due to the structural similarities of INH and pyridine nucleotides.[22] INH probably blocks the conversion of lactate to pyruvate in the Krebs cycle, which is dependent on the competence of the enzyme lactic dehydrogenase (LDH) and on nicotinamide-adenine dinucleotide (NAD), formerly known as diphosphopyridine nucleotide (DPN).[12]

Patiala and Goldman also observed structural similarities of the pyridine nucleotide in NAD to INH and suggested that it was possible to replace nicotinamide with INH in this molecule.[23,24] When this is done, NAD is inactivated. These phenomena, although observed in the course of longterm therapy or in vitro systems, nevertheless point to NAD-NADH interconversion and related steps in the Krebs cycle as likely points of INH toxicity.[12] This could explain the clinical manifestations and laboratory findings of the lactic acidosis present in our patient.

LABORATORY TESTS

In the evaluation of any comatose patient, a standard battery of tests is needed. These include glucose, electrolytes, blood urea nitrogen, serum creatinine, complete blood count, liver functional tests, and arterial blood gases if the respiratory status is depressed. Furthermore, depending on the patient's clinical condition, a 12-lead EKG and roentgenogram should be performed.

Because of the nature of INH, few laboratories routinely perform quantitative serum determinations. The majority of the laboratories that are capable of assaying INH quantitatively do so for research purposes, and INH serum levels in an acute situation are not usually available. For rapid qualitative detection of INH and its metabolites, the urine may be tested with commercially available reagent-impregnated paper strips.[25]

Treatment should not await the results of quantitative tests. In cases where the laboratory facilities are available for assaying INH quantitatively, it is important to be aware that the serum concentrations are significantly higher in acute intoxications than those occurring with therapeutic doses. Normal daily doses of INH (3 to 5 mg/kg/day) produce peak serum levels ranging from 1 to 7 μg/ml, and intermittent INH therapy (14 mg/kg biweekly) may produce levels in the range of 16 to 32 μg/ml.[1] Retrospective analysis of serum INH levels in acute intoxication shows that levels have ranged from 20 μg/ml to greater than 480 μg/ml.[10,12]

In the present case, the use of toxicologic screening was probably more im-portant than quantification of an INH serum level. Thus, during the initial assessment of the patient's clinical status, a number of potential toxicologic causes could be ruled out, and an appropriate therapeutic regimen could be instituted at the same time.

INDICATED THERAPEUTIC MEASURES

With the high morbidity and mortality rates associated with INH intoxication, careful consideration should be given to the immediate diagnostic workup of suspected INH overdosages. Generally, the management of these patients is divided into three basic categories: (1) correction of life-threatening symptoms, (2) administration of pyridoxine, and (3) nonspecific, symptomatic, and supportive care.

Correction of Life-Threatening Symptoms

The most common life-threatening symptoms associated with INH overdosage are the CNS and metabolic disturbances. After preliminary steps have been taken to assure adequate vital signs, the patient's metabolic status should be assessed by arterial blood gas determination. If the patient is seizing, intravenous diazepam should be administered at a dosage of 5 to 10 mg, at a rate not to exceed 5 mg/min.[3,12] Barbiturates, hydantoins, and diazepam have each been found to raise CNS GABA levels of animals whose GABA had been depleted by INH administration, as well as in animals with normal amounts of GABA.[26,27]

An apparent superiority of diazepam in controlling INH-induced convulsions may reflect its capacity, greater than that of other anticonvulsants, for increasing GABA levels in the CNS.[26,27] When metabolic acidosis is present, sodium bicarbonate should be administered by intravenous injection. Initially, one or two ampules (50 mEq/ampule) of sodium bicarbonate are given with further administration, based on clinical and laboratory evaluation.

Administration of Pyridoxine

The use of pyridoxine in the treatment of INH overdosages has been recommended by many investigators,[1,3,4,6,7–14,21,28] in attempts to accelerate the formation of the active coenzyme, pyridoxal phosphate, which is specifically inhibited by INH. It is believed that effective therapy depends on early administration of pyridoxine, along with other supportive measures.

The optimal dose of pyridoxine should at least be equal to the estimated maximum amount of INH ingested. An initial dose of up to 5 g (5 g/50 ml) may be administered IV over 3 to 4 minutes.[1] The dose may be repeated at 5- to 10-minute intervals until the dose of INH ingested is exceeded, seizures cease, or consciousness is regained.[1,14] Alternatively, an intravenous infusion of 5 g of pyridoxine HCl in 500 ml of fluid may be given over a 2-hour period and repeated as needed to control manifestations of INH toxicity.[1] Experimental studies indicate that pyridoxine is toxic only in doses of 4 to 5 g/kg of body weight.[29]

Nonspecific, Symptomatic, and Supportive Care

After initial stabilization of life-threatening symptoms, steps should be taken to evacuate the stomach, prevent further absorption, and enhance excretion of INH. If the patient comes to the ER soon after ingestion, and if contraindications to induction of emesis are not present, syrup of ipecac should be given, with copious amounts of fluid. It should be kept in mind that seizures may spontaneously occur early in the course, thereby contraindicating induction of emesis. If needed, gastric lavage with the largest tolerable nasogastric tube should be performed. After gastric evacuation is complete, activated charcoal, 5 to 10 times the estimated ingested dose or 25 to 50 g in a water slurry, should be administered orally or via the nasogastric tube. The activated charcoal should be followed by a saline cathartic.

To enhance excretion, several authors have recommended forced diuresis, initiated by fluids, osmotic diuretics, or furosemide, with a goal of 3 to 6 ml/kg/hr of urine output.[1,3,10,12–14,15] Forced diuresis should be continued as long as the patient is under therapy and for 6 to 12 hours beyond apparent clinical recovery, to assure complete clearance of the drug and to prevent relapse.[30] In severe INH intoxications and in patients with renal insufficiency, dialysis is recommended. Successful use of treatment with hemodialysis and peritoneal dialysis has been reported.[10,31,22] This treatment modality may also be the only method of correcting serious acid-base disturbances.[8]

Treatment of life-threatening symptoms in the patient presented included diazepam for convulsions and sodium bicarbonate for metabolic acidosis. Pyridoxine therapy was begun with an intravenous injection of 5 g over 2 to 3 minutes. The patient's blood gases normalized after intensive sodium bicarbonate therapy (222 mEq in 4 hours) and continued administration of pyridoxine, of fluids, and furosemide, and successful treatment was accomplished without the use of dialysis.

GENERAL PROGNOSIS

Prognosis in acute INH intoxication is largely dependent on early recognition and treatment of complications. Specific factors that influence the prognosis include age, pre-existing seizure disorder, decreased renal function, and degree of metabolic acidosis. Untreated INH intoxications are uniformly associated with a high mortality rate.[3] Early pyridoxine administration has produced encouraging results, and its use even in doubtful circumstances is recommended because of its relative nontoxicity and potential benefit.

High INH serum levels have been documented in cases of intoxications, but the significance of these levels in determining prognosis has not been defined. Retrospective analysis of serum INH in the patient presented in this case report revealed a level of 110 mEq/ml, yet the importance of this finding was the documentation of the presence of INH rather than the quantity.

REFERENCES

1. Sievers ML, and Herrier RN: Treatment of acute isoniazid toxicity. *Am J Hosp Pharm, 32*:202–206, 1975.
2. Nelson LG: Grand mal seizures following overdose of isoniazid. *Am Rev Respir Dis, 91*:600–604, 1965.
3. Brown CV: Acute isoniazid poisoning. *Am Rev Respir Dis, 105*:206–216, 1972.
4. Cameron WM: Isoniazid overdose. *Can Med Assoc J, 118*:1413–1415, 1978.
5. Sievers ML, Cynamon MH, and Bittker TE: Intentional isoniazid overdose among Southwestern American Indians. *Am J Psychiatry, 132*:662–665, 1975.
6. Goldfrank L, and Osborn H: INH toxicity. *Hosp Physician, Oct.*:32–35, 1977.
7. Coyer JR, and Nicholson DP: Isoniazid-induced convulsions: Part II-experimental. *South Med J, 69*:296–297, 1976.
8. Bears ES, et al: Suicidal ingestion of isoniazid: An uncommon cause of metabolic acidosis and seizures. *South Med J, 69*:81–83, 1974.
9. Mottram PE, Johnson PB, and Hoffman JE: Isoniazid toxicity. Reversal with pyridoxine. *Minn Med, 57*:81–83, 1974.
10. Sitprija V, and Holmes JH: Isoniazid intoxication. *Am Rev Respir Dis, 90*:248–254, 1964.
11. Whitefield CL, and Klein RG: Isoniazid overdose: Report of 40 patients with a critical analysis of treatment and suggestions for prevention. *Am Rev Respir Dis, 103*:887, 1971.
12. Terman DS, and Teitelbaum DT: Isoniazid self-poisoning. *Neurology, 20*:299–304, 1970.
13. Aach R, and Kissane J: Generalized seizures following isoniazid therapy for tuberculosis in a patient with uremia. *Am J Med, 53*:765–775, 1972.
14. Coyer JR, and Nicholson DP: Isoniazid-induced convulsions: Part I-clinical. *South Med J, 69*:294–296, 1976.
15. Katz BE, and Carver MW: Acute poisoning with isoniazid treated by exchange transfusion. *Pediatrics, 18*:72–76, 1956.
16. Moulding T, Iseman M, and Sbarbaro J: Preventing isoniazid hepatotoxicity. *Ann Intern Med, 85*:398–399, 1976.
17. Freinkel N, et al: The hypothermia of hypoglycemia. *N Engl J Med, 287*:841, 1972.
18. Holtz P, and Palm D: Pharmacological aspects of vitamin B₆. *Pharmacol Rev, 16*:113–178, 1964.
19. Wood JD, and Peesker SJ: A correlation between changes in GABA metabolism and isonicotinic acid hydrazide induced seizures. *Brain Res, 45*:489–498, 1972.
20. Wood JD, and Peesker SJ: The effect on GABA metabolism in brain of isonicotinic acid hydrazide and pyridoxine as a function of time after administration. *J Neurochem, 19*:1527–1537, 1972.
21. Reilly RH, et al: Convulsant effects of isoniazid. *JAMA, 152*:1317–1321, 1953.
22. Peters JH, Miller KS, and Brown P: Studies on the metabolic basis for the genetically determined capacities for isoniazid inactivation in man. *J Pharmacol Exp Ther, 150*:298–304, 1965.
23. Patiala J: The amount of pyridine nucleotides (coenzymes I and II) in blood in experimental tuberculosis before and during isoniazid treatment. *Am Rev Tuberc, 70*:453–464, 1954.
24. Goldman DS: On the mechanism of action of isonicotinic acid hydrazide. *J Am Chem Soc, 76*:2841, 1954.
25. Kilburn JO, et al: Reagent-impregnated paper strip for detection of metabolic products of isoniazid in urine. *Am Rev Respir Dis, 106*:923–924, 1972.
26. Saad SF: Effect of diazepam on gamma-aminobutyric acid (GABA) content of mouse brain. *J Pharm Pharmacol, 24*:839–840, 1972.
27. Saad SF, el-Masry AM, and Scott PM: Influence of certain anticonvulsants on the concentration of gamma-aminobutyric acid in the cerebral hemisphere of mice. *Eur J Pharmacol, 17*:386–392, 1972.
28. Biehl JP, and Vilter RW: Effect of isoniazid on vitamin B₆ metabolism: Its possible significance in producing isoniazid neuritis. *Proc Soc Exp Biol Med, 85*:389, 1954.
29. Goodman LS, and Gilman A: *The Pharmacological Basis of Therapeutics.* New York, Macmillan, 1975, pp. 1556–1558.
30. Jacobziner H, and Rayrin RW: Isoniazid intoxication. *NY State J Med, 64*:664–666, 1964.
31. Jorgensen HE, and Wieth JO: Dialysable poisons: Hemodialysis in the treatment of acute poisoning. *Lancet, 1*:84–84, 1963.

Index

Page numbers in *italics* refer to illustrations; page numbers followed by "t" refer to tables.

Absorption prevention, 6–7, 12–13, 12t
Acetaminophen intoxication, 259–270
  case report of, 259–260
  clinical assessment and management in, 260–268
  manifestations of, 260–262
    cardiac abnormalities as, 262
    hepatotoxicity as, 261–262, *261*
    renal toxicity as, 262
    three phases of, 260–261
    metabolic pathways of, *261*
  prognosis in, 268
  recorded incidence of, *260*
  severity assessment in, 262–264
    dose in, 263
    half-life and, 264
    hepatic enzyme concentrations and, 263
    nomogram for, 263–264, *263*
    physical examination for, 263
  therapy in, 266–267, 266t
    endpoint of, 267–268
    nonspecific, 267
    protective, 267
  toxicity of, 265–266
    decreased, 265–266
    increased, 265
    unaltered, 266, 266t
  unclarified aspects of, 268
Activated charcoal, 6
Adenyl cyclase, 159t
Amphetamine(s), abuse of, 183–184
  chemical structure of, *184*
  common products of, 184t
  illicit production of, 185
  uses of, 183
Amphetamine intoxication, 183–199
  cardiovascular effects of, 190, 196
  case report of, 185
  central nervous system effects of, 188–189, 196–197
    euphoria as, 189
    mechanism of action of, 188
    psychosis as, 189
    severity rating of, 186t, 188

    stereotypic behavior as, 188
  clinical assessment and management in, 185–197
  diagnosis of, 185
  hyperthermia in, 189–190
  laboratory data in, 187–188
  possible substances in, 185–187
  prognosis in, 197
  pupil reaction in, 190
  respiratory rate in, 190
  symptomatic assessment in, 186t
  therapeutic endpoint in, 197
  therapeutic measures in, 190–196
    absorbed drug removal as, 194–195
      dialysis for, 195
      forced acidic diuresis for, 194–195
      pharmacokinetics and, 194
    absorption prevention as, 192–194
      dosage forms and, 193–194
      dose in, 193
      symptoms and, 192–193
      time since ingestion and, 193
    life-threatening symptoms and, 190–192
      butyrophenones for, 191
      chlorpromazine for, 190–192
      convulsions as, 190–191
      curarization for, 192
      diazepam for, 191
      haloperidol for, 191
      hypertension as, 192
      hyperthermia as, 191–192
    symptomatic and supportive care as, 196
Anticholinergic agents, 186–187
Anticholinergic syndrome, 129–131
  central and peripheral signs and symptoms of, 129t
  common drugs and plants producing, 130t
  physostigmine salicylate in, 129–131
  substances capable of producing, 129
Anticholinesterase agents, reversible, *131*
Anticonvulsant intoxication, 171–182. See also individual drugs
  acute management of, 172
  case report of, 171–172

Anticonvulsant intoxication, *continued*
  clinical assessment and management in, 172–180
  diagnosis of, 172
  laboratory tests in, 173–175
  prognosis in, 177
  symptoms and complications of, 172–173
  therapeutic measures in, 175–177
Antidepressants, tricyclic, 187. See also *Tricyclic antidepressant intoxication*
Antidotes, 9–12, 10t–11t
  universal, 9, 12
Apomorphine, 6
  barbiturate poisoning and, 67–68
Atomic absorption spectrophotometry, 31–32
Atropinism, 132
Automatism, 61

Barbiturate intoxication, 61–75
  assessment and management in, 62–74
  automatism in, 61
  cardiovascular effects of, 64
  case report of, 62
  central nervous system effects of, 64
  clinical diagnostic considerations in, 62
  coma evaluation in, 65t
  complications of, 72–73
    hypothermia as, 73
    pneumonitis as, 73
    renal shutdown as, 73
    shock as, 72–73
    skin blisters as, 73
    thrombophlebitis and pulmonary embolism as, 73
    withdrawal symptoms as, 73
  drug tolerance in, 64
  gastrointestinal effects of, 64
  hypothermia in, 64
  incidence of, 61
  laboratory findings in, 63t
  laboratory results assessment in, 64–65
  prognosis in, 74
  respiratory effects of, 64
  successful therapy in, 73–74
  therapeutic measures in, 65–72, 63t
    activated charcoal and cathartics as, 68
    forced diuresis as, 70
    history of, 65–66
    lavage and/or emesis as, 67–68
    life-threatening symptoms and, 66–67
    patient management for, 66
    peritoneal dialysis, hemodialysis, hemoperfusion as, 71–72
    pharmacokinetics and, 68–70, 69t
    Scandinavian Method of, 66
    symptomatic and supportive care as, 72
    urinary alkalinization as, 70–71
Benzodiazepine derivatives, 82–85
  absorption of, 83
  addiction and withdrawal and, 85
  drugs included in, 82
  intoxication treatment and, 83–85
  overdosage of, 83
  pharmacokinetics of, 83, 84t
  structure of, 82

  substitution salts of, 83t
Benzoylecgonine, 210
Benzylisoquinolines, 103
Biliary excretion of intoxicants, 13
Biologic fluids, for laboratory analysis, 21–25, 22t–24t
Blood analysis, 21, 25
Body surface decontamination, 7
Bromides, 90–91
  intoxication symptoms in, 90–91
  intoxication treatment in, 91
Bromism, 91
Butyrophenones, 191

cAMP, 159t
Caffeine, 186
Carbamazepine intoxication, 179
Cardiovascular function in semicomatose patient, 8, 9t
Catharsis, 6–7
Celontin, 179
Central nervous system stimulant intoxication, 183–199. See also *Amphetamine intoxication*
Children, neuroleptic intoxication in, 141, 143
Chloral derivatives, 88–90
Chloral hydrate, 89–90
  intoxication symptoms in, 89
    treatment of, 89
  pharmacokinetics of, 89
  tolerance and dependence on, 89
  withdrawal from, 89–90
Chlorpromazine, 190–192
Chromatography, 28–30
  gas-liquid, 29–30
  thin layer, 28–29
Clearance, dialysis, 45
  total body, 53–54
Clonazepam intoxication, 179
Clonopin intoxication, 179
Cocaine, 187
  abuse of, 202–203
    chronic, effects of, 211–213
      hallucinations as, 212
      psychosis as, 212–213
      tolerance and dependence in, 213
  cost of, 202
  free base, 203
  illicit importation of, 201–202
  legitimate manufacture of, 201
  metabolism of, *211*
  oral use of, 203
  pharmacokinetics of, 210–211, *211*
  slang names for, 202
  structure of, *202*
Cocaine intoxication, 201–215
  autonomic nervous system effects of, 205–206
  cardiovascular effects of, 206
  case report of, 203
  central nervous system effects of, 204–205
  clinical assessment and management in, 204–213
  gastrointestinal reactions to, 207
  hyperpyrexia in, 207
  manifestations and mechanisms of, 204–207, 205t
  prognosis in, 213

pupil reaction in, 207
respiratory effects of, 206
therapeutic measures in, 208–211
   absorption prevention as, 209–210
   excretion facilitation as, 210–211
   life-threatening symptoms and, 208–209
   toxicology laboratory in, 207–208
Color tests, 25–26
Coma evaluation, 65t
Comatose patient, principles of treatment of, 8–17
Corrosives, commonly ingested, 5t
Cylert, 186

Dialysis, assessing effectiveness of, 44–52
   clinical status in, 44
   dialysis clearance in, 45
   extraction ratio in, 42t, 45, 52
   pharmacokinetic parameters in, 44
   volume of drug eliminated in, 45
   clinical choice of, 43–44
      drug criteria in, 43–44
         distribution phase and, 44
         fraction excreted and, 44
         particle size and, 43
         protein binding and, 43
         volume of distribution and, 43–44
      patient criteria in, 43
   common intoxicants and, 46t–51t
   lithium intoxication and, 165
   peritoneal, 15, 39–41
      complications of, 40–41
      efficacy of, 40
      procedure in, 39–40, 40
      solutions for, 40
   predicting effectiveness of, 52–54
      total body clearance in, 53–54
      volume of distribution in, 46t–51t, 52–53, 52
Dialysis clearance, 45
Diazepam, 191
Decontamination, body surface, 7
Deferoxamine color test, 275
Depakene intoxication, 177–179
Digitoxin, 246t
Digoxin, digitoxin vs., 246t
   history of, 245
   pharmacokinetics of, 246t
Digoxin intoxication, 246–257
   case report of, 246
   chronic vs. acute, 252–253, 252t
   clinical assessment and management in, 247–256
   prognosis in, 255
   severity assessment in, 248–249
      dose in, 248
      half-life and, 249, 250
      physical examination in, 248
      serum potassium concentrations in, 248
   therapeutic endpoints in, 255
   therapeutic measures in, 253–255
      absorption decrease as, 253
      protective therapy as, 253–255
         atropine for, 254
         cardioversion for, 254–255
         lidocaine for, 254
         overdrive suppression for, 254

phenytoin sodium for, 254
serum potassium elevation and, 254
   toxicity manifestations in, 247–248
   toxicity reduction in, 249–252
      dialysis and hemoperfusion in, 251
      digoxin-specific antibodies in, 251–252
      renal elimination in, 249–251
   unclarified aspects of, 255–256
Diphenylheptane derivatives, 106, 106
Diuresis, osmotic, 14

Ecgonine methyl ester, 210–211
Electron-spin resonance spectra, 27
Emergencies, toxic, principles of treatment in, 3–18
Emesis, in intoxicated patient, 5–6
Enzyme multiplied immunoassay, 26–27
Ethchlorvynol, 87–88
   intoxication with, complications in, 88
      symptoms in, 87–88
      treatment in, 88
   pharmacokinetics of, 88
   tolerance and dependence on, 88
   withdrawal and, 88
Ethinamate, 85–86
Ethosuximide, 179
Ethotoin intoxication, 177
Extraction ratio, 42t, 45, 52
Eye irrigation, 7

Fenfluramine, 186
Fluorometry, 31
Forrest test, 25–26, 147t
Free base, 203
Free radical assay technique, 27

Gagging, mechanical, 6
Gas-liquid chromatography, 29–30
Gastric lavage, 12–13, 12t
   intoxicated patient and, 4–5
   laboratory analysis in, 21
Gastrointestinal absorption, 13
Gemonil, 179
Glutethimide, 92–93
   autopsy findings in toxicity with, 93
   cyclic coma and, 92
   intoxication treatment in, 93
   overdosage symptoms of, 92
   pharmacokinetics of, 92
   tolerance and dependence with, 93
   withdrawal from, 93
Green soap tincture, 7

Hallucinogens, 187
Haloperidol, 191
Hemagglutination inhibition, 27–28
Hemodialysis, 15, 37–39
   complications of, 39
   efficacy of, 39
   principles of, 38
   procedure in, 38–39

Hemoperfusion, charcoal or resin, 15, 41–43
  circuit for, *41*
  complications of, 42–43
  efficacy of, 42, 42t
  plasma extraction ratio in, 42t
  sorbents in, 41t
Hydantoin intoxication, 177

Immunoassay, 26–28
  disadvantages of, 26
  enzyme multiplied, 26–27
  free radical, 27
  hemagglutination inhibition, 27–28
  radio-, 28
  types of, 26
Infant, narcotic withdrawal in, 120
Infrared absorption spectrophotometry, 31
INH. See *Isoniazid*
Intoxicants, biologic fluids and, 22t–24t
  dialyzability of, 46t–51t
Intoxicated patient, 1–57
  asymptomatic, 4
  awake, 4–8
    absorption prevention in, 6–7
      activated charcoal for, 6
      catharsis for, 6–7
    decontamination of, 7
    discharge of, 7–8
    emesis in, 5–6
      apomorphine in, 6
      mechanical gagging in, 6
      syrup of ipecac for, 5–6
    eye irrigation in, 7
    gastric lavage in, 4–5
    skin decontamination in, 7
    work-up and history of, 4
  incidence of death in, 3, 4t
  semicomatose or comatose, 8–17
    absorption prevention in, 12–13, 12t
    antidotes for, 9–12, 10t–11t
    biliary excretion of intoxicant in, 13
    cardiovascular function in, 8, 9t
    dialysis and hemoperfusion in, 15
    gastrointestinal absorption and, 13
    history in, 9
    lavage solutions for, 12t
    lung excretion of intoxicant in, 13
    physiologic disturbances in, 16t
    respiratory function in, 8
    supportive and symptomatic care of, 15–17
    urinary catheterization in, 8
    urinary excretion of intoxicant·in, 13–15
      osmotic diuresis and, 14
      urinary pH and, 14
    vasopressor agents for, 9t
Ipecac, syrup of, 5–6
Iron intoxication, 271–278
  case report of, 272
  cause of toxic effects in, 273
  clinical assessment and management in, 272–278
  incidence of, 271
  laboratory tests in, 275–276
    abdominal roentgenogram in, 275
    qualitative deferoxamine color test in, 275

    serum iron determination in, 275
  prognosis in, 277
  quantity of iron in, 273–275, 274t
  stages of, 272t
  therapeutic endpoints in, 277
  therapeutic measures in, 276–277
    abdominal roentgenogram in, 276
    deferoxamine as, 276–277
    dialysis as, 277
    exchange transfusion as, 277
    gastric lavage as, 276
  toxic manifestations of, 272–273, 272t
Iron preparations, common, iron content of, 274t
Isoniazid, structure of, *280*
Isoniazid intoxication, 279–286
  case report of, 279–280
  causes of toxicity in, 281–282, 282t
  clinical assessment and management in, 280–286
  diagnosis of, 280–281
  laboratory tests in, 284
  manifestations of, 282–284
    central nervous system effects as, 283
    laboratory studies and, 282
    metabolic acidosis as, 281, 282t, 283–284
  prognosis in, 285–286
  therapeutic measures in, 284–285
    life-threatening symptoms and, 284–285
    nonspecific care as, 285
    pyridoxine as, 285

Laboratory, toxicology, 19–35
  analysis techniques of, 25–33
    chromatography as, 28–30
    color tests as, 25–26
    immunoassay as, 26–28
    mass spectrometry as, 32
    spectrophotometric methods for, 30–32
  assessment by, 20
  biologic fluids for, 21–25, 22t–24t
    blood as, 21, 25
    gastric contents as, 21
    urine as, 21
  role and use of, 19–20
    in cocaine overdosage, 207–208
    in lithium intoxication, 154t, 157–159, *158*
    in narcotic analgesic intoxication, 109–110
    in neuroleptic intoxication, 145–148, 147t
    in tricyclic antidepressant intoxication, 132
  turn around time of, 20–21
Lavage solutions, 12t
Levallorphan, 112
Lithium intoxication, 153–169
  cardiovascular system and, 160
  case report of, 154–155
  central nervous system and, 160–161
  clinical assessment and management in, 155–167
  differential diagnosis in, 156–157
  gastrointestinal system and, 160
  general prognosis in, 166
  hemodialysis in, 158, *158*
  history in, 156
  hormone responses and, 159t
  laboratory findings in, 154t, 157
  laboratory results in, 157–159, *158*

manifestations and mechanisms of, 159–162
neurophysiology in, 159
physical examination in, 156
prevention of, 166–167
  fetus and neonate and, 167
  patient selection in, 166
  serum concentrations and, 166–167
  thyroid function and, 167
renal system and, 161–162
side effects of, 155t
symptomatic and supportive care in, 165
therapeutic interventions in, 155–156
treatment in, 162–165
  absorbed drug removal as, 163–165
  dialysis in, 165
  emesis or lavage as, 162–163
  forced alkaline diuresis in, 164–165
  pharmacokinetics and, 163
  renal handling and, 163–164
  saline cathartics as, 163
LSD, 187
Lung excretion of intoxicants, 13
Lysergic acid diethylamide, 187

Magnesium citrate, 7
Magnesium sulfate, 7
Mass spectrometry, 32
Mazindol, 186
Mebaral, 179
Medicaid, 152
Meperidine, *105*
Mephenytoin intoxication, 177
Mephobarbital, 179
Meprobamate intoxication, 86–87
Mesantoin intoxication, 177
Methadone, detoxification with, 118–119
  maintenance with, 119–120
Methaqualone intoxication, 93–95
  pharmacokinetics of, 94
  symptoms of, 93–94
  treatment of, 94
  withdrawal in, 94–95
Metharbital, 179
Methsuximide intoxication, 179–180
Methylphenidate, 186
Methyprylon, 91–92
Mickey Finn, 89
Milontin, 179
Morphine, *104*, 104t
Mysoline intoxication, 179

Nalorphine, 112
Naloxone, 112–113
Narcotic analgesic intoxication, 101–125
addiction and, 117–118
cardiovascular system and, 108
case report of, 102
central nervous system in, 106–108
  analgesic and/or euphoric effects on, 107
  bradycardiac effects and, 108
  endocrinologic effects on, 107–108
  excitatory effects and, 108
  nausea and emetic effects on, 108

  pupil reaction in, 108
  respiratory effects on, 107
  sedative-hypnotic effects on, 107
clinical assessment and management in, 102–121
complications in, 113–117
  cardiac, 114–115
    arrhythmias as, 114
    endocarditis as, 114–115
  gastrointestinal, 115–116
    duodenal ulcers and intestinal hemorrhage
      as, 116
    hepatitis as, 115–116
  miscellaneous, 117
  pulmonary, 113–114
    aspiration pneumonia as, 114
    edema as, 113–114
    embolization as, 114
  renal, 116–117
    acute nephritis as, 117
    acute tubular necrosis and renal failure as,
      116
    nephrotic syndrome as, 116–117
    urinary tract infections as, 117
detoxification in, 117–120
  methadone, 118–119
  methadone maintenance and, 119–120
drug classification in, 102–106
  natural opium alkaloids in, 103, 103t, *104*, 104t
  semisynthetic opiate derivatives in, 103–105,
    104t
  synthetic narcotic analgesics in, 105–106, *106*
gastrointestinal system and, 108–109, 115–116
infant withdrawal and, 120
pharmacokinetics in, 109
prognosis in, 120–121
therapeutic measures in, 110–120
  emergency, 110–111
  nonspecific, 111
  specific, 111–113
    nalorphine and levallorphan as, 112
    naloxone, 112–113
toxicology laboratory in, 109–110
withdrawal and, 118
Neuroleptic intoxication, 137–151
autonomic nervous system in, 144
cardiovascular system in, 143–144
  arrhythmias in, 143–144
  blood pressure and pulse and, 143
  EKG abnormalities and, 143
case report of, 138–140
central nervous system in, 140–143, 142t
  basal ganglia and, 141–143, 142t
  extrapyramidal symptoms and, 142t
  hypothalamus and, 141
  limbic system in, 141
  reticular activating system and, 140–141
chemical classes, 138, *138*
clinical assessment and management in, 140–150
common drugs in, 139t
Forrest tests for, 147t
general prognosis in, 150
laboratory in, 145–148, 147t
manifestations and mechanisms of, 140–144
severity of, 144–145
  dosage considerations in, 145

Neuroleptic intoxication, *continued*
  life-threatening symptoms and, 144–145
  physical examination in, 144
  therapeutic measures in, 148–149
    activated charcoal as, 148
    catharsis as, 148
    emesis as, 148
    lavage as, 148
    symptomatic and supportive care as, 148–149
  therapy endpoint in, 150
  toxicity decrease in, 149–150
    charcoal perfusion as, 150
    forced diuresis as, 149–150
    hemodialysis as, 149
Nonbarbiturate intoxication, 77–99
  case report of, 78
  clinical assessment and management in, 78–95
  general prognosis in, 95
  incidence of, 77
  laboratory results in, 81, 81t
  manifestations and mechanisms of, 80–81
  progressive dose-related effects of, 80
  representative drugs in, 78–80, 79t
  therapeutic measures in, 81–95
    general supportive, 81–82
    nonspecific, 82
    specific, 82–95
      for benzodiazepine derivatives, 82–85, *82*, 83t–84t
      for bromides, 90–91
      for chloral derivatives, 88–90
      for ethchlorvynol, 87–88
      for ethinamate, 85–86
      for glutethimide, 92–93
      for meprobamate, 86–87
      for methaqualone, 93–95
      for methyprylon, 91–92
      for paraldehyde, 90
  toxic doses in, 81t
Norcocaine, 210

Opiate derivatives, semisynthetic, 103–105, 104t
Opium alkaloids, 103, 103t, *104*, 104t
Osmotic diuresis, 14

Paraldehyde, 90
PCP. See *Phencyclidine*
Peganone intoxication, 177
Pemoline, 186
Petroleum distillates, commonly ingested, 5t
Pharmacokinetics, of barbiturates, 68–70, 69t
  of benzodiazepine derivatives, 83, 84t
  of chloral hydrate, 89
  of ethchlorvynol, 88
  of glutethimide, 92
  of lithium, 163
  of meprobamate, 86
  of methaqualone, 94
  of narcotic analgesics, 109
Phenanthrenes, 103, *104*
Phencyclidine, 187
  illicit use of, 217–218
  side effects of, 217
  structure of, *218*
  uses of, 217
Phencyclidine intoxication, 218–225
  acute renal failure in, 221
  anticholinergic effects in, 220–221
  assessment and treatment in, 219–225
  blood pressure in, 220
  case report of, 218–219
  clinical manifestations of, 219–220
    high dose and, 220
    low dose and, 219
    moderate dose and, 219
  clinical pharmacology in, 223
  diagnosis of, 221–222
  neuropsychiatric disturbances in, 220
  prognosis in, 225
  respiratory effects of, 221
  therapeutic measures in, 222–224
    constant gastric suction as, 224
    emergency procedures as, 222–223
    urinary acidification as, 224
  tolerance or dependence in, 224–225
  toxic effects in, mechanism of, 220–221
  urine and serum level determinations in, 222
Phensuximide, 179
Phenylpiperidine derivatives, *105*, 106
Phenytoin intoxication, autonomic and endocrinologic symptoms of, 173
  case report of, 171–172
  classic symptoms of, 172
  extrapyramidal symptoms in, 173
  history in, 173
  laboratory tests in, 173–175
    assay as, 175
    interpretation of, 175
  misdiagnosis of, 173
  movement disorders in, 173
  neurologic symptoms of, 172–173
  other drugs in, 173
  pharmacokinetics in, 174, *174*
  prognosis in, 177
  therapeutic measures in, 175–177
    absorption minimization as, 175–176
    life-threatening symptoms and, 175
    removal of absorbed drug as, 176–177
      hemodialysis as, 176
      peritoneal dialysis in, 176
    summary of, 177
  total/free phenytoin ratio and, 175
Physostigmine salicylate, 129–131
Plasma extraction ratios, 42t
Pondimin, 186
Primidone intoxication, 179
Pyridoxine, 285

Radioimmunoassay, 28
Reinsch test, 25–26
Respiratory function in semicomatose patient, 8
Ritalin, 186

Salicylate intoxication, 227–243
  assessment and management in, 228–242
  case report of, 228

history in, 228–229
laboratory tests in, 230
management of, 236t
nomogram for severity of, 231, *231*
prognosis in, 242
serum salicylate levels in, 232t
severity of, 229–232, 229t, *231*, 232t
therapeutic measures in, 236–242
  elimination as, 240–242
    dialysis and hemoperfusion as, 241–242
    diuresis for, 240–241
  exposure termination as, 236–238
    activated charcoal in, 237
    cathartic in, 237–238
    forced emesis in, 237, 237t
    gastric lavage in, 237
  supportive care as, 238–240
    dehydration and, 238–239, 239t
    hemorrhage and, 240
    hyperpnea and, 239
    hyperthermia and, 239
    hypoglycemia and, 239
    seizures and, 239–240
    tetany and, 240
toxic manifestations in, 232–236
  acid-base disturbance as, 232–233
  CNS toxicity as, 236
  fluid and electrolyte imbalance as, 234–235, 235t
  glucose metabolism as, 234, 234t
  hematologic manifestations as, 235
  hyperthermia as, 236
  metabolic acidosis as, 233t
  metabolic defects as, 233–234, 233t
  pulmonary edema as, 236
  renal failure as, 236
  respiratory response as, 232–233
Saline cathartics, 6–7
Sanorex, 186
Semicomatose patient, 8–17
Skin decontamination, 7
Sodium sulfate, 7
Spectrophotometry, 30–32
  atomic absorption, 31–32
  fluorometry as, 31
  infrared absorption, 31
  mass, 32
  ultraviolet, 31
  visual, 30–31

Spot tests, 25–26
Succinimide intoxication, 179
Syrup of ipecac, 5–6

Tegretol intoxication, 179
Theobromine, 186
Theophylline, 186
Thin layer chromatography, 28–29
Total body clearance, 53–54
Tricyclic antidepressant intoxication, 127–136
  anticholinergic syndrome in, 129–131, 129t, 130t, *131*
  cardiovascular system and, 131–132
    cardiac conduction and, 131
    hypertension or hypotension and, 131–132
    tachyarrhythmias and, 131
  case report of, 127–128
  central nervous system in, 131
  chemical structure, *128*
  clinical assessment and management in, 128–135
  diagnostic considerations in, 128–129, 129t
  general prognosis in, 135
  laboratory tests in, 132
  peripheral anticholinergic effects in, 132
  therapeutic measures in, 132–135
    absorbed drug removal as, 134
    further drug absorption and, 134
    life-threatening symptoms and, 132–133
    symptomatic and supportive care as, 134–135
    unabsorbed drug removal as, 133–134
  therapy endpoint in, 135

Ultraviolet spectrophotometry, 31
Universal antidote, 9, 12
Urinary catheterization in semicomatose patient, 8
Urinary excretion of intoxicants, 13–15
Urine, laboratory analysis of, 21
  pH of, 14

Valproic acid intoxication, 177–179
Vasopressor agents, 9t
Volume of distribution, 46t–51t, 52–53, *52*

Zarontin, 179

WARNER MEMORIAL LIBRARY
EASTERN COLLEGE
ST. DAVIDS, PA. 19087